HEALTH PROBLEMS OF U.S. & NORTH AMERICAN INDIAN POPULATIONS

Papers by
David Rabin, Bascom Anthony, Saul Harrison, et al

MSS Information Corporation
9 East 48th Street New York, N.Y. 10017

TABLE OF CONTENTS

CREDITS AND ACKNOWLEDGEMENTS

Anthony, Bascom F.; G. Scott Giebink; and Paul G. Quie, "Neomycin-Resistant Staphylococci in a Rural Outpatient Population," *American Journal of Diseases of Children*, June, 1967, 113:666-669.

Anthony, Bascom F.; Lawrence V. Perlman; and Lewis W. Wannamaker, "Skin Infections and Acute Nephritis in American Indian Children," *Pediatrics*, February, 1967, 39:263-279.

Balke, Bruno; and Clyde Snow, "Anthropological and Physiological Observations on Tarahumara Endurance Runners," *American Journal of Physical Anthropology*, September, 1965, 23:293-301.

Blodi, Frederick C.; and William S. Hunter, "Norrie's Disease in North America," *Documents of Ophthalmology*, 1969, 26:434-450.

Blumberg, Baruch S.; John R. Martin; and Liisa Melartin, "Alloalbuminemia: Albumin Naskapi in Indians of the Ungava," *The Journal of the American Medical Association*, January 15, 1968, 203:180-185.

Brody, Jacob A.; Irvin Emanuel; Robert McAlister; and E. Russell Alexander, "Measles Vaccine Field Trials in Alaska: II. Vaccination on St. Paul Island, Pribilofs, Where Measles Had Been Absent for 21 Years," *The Journal of the American Medical Association*, December 14, 1964, 190:965-968.

Brody, Jacob A.; Theresa Overfield; and Robert McAlister, "Draining Ears and Deafness Among Alaskan Eskimos," *The Archives of Otolaryngology*, January, 1965, 81:29-33.

Brown, James E.; and Chris Christensen, "Biliary Tract Disease Among the Navajos," *The Journal of the American Medical Association*, December 11, 1967, 202:138-140.

Burch, Thomas A., "Epidemological Studies on Rheumatic Diseases," *Military Medicine*, June, 1966, 131:507-511.

Cameron, Thomas W. M., "Northern Sylvatic Helminthiasis," *Archives of Environmental Health*, October, 1968, 17:614-621.

Comstock, George W.; Shirley H. Ferebee; and Laurel M. Hammes, "A Controlled Trial of Community-Wide Isoniazid Prophylaxis in Alaska," *American Review of Respiratory Disease*, June, 1967, 95:935-943.

Corbett, Thomas H.; and Jacob A. Brody, "An Epidemic in an Eskimo Village Due to Group-B Meningococcus: Part 2. Clinical Features," *The Journal of the American Medical Association*, May 2, 1966, 196:388-390.

Dawson, Chandler R.; Lavelle Hanna; T. Rodman Wood; Virginia Coleman; Odeon C. Briones; and Ernest Jawetz, "Controlled Trials with Trisulgapyrimidines in the Treatment of Chronic Trachoma," *The Journal of Infectious Diseases*, June, 1969, 119:581-590.

Drevets, Curtis C., "Diabetes Mellitus in Choctaw Indians," *The Journal of the Oklahoma State Medical Association*, July, 1965, 322-329.

Gregg, John B.; James P. Steele; and Ann Holzhueter, "Roentgenographic Evaluation of Temporal Bones from South Dakota Indian Burials," *American Journal of Physical Anthropology*, March, 1965, 23:51-61.

Harrison, Saul I; John H. Hess, Jr.; and Joel P. Zrull, "Paranoid Reactions in Children," *Journal of the American Academy of Child Psychiatry*, October, 1963, 2:677-692.

Healy, George R.; Neva N. Gleason; Robert Bokat; Harry Pond; and Margaret Roper, "Prevalence of Ascariasis and Amebiasis in Cherokee Indian School Children," *Public Health Reports*, October, 1969, 84:907-914.

Hesse, Frank G., "Incidence of Disease in the Navajo Indian," *Archives of Pathology*, May, 1964, 77:553-557.

Jarcho, Saul, "Anomaly of the Vertebral Column, (Klippel-Feil Syndrome) in American Aborigines," *Journal of the American Medical Association*, September 6, 1965, 193:187-188.

Kravetz, Robert E.; and Alfred S. Gilmore, "Cholecysto-Gastric Fistula Masquerading as Carcinoma of the Stomach," *Annals of Surgery*, March, 1964, 159:461-464.

Leon, Robert L. Harry W. Martin; and John H. Gladfelter, "An Emotional and Educational Experience for Urban Migrants," *American Journal of Psychiatry*, September, 1967, 124:381-384.

Lutwak, Leo; Leonard Laster; Hillel J. Gitelman; Maurice Fox; and G. Donald Whedon, with Dorothy E. Wolfe; and Minnie L. Woodson, "Effects of High Dietary Calcium and Phosphorus on Calcium, Phosphorus, Nitrogen and Fat Metabolism in Children," *American Journal of Clinical Nutrition*, February, 1964, 14:76-82.

Mandell, Gerald Lee; and Leonard R. Prosnitz, "Peritonsillar Abscess and Cellulitis: Observations from Cases on Navaho Reservation," *New York State Journal of Medicine*, October 15, 1966, 66:2667-2669.

Mayberry, Ruben H.; and Robert D. Lindeman, "A Survey of Chronic Disease and Diet in Seminole Indians in Oklahoma," *The American Journal of Clinical Nutrition*, September, 1963, 13:127-134.

Maynard, James E.; Elmer T. Feltz; Herta Wulff; Robert Fortuine; Jack D. Poland; and Tom D. Y. Chin, "Surveillance of Respiratory Virus Infections Among Alaskan Eskimo Children," *The Journal of the American Medical Association*, June 12, 1967, 200:124-125.

Maynard, James E.; and Irving G. Kagan, "Intradermal Test in the Detection of Trichinosis," *The New England Journal of Medicine*, January 2, 1964, 270:1-6.

McMahan, C. A., "Autopsied Cases by Age, Sex and 'Race'," *Laboratory Investigation*, 1968 18:468-478.

Mouratoff, George J.; Nicholas V. Carroll; and Edward M. Scott, "Diabetes Mellitus in Eskimos," *The Journal of the American Medical Association*, March 27, 1967, 199:107-112.

Pelner, Louis, "Peyote Cult, Mescaline Hallucinations, and Model Psychosis," *New York State Journal of Medicine*, November 1, 1967, 67:2833-2843.

Rabin, David L.; Clifford R. Barnett; William D. Arnold; Robert H. Freiberger; and Gyla Brooks, "Untreated Congenital Hip Disease: A Study of the Epidemiology, Natural History and Social Aspects of the Disease in a Navajo Population," *American Journal of Public Health*, Supplement to February, 1965, 55:1-44.

Sievers, Maurice L., "Disease Patterns Among Southwestern Indians," *Public Health Reports*, December, 1966, 81:1075-1083.

Wallach, Edward E.; Alan E. Beer; and Celso-Ramon Garcia, "Patient Acceptance of Oral Contraceptives: I. The American Indian," *American Journal of Obstetrics and Gynecology*, April 1, 1967, 97:984-991.

Neomycin-Resistant Staphylococci in a Rural Outpatient Population

Bascom F. Anthony, MD; G. Scott Giebink; and Paul G. Quie, MD, Minneapolis

THE OCCURRENCE of neomycin-resistant staphylococci, sometimes in epidemic proportions, is now a well-documented finding in the hospital environment. However, the existence of such strains in outpatient populations in the United States has not been previously described. The identification of *Staphylococcus aureus* with resistance to multiple antibiotics, including neomycin and bacitracin, in the infected skin lesions of the children of two Minnesota Indian reservations is the subject of the present report.

Materials and Methods

Coagulase-positive staphylococci isolated from skin lesions of Indian children living on the Red Lake and Cass Lake Reservations in northern Minnesota were examined for antibiotic sensitivity. The rural nature of these communities as well as the problem of superficial skin infections and associated acute nephritis were described over a decade ago by Kleinman.[1] More recently, the continuing prevalence of pyoderma and the identification of group A streptococci and coagulase-positive staphylococci in the majority of skin lesions in this population have been reported.[2,3]

The reservations were visited at regular three-week intervals as part of a prospective epidemiological study.[3] Skin lesions were cultured after thorough cleansing of the surface with 70% alcohol and puncturing the pustules or lifting the crusts with sterile hypodermic

Reprint requests to Department of Pediatrics, University of Minnesota Medical School, Minneapolis 55455 (Dr. Anthony).

needles. Sheep blood agar plates were inoculated immediately with swabs obtained from lesions. After overnight incubation, colonies resembling *S aureus* were tested by the Cadness-Graves[4] slide-agglutination method and, when negative, by the plasma-clot method for coagulase. Coagulase-positive strains were phage-typed by the method of Blair and Williams[5] using 22 bacteriophages and including the following: group 1—29, 52, 52A, 79, 80; group 2—3A, 3B, 3C, 55, 71; group 3—6, 7, 42E, 47, 53, 54, 75, 77, 83A; group 4—42D; and miscellaneous—81 and 187. Staphylococci which failed to type with phages in routine test dilution (RTD) were tested with concentrated phage (RTD × 10³).

Antibiotic sensitivity tests were performed on all coagulase-positive strains by a modification of the single, high-potency disc technique.[6] Several colonies were picked from the primary culture or first subculture and inoculated into trypticase soy broth. After overnight incubation, a 1:100 dilution was flooded over the surface of Mueller-Hinton agar poured to a standard depth. When the plates had thoroughly dried antibiotic discs were applied. The concentrations of drug in the discs were as follows: penicillin, 10 units; neomycin, 30γ; streptomycin, 10γ; kanamycin, 30γ; bacitracin, 10 units; tetracycline, 30γ. The plates were incubated overnight at 37 C and the diameters of the inhibition zones were measured and recorded in millimeters. Tube-dilution antibiotic sensitivities were determined on selected strains by a standard technique.[7]

Results

The 442 staphylococcal isolates described in this report were recovered exclusively from infected skin lesions between June 1964 and August 1965. Neomycin-resistant staphylococci were isolated throughout this period. The 442 strains were cultured from 213 patients, representing 133 families. Neomycin-resistant organisms were isolated from 18 of the 213 patients (9%), representing 13 of the 133 families (10%). Neomycin-resistant staphylococci were recovered repeatedly (two to four occasions) from seven patients and on only one occasion from the remaining 11.

A striking bimodal distribution of inhibition zones was found with the 30γ neomycin discs (Fig 1). Corresponding tube-dilution sensitivity tests performed on selected strains are shown in the lower half of the figure. Representatives of the predominant group with zones of 20 mm or more were consistently sensitive to neomycin by tube-dilution minimal inhibitory concentration (MIC of 12.5γ/ml or less). All 32 strains with inhibition zones of 10 to 16 mm were highly resistant (MIC, 200γ/ml or greater).

Similar distributions were found when staphylococci were tested with the tetracycline and streptomycin discs (Fig 2). Although the relationship between inhibition zone diameters and tube-dilution sensitivities is not shown in this figure, resistance and sensitivity to tetracycline and streptomycin were confirmed by sample tube-dilution tests.

A bimodal distribution of inhibition zones also occurred with the 10-unit penicillin discs, but the predominant population was resistant (Fig 3). All tested strains with zones of 27 mm or less were, with one exception, highly resistant to penicillin (MIC, 100 units/ml or greater). Strains with zones of 40 mm or more were highly sensitive (MIC, less than 0.1 unit/ml). Strains with zones of intermediate diameter of initial testing often fell into the sensitive or resistant group on retesting, but the few strains with persisting intermediate zone diameters proved to be moderately sensitive (MIC, 0.2 to 0.4 unit/ml).

In contrast to the above findings, a bimodal distribution of inhibition zones did not occur on testing with 10-unit bacitracin discs (Fig 4). Instead a single population of strains was found, consisting of both resistant and sensitive strains, as indicated by tube-dilution tests performed on 51 selected strains (Fig 4).

Table 1 summarizes the frequency of re-

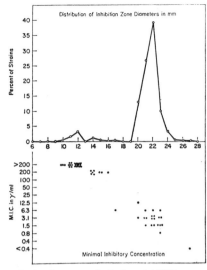

Fig 1.—Percentage distribution of inhibition zone diameters of 422 strains of S aureus tested with 30γ-discs of neomycin. Corresponding tube-dilution sensitivities (MIC) of 54 individual selected strains are shown in the lower portion.

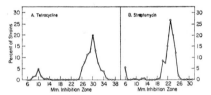

Fig 2.—Percentage distribution of inhibition zone diameters of 442 strains of S aureus tested with 30γ-discs of tetracycline (A) and with 10γ-discs of streptomycin (B).

sistance of S aureus as indicated by inhibition zone diameters. Approximately 92% of the 442 strains were highly resistant to penicillin while a minority were resistant to neomycin (7%), streptomycin (7%), and tetracycline (12%).

The sensitivity patterns of the 32 strains resistant to 200γ/ml or more of neomycin are summarized in Table 2. All strains exhibited the expected cross-resistance to kanamycin (MIC, > 25γ/ml) and were also highly resistant to penicillin. Twenty-six of the 32 neomycin-resistant strains were resistant to greater than 25 units/ml of bacitracin.

8

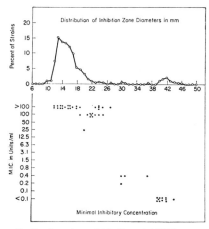

Fig 3.—Percentage distribution of inhibition zone diameters of 442 strains of S aureus tested with 10-unit discs of penicillin G. Corresponding tube-dilution sensitivities (MIC) of 49 individual selected strains are shown in the lower portion.

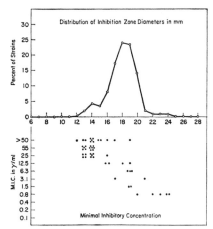

Fig 4.—Percentage distribution of inhibition zone diameters of 442 strains of S aureus tested with 10-unit discs of bacitracin shown in upper portion. Corresponding tube-dilution sensitivites (MIC) of 51 individual selected strains are shown in the lower portion.

The exact frequency of bacitracin-resistance is unknown since tube-dilution sensitivities for this antibiotic were performed on only 51 selected strains. These strains included all of the neomycin-resistant staphy-

Table 1.—The Percentage of 442 Staphylococcal Strains Resistant to the Antibiotics Examined

Antibiotic	Percent	Inhibition Zone Diameter, mm	MIC*
Penicillin	92.4	6 to 27	100 units/ml or more
Neomycin	7.3	6 to 16	200γ/ml or more
Tetracycline	11.8	6 to 14	25γ/ml or more
Streptomycin	7.3	6 to 13	200γ/ml or more

*MIC indicates minimal inhibitory concentration by tube-dilution performed on sample strains.

Table 2.—Pattern of Antibiotic Sensitivities of 32 Neomycin-Resistant

Kanamycin	Penicillin	Tetracycline	Streptomycin	Bacitracin†	No. of Strains
R*	R	R	R	R	23
R	R	R	R	S*	1
R	R	S	S	R	3
R	R	S	S	S	5
				Total	32

*R indicates resistant and S, sensitive.
†Resistance to bacitracin was defined as MIC of 25 units/ml or greater determined by tube-dilution sensitivities.

Table 3.—Frequency of Reaction of 294 Staphylococcal Strains With Concentrated Suspensions (RTD × 10³) of Group 3 Phages and of Phage 54

	No. of Strains	No. Reacting With Group 3 Phages (RTD x 10³)	No. Reacting With Phage 54 (RTD x 10³)
Neomycin-resistant	32	31	28
Neomycin-sensitive	262	114	20
Total	294	145	48

lococci, and 26 of these 32 strains were resistant to bacitracin. There may be additional strains sensitive to neomycin but resistant to bacitracin which have not been tested by bacitracin tube-dilutions.

Results of phage-typing of 294 of the 442 staphylococcal isolates, including the 32 neomycin-resistant strains, are summarized in Table 3. All neomycin-resistant staphylococci were nontypable at the RTD, but 31 of the 32 strains reacted with group 3 phages at RTD × 10³. This was the most frequently encountered phage pattern of staphylococci in the population under study and was also found in 114 of 262 neomycin-sensitive

9

strains (44%). However, 28 (90%) of the group 3 (RTD × 10³) neomycin-resistant staphylococci reacted with concentrated phage 54 at RTD × 10³, while only 20 (18%) of the 114 neomycin-sensitive strains in this group reacted with phage 54 at RTD × 10³. The difference in frequency of reactions with concentrated phage 54 between neomycin-sensitive and neomycin-resistant strains was statistically significant ($P < .001$). Application of multiple tenfold dilutions of phage 54 to these strains indicated that these reactions with concentrated phage 54 were invariably the result of inhibition rather than true phage lysis.

The medical records of the above 18 patients and of 100 randomly selected Indian children with pyoderma at Red Lake were reviewed to determine the nature of therapy for pyoderma during the 12 months preceding isolation of the reported strains. Of the randomly selected patients, almost 50% received some form of penicillin, while 20% received bacitracin ointment and 15% received neomycin ointment (Fig 5). Therapy received by the 18 individuals with skin lesions harboring neomycin-resistant staphylococci did not appear to differ significantly from the regimens employed in the other patients: 10 of the 18 (55%) received penicillin therapy, four (22%) received topical bacitracin, and an equal number were treated with topical neomycin.

Comment

The capacity of certain strains of *S aureus*, capable of multiplication in the presence of antibiotics, to become the predominant strains in hospitals has been widely recognized. The appearance of such strains of staphylococci has been reported after the introduction of many new antibiotics, often within the first few months of general use of these agents. Neomycin, for a time, appeared exempt from this phenomenon; for 11 years following its introduction there were no known epidemic strains with resistance. Since 1960, however, outbreaks of disease associated with neomycin-resistant staphylococci have been reported from hospitals in the United States, England, and other nations.[8-17]

This report documents, for the first time in the United States, the occurrence of neo-

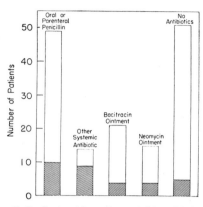

Fig 5.—Treatment for pyoderma administered during the 12 months preceding isolation of reported strains in 18 patients yielding neomycin resistant staphylococci and in 100 control pyoderma patients; note control patients whose lesions did not contain neomycin-resistant staphylococci (**white bars**) and patients with lesions containing neomycin-resistant staphylococci (**shaded bars**).

mycin-resistant staphylococci in an outpatient population. That such an occurrence may be more common than is generally appreciated is suggested by a recent survey of staphylococcal strains in Poland, in which neomycin-resistance was common in both hospital and outpatient isolates according to J. Jeljaszewicz.[18]

Only one report has described the occurrence of bacitracin-resistance in neomycin-resistant strains in a hospital outbreak.[17] This is the only report, to our knowledge, of a significant frequency of bacitracin-resistant staphylococci in an outbreak or a survey. Resistance of *S aureus* to bacitracin has been induced in vitro[19] and naturally occurring resistance has also been observed.[20] However, staphylococci in most clinical situations are believed to be almost uniformly sensitive to this antibiotic.[21,22]

The factors promoting the emergence of neomycin-resistant staphylococci are unknown, although several studies have suggested that the widespread clinical use of topical and oral neomycin has operated as a selective factor.[9,15,17] In addition, Jevons and Parker[23] have suggested that the transfer of genetic material between staphylococcal strains by lysogenizing bacteriophage (transduction) may be responsible for the appearance of new phage patterns and possibly of other characteristics in hospital epidemic strains. A possible role for transduction in the acquisition of antibiotic resistance is supported by the recent demonstration in vivo transfer of antibiotic resistance by this mechanism in experimental staphylococcal infections.[24] In the present study, the factors responsible for the occurrence of neomycin resistance are unknown. Although topical antibiotics are freely employed to treat pyoderma in this population, their use in patients subsequently found to harbor neomycin-resistant strains did not appear to be significantly more common than in other patients.

Reports concerning outbreaks of disease associated with neomycin-resistant staphylococci in hospitals in the United States have indicated the responsible strains to be nontypable with RTD of the standard phages but typable when tested with concentrated phage 54.[9-11] Workers in other countries have emphasized that staphylococci isolated in similar outbreaks manifested inhibition rather than true lysis by concentrated suspensions of phage 54 and other group 3 phages.[12-17] In addition, Rountree and Beard[17] reported that their neomycin-resistant strains were lysed by additional new phages (B5 and 77Ad). This study confirms that inhibition by phage 54 at RTD $\times$ 10^3 is a common characteristic of neomycin-resistant staphylococci in the United States; this reaction distinguishes them from neomycin-sensitive strains which commonly react with other group 3 phages at RTD $\times$ 10^3, but seldom with phage 54. Ten of the neomycin-resistant strains were tested at the Communicable Disease Center, Atlanta, against new phages by Dr. P. B. Smith. One was lysed by B5/77Ad/D at RTD and one by UC18 at RTD $\times$ 10^3.

Some of the shortcomings in the performance and interpretation of antibiotic-disc sensitivities have been reviewed.[6,25] Our experience clearly confirms the validity of the recommendations concerning the standardization of bacterial inoculum, the employment of high-potency discs and the careful measurement and recording of inhibition-zone diameters. Using these precautions, it was found that staphylococci were divided by the zone diameters into distinct populations of resistant and sensitive strains and that a particular zone size could be generally related to an approximate MIC by tube-dilution testing, confirming earlier reports.[6,25] For unknown reasons, the 10-unit bacitracin discs did not resolve the staphylococcal population into distinct groups of sensitive and resistant strains; resistance could be determined only by the use of tube-dilution techniques.

The predominance in this study of staphylococci highly resistant to penicillin and the occurrence of strains also resistant to other antibiotics indicate that it is increasingly hazardous for the physician to assume that staphylococci isolated from nonhospital sources will be sensitive to antibiotics in common use. This is true even of agents such as neomycin and bacitracin which are usually effective against staphylococci in vitro and which, because of their systemic toxicity, are used primarily for topical administration.

Summary

The antibiotic sensitivites of 442 strains of S aureus isolated from the pyoderma lesions of Indian children from two Minnesota reservations were determined. Single, high-potency discs of penicillin, neomycin, tetracycline, and streptomycin yielded a clear separation of resistant and sensitive strains as confirmed by tube-dilution testing. High-potency discs of bacitracin, however, failed to resolve the staphylococci into resistant and sensitive populations, although both bacitracin-resistant and sensitive strains were identified by tube-dilution tests.

Approximately 90% of the staphylococci were highly resistant to penicillin, and a smaller proportion was resistant to the other antibiotics tested. Thirty-two neomycin-resistant strains were isolated and these were invariably resistant to penicillin and kanamycin. Resistance to bacitracin, tetracycline, and streptomycin was demonstrated by the majority of the neomycin-resistant strains.

Reaction with concentrated suspensions of group 3 phages was a common characteristic of the staphylococcal skin isolates, while inhibition by concentrated phage 54 was significantly more common in neomycin-resistant strains than in sensitive strains.

11

These findings emphasize the danger of presumptions concerning the antibiotic sensitivity of *S aureus* encountered in outpatient populations.

This study was supported by research grant CD-00151 from the US Public Health Service and conducted under the sponsorship of the Commission on Streptococcal and Staphylococcal Diseases, Armed Forces Epidemiological Board, and was supported by the Offices of the Surgeon General, Department of the Army, Washington, DC. Mrs. JoAnn Watson phage-typed the staphylococci. The 22 bacteriophages were provided by the Communicable Diseases Center, Atlanta.

References

1. Kleinman, H.: Epidemic Acute Glomerulonephritis at Red Lake, *Minnesota Med* 37:479-483, 489, 1954.

2. Perlman, L.V., et al: Post-Streptococcal Glomerulonephritis, *JAMA* 194:63-70, 1965.

3. Anthony, B.F.; Perlman, L.V.; and Wannamaker, L.W.: Skin Infections and Acute Nephritis in American Indian Children, *Pediatrics* 39:263-279, 1967.

4. Cadness-Graves, B.: Slide-Test for Coagulase-Positive Staphylococci, *Lancet* 1:736-738, 1943.

5. Blair, J.E., and Williams, R.E.O.: Phage Typing of Staphylococci, *Bull WHO* 24:771-784, 1961.

6. Petersdorf, R.G., and Sherris, J.C.: Methods and Significance of In Vitro Testing of Bacterial Sensitivity to Drugs, *Amer J Med* 39:766-779, 1965.

7. Rammelkamp, C.H., and Maxon, T.: Resistance of *Staphylococcus aureus* to the Action of Penicillin, *Proc Soc Exper Biol Med* 51:386-389, 1942.

8. Finegold, S.M., and Gaylor, D.W.: Enterocolitis Due to Phage Type 54 Staphylococci Resistant to Kanamycin, Neomycin, Paramomycin and Chloramphenicol, *New Eng J Med* 263:1110-1116, 1960.

9. Quie, P.G.; Collin, M.; and Cardle, J.B.: Neomycin-Resistant Staphylococci, *Lancet* 2:124-126, 1960.

10. Griffith, L.J., et al: Appearance of Kanamycin Resistance in a Single Phage Type of Staphylococcus, *J Bact* 81:157-159, 1961.

11. Cohen, L.S.; Fekety, F.R.; and Cluff, L.E.: Studies of the Epidemiology of Staphylococcal Infection: IV. The Changing Ecology of Hospital Staphylococci, *New Eng J Med* 266:367-372, 1962.

12. Comtois, R.D., and Bynoe, E.T.: Report on a Particular Phage-Type of Staphylococcus Isolated in Some Hospitals in Canada, *Canad J Public Health* 54:357-363, 1963.

13. Jacobs, S.I., and Willis, A.T.: Neomycin Resistance in Newly Recognized Strains of *Staphylococcus aureus*, *Lancet* 2:459-460, 1963.

14. Robertson, J.J.: Neomycin Resistance in a Newly Recognized Strain of *Staphylococcus aureus*, *Lancet* 2:333-334, 1963.

15. Lowbury, E.J.L., et al: Neomycin-Resistant *Staphylococcus aureus* in Burns Unit, *J Hyg* 62:221-228, 1964.

16. Mitchell, A.A.B.: New Epidemic Strains of *Staphylococcus aureus*: Emergence and Spread in a General Hospital, *Lancet* 1:859-862, 1964.

17. Rountree, P.M., and Beard, M.A.: The Spread of Neomycin-Resistant Staphylococci in a Hospital, *Med J Aust* 1:498-502, 1965.

18. Jeljaszewicz, J., and Hawiger, J.: The Resistance to Antibiotics of Strains of Staphylococci Isolated in Poland, *Bull WHO* 35:231-241, 1966.

19. Stone, J.L.: Induced Resistance to Bacitracin in Cultures of *Staphylococcus aureus*, *J Infect Dis* 85:91-96, 1949.

20. Jawetz, E.: *Polymixin, Neomycin, Bacitracin,* New York: Medical Encyclopedia Inc., 1956, p 96.

21. Gill, F.A., and Hook, E.W.: Changing Patterns of Bacterial Resistance to Antimicrobial Drugs, *Amer J Med* 39:780-795, 1965.

22. Shinefield, H.R., and Ribble, J.C.: Current Aspects of Infections and Diseases Related to *Staphylococcus aureus*, *Ann Rev Med* 16:263-284, 1965.

23. Jevons, M.P., and Parker, M.T.: The Evolution of New Hospital Strains of *Staphylococcus aureus*, *J Clin Path* 17:243-250, 1964.

24. Novick, R.P., and Morse, S.I.: In Vivo Transmission of Drug Resistance Factors Between Strains of *Staphylococcus aureus*, *J Exp Med* 125:45-59, 1966.

25. Petersdorf, R.G., and Plorde, J.J.: The Usefulness of In Vitro Sensitivity Tests in Antibiotic Therapy, *Ann Rev Med* 14:41-56, 1963.

SKIN INFECTIONS AND ACUTE NEPHRITIS IN AMERICAN INDIAN CHILDREN

Bascom F. Anthony, M.D., Lawrence V. Perlman, M.D., and
Lewis W. Wannamaker, M.D.

IN THE summer and fall of 1953, the Red Lake Indian Reservation in northern Minnesota was the scene of an epidemic of acute nephritis involving 63 children. A notable feature of this outbreak, first described by Kleinman, was the presence of pyoderma in a majority of the nephritic children.[1,2] A previously unrecognized strain of group A streptococcus was isolated from the throats and skin lesions of nephritic children and also from children without evidence of nephritis.[3] Simultaneously, a serologically identical streptococcus was isolated in an epidemiologically related family outbreak of acute nephritis in Minneapolis.[4] The nephritogenic strain associated with these two incidents has subsequently been designated as type 49.

A decade after the Red Lake epidemic, the survivors were examined by Perlman, et al. and found to be free of chronic nephritis.[5] At this time, the prevalence of pyoderma and the occurrence of endemic acute nephritis was observed, not only at Red Lake but also on the nearby Cass Lake Reservation which was not involved in the nephritis outbreak of 1953. Since these populations presented an unusual opportunity to examine the epidemiology of skin infec-

tions and the relationship of pyoderma to acute nephritis, a study was initiated in early 1964. The purpose of this report is to present preliminary observations gathered in the first 18 months.

MATERIALS AND METHODS

From February 1964 through August 1965, 25 field trips were made at 3-week intervals by a team of investigators to two Minnesota Indian reservations. The Red Lake Reservation, with a population of approximately 2,500, and the Cass Lake Reservation, with a population of about 1,000, are inhabited by Chippewa Indians and are located approximately 45 miles apart in north central Minnesota.

All children known to have skin lesions were screened and those with lesions judged to be possibly infected were enrolled in the study. Children remained in the study until the lesions were either healed or were negative for β-hemolytic streptococci and coagulase-positive staphylococci on two successive examinations. On every examination, children were inspected for skin lesions and for signs of acute nephritis. The nature, location and extent of lesions were recorded and the parent, if

This investigation was conducted under the sponsorship of the Commission on Streptococcal and Staphylococcal Diseases, Armed Forces Epidemiological Board, and was supported by the offices of the Surgeon General, Department of the Army, Washington, D.C., and by a research grant from the U.S. Public Health Service (CD-00151). Support for the initial phases of some of the investigations cited here was obtained from the Heart Disease Control Branch, Bureau of State Services, U.S. Public Health Service, through the Minnesota Department of Health.

available, or the child was specifically questioned regarding hematuria and other manifestations of acute nephritis and also of acute rheumatic fever. If clinical or laboratory findings suggested the existence of acute nephritis, patients were hospitalized at the University of Minnesota Hospitals for more thorough evaluation, which usually included percutaneous renal biopsy.*

The therapy for pyoderma was under control of the local Public Health Service physicians. Of the first 101 children to complete the study, 8 received parenteral penicillin, 6 oral antibiotics, 10 topical antibiotics, and 30 received various combinations of these agents.

At each examination, cultures of the anterior nares and posterior pharynx were obtained on sheep blood agar. Skin lesions, if present, were cultured after cleansing the skin with 70% alcohol and puncturing pustules or lifting the crusts with hypodermic needles; culture swabs were plated directly onto sheep blood agar and onto duplicate blood agar plates containing crystal violet (1:1,000,000), a medium which inhibits staphylococcal growth and allows selective growth of streptococci. Streaking of the inoculum included a stab into the medium to demonstrate subsurface hemolysis. Urine was tested for hemoglobin, protein, and sugar with the Hemacombistix† and, if positive for hemoglobin or protein, the sediment was examined microscopically. On approximately 150 urine samples, the Hemacombistix was performed in conjunction with a semiquantitative microscopic examination described by Stetson, et al.[6] and the hemoglobin reaction was found sufficiently sensitive to detect the presence of more than 10 erythrocytes per cubic millimeter. Blood was collected and the separated serum was stored by freezing. Antistreptolysin O (ASO) was determined by a modification of the method of Rantz and Randall[7] in which a 0.1 log dilution scheme

was used. Anti-desoxyribonuclease B (anti-DNAse B) titers were determined by the method of McCarty[8] as modified by Ayoub and Wannamaker.[9] Antibody titers on all sera from each patient were determined simultaneously for each test.

After overnight incubation at 37°C, blood-plates were examined under a colony microscope for identification of β-hemolytic streptococci and for variations in the morphology of colonies. A single suspicious colony, or multiple colonies if morphologically different, was subcultured for grouping and M-protein typing by the precipitation technique.[10,11] Group A streptococci‡ were also classified by the agglutination technique for T-protein.[12] Interpretation of the T-agglutination results conformed with that of Parker.[13]

Staphylococci were subcultured as necessary until pure and were tested for clumping factor by the slide test. When negative, the coagulase tube test was done. Typing was performed by standard techniques[14] with a regular set of 22 phages provided by the Communicable Disease Center, which includes the following: 29, 52, 52A, 79, 80 in group I; 3A, 3B, 3C, 55, 71 in group II; 6, 7, 42E, 47, 53, 54, 75, 77, 83A in group III; 42D in group IV; 187 and 81 in miscellaneous group. If no reaction occurred at routine test dilution (R.T.D.), concentrated phage was applied (R.T.D. × 10³). Antibiotic sensitivities of staphylococci were determined by a modification of the single, high-potency disc method of Kirby and Bauer.[15] Utilizing Mueller-Hinton medium (Difco), the following antibiotic discs were used: penicillin G 10 units, streptomycin 10γ, tetracycline 30γ, neomycin 30γ and bacitracin 10 units.§ Tube-dilution sensitivities[16] were performed on selected strains showing varying inhibition zone sizes.

---

* Kidney biopsies were performed by Dr. Alfred F. Michael and his associates and were interpreted by Dr. Barbara Burke.

† Ames Company, Inc., Elkhart, Indiana.

‡ Streptococcal grouping and anti-M typing serum were provided by the Communicable Disease Center, Atlanta, Georgia, and anti-T serum by Dr. M. T. Parker and Mr. W. R. Maxted of the Public Health Laboratory, Colindale, London, England.

§ Baltimore Biological Laboratories, Baltimore, Maryland.

14

For comparison of rates of respiratory carriage of streptococci, a group of Indian children without skin lesions was cultured. The group consisted of 72 school children (mean age 10.4 years) surveyed in February 1964 and 73 school and preschool children (mean age 5 years) examined in October 1965 in two villages on the Red Lake Reservation. The results of the two surveys did not differ significantly and were combined. The mean age of the combined control group was 7.7 years.

RESULTS

During the 18 months of the study covered by this report, 270 children and adolescents were enrolled. There were 127 males and 143 females. Age distribution is shown in Figure 1.

In 83% of the children, lesions were present on the extremities, in 20% the face and scalp were involved, and in 11% lesions were present on the trunk. Skin lesions were usually covered by a thick, tenacious crust which surprisingly often concealed pus. One hundred forty children (51%) had frankly purulent lesions on the initial examination, while vesicular lesions were distinctly rare (3%). Regional lymphadenitis was not impressive and cellulitis was uncommon. There was definite evidence of infected chronic eczema in 17 children (6%), and in 7 children (2.5%) there was secondary infection of a second-degree burn. Over half of the children were suspected of having scabies with secondary infection. A history was often obtained that lesions were initiated by mechanical trauma and by insect bites. Less commonly reported incidents were animal bites and poison ivy. It was apparent that most of the pyoderma observed resulted from secondary infection of a variety of insults to the skin and that primary infection of the intact skin was probably relatively uncommon in this population.

Of the 270 children enrolled, 165 completed the study during the time covered in this report. Eighteen (11%) of these children experienced a known recurrence of

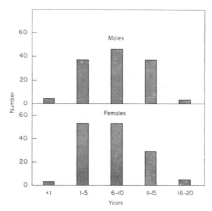

FIG. 1. Distribution by sex and age of 270 Indian children included in the study.

skin lesions and were re-enrolled; 12 of these completed a second course of observation. The 6-week follow-up rate at Red Lake was approximately 90% and at Cass Lake approximately 70%.

Bacteriology of Skin Lesions

From the 270 initial skin cultures (Fig. 2), β-hemolytic streptococci were recovered in a total of 222 (82%), in pure culture in 67 (25%). Coagulase-positive staphylococci were present in 183 cultures (68%), of which 28 (10%) were pure. By comparison, the results of all subsequent skin cultures indicate no significant change in the frequency of bacterial species in skin cultures at the time of follow-up (Fig. 2).

CLASSIFICATION OF STREPTOCOCCI (Fig. 3): Of the 222 cultures positive for β-hemolytic streptococci, 216 (98%) contained Group A organisms. In six of these, a second streptococcal group was present (group G in 3, B in 2, C in 1). In six cultures only non-group A strains were found (group G in 5 and group B in 1). Seventeen percent of the group A strains were typable by the M-protein precipitation method, but 94% yielded recognizable and reproducible agglutination patterns with T-protein antisera. Of the 13 strains not agglutinated by the T-protein method, 7 were type 31-M, so that

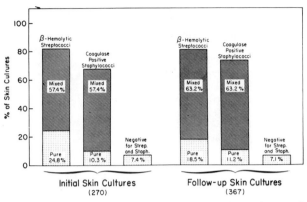

FIG. 2. Frequency of isolation of streptococci and staphylococci from initial and subsequent skin cultures.

only 3% of the group A strains could not be classified by either method.

By far the most common group A streptococcal strains were those reacting with various combinations of the 3, 13, and B3264 T-antisera (Table I), comprising almost 43% of the initial group A isolates. Next in frequency were the 8/25/Impetigo 19 strains (approximately 16%), while the 17/23/47, 5/27/44, and 11/12/27/28 T-patterns occurred in a smaller proportion. The most frequent M-type was type 41, which occurred in approximately 30% of the 3/13/B3264 strains. Most of the remaining

M-typable strains were type 31. Several of the type 41 strains and one of the type 31 strains were confirmed by bactericidal tests.

A comparison of the streptococcal types isolated from lesions at Red Lake and at Cass Lake (Fig. 4) suggests some differences between the bacterial populations in the two reservations. While strains with the T-pattern 3/13/B3264 were equally common in both locales, the frequency with which these strains were found to possess the type 41 M-protein was significantly greater at Cass Lake than at Red Lake (66% vs 2%). The difference was equally

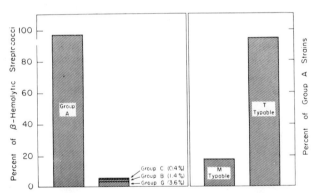

FIG. 3. Groups of β-hemolytic streptococci (left) and frequency of classification of Group A streptococci (right) isolated from initial skin cultures.

16

TABLE I

CLASSIFICATION OF 217 GROUP A STREPTOCOCCAL
STRAINS RECOVERED FROM INITIAL SKIN CULTURES*

T-Pattern	Number	% of All Group A Strains	M-Type	Number	% of Corresponding T-Pattern Which were M-Typable
3/13/B3264	93	42.9	41	28	30.1
8/25/Impetigo 19	34	15.7	—	—	—
5/27/44	16	7.4	—	—	—
17/23/47	20	9.1	—	—	—
11	8	3.7	—	—	—
12	6	2.8	12	2	33.3
11/12/27/28	17	7.8	—	—	—
4	3	1.4	—	—	—
14	1	0.5	—	—	—
Miscellaneous	6	2.7	⊥	—	—
No agglutination	13	6.0	31	7†	53.8
Total	217	100		37	

* One of the 216 initial cultures contained two different group A streptococci, 3/13/B3264 and a strain which was unclassified by T-agglutination.

† The remaining six strains (unclassified by T-agglutination) were also non-typable for M-protein.

apparent in the follow-up cultures. At Cass Lake, the tendency was for strains giving both reactions (41 M-reaction + 3/13/B3264 T-pattern) to occur in members of the same family and repeatedly in the same patient, suggesting that this was a valid and not a spurious finding. The other notable differences were the absence of type 17/23/47 T-patterns from Cass Lake and the absence of the 31-M strain from Red Lake during this period, in skin as well as in respiratory cultures.

CLASSIFICATION OF STAPHYLOCOCCI: Of the 183 strains of *Staphylococcus aureus* isolated from the initial skin cultures, 154 were phage-typed (Table II). Seventy percent of the strains could be typed with the routine test dilution (R.T.D.) or with concentrated phage (R.T.D. x 10^3). The most frequent reaction (38%) was with multiple phages of group III at R.T.D. x 10^3. The distribution of phage reactions was not sig-

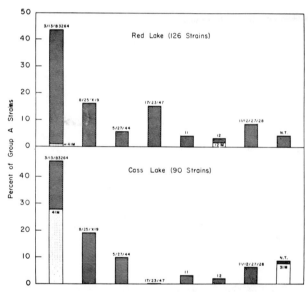

FIG. 4. Comparison of the distribution of group A streptococcal strains in initial skin cultures at Red Lake and at Cass Lake Reservations. (Numbers in bars designated "M" indicate M-type. Numbers over bars indicate T-pattern N.T. indicates no T-agglutination. 8/25/x19 = 8/25/Impetigo 19.)

17

TABLE II

PHAGE TYPES OF *STAPH. AUREUS* ISOLATED
FROM INITIAL SKIN CULTURES

Phage Pattern	Number	%
Group I, including 80/81	16	10.3
Group II, including 71	9	5.8
Group II (R.T.D.$\times 10^3$)	2	1.3
Group III	8	5.2
Group III (R.T.D.$\times 10^3$)	59	38.3
Other	14	9.1
N.T. (R.T.D. and R.T.D.$\times 10^3$)	46	30.0
Total	154	100

R.T.D. refers to routine test dilution of phage.

nificantly different in mixed cultures of streptococci and staphylococci than in pure staphylococcal cultures.

ANTIBIOTIC SENSITIVITIES OF STAPHYLO-COCCI: By determination of the sizes of inhibition zones around antibiotic discs, the staphylococci were divided for each antibiotic into two distinct groups which, on the basis of tube-dilution sensitivity determinations performed on sample strains from each group, represented resistant and sensitive strains (Table III). The strains of intermediate zone size were usually found on retesting to give zones diameters of either resistant or sensitive strains in the case of penicillin, tetracycline, and neomycin. The intermediate strains for streptomycin, however, persisted on retesting; the only one of these examined by the tube-dilution test required 25γ/ml for inhibition. A bimodal distribution was not found in the case of the 10-unit bacitracin discs, which gave a single peak of zone diameters on a distribution curve. At least 85% of the strains were sensitive to streptomycin, tetracycline, and neomycin, but almost 90% were highly resistant to penicillin.

SERIAL CHANGES IN STEPTOCOCCAL STRAINS: The results of serial cultures from each patient who completed the study during the period of this report were analyzed to determine the stability of the streptococcal flora recovered from his skin lesions (Table IV). In none of the 78 chil-

dren with only one positive skin culture for group A streptococci was more than one strain identified by M-protein and T-pattern, while, of the 40 patients with two positive cultures, 21 had the same strain on the second examination, 18 had a different strain from the first culture, and 1 patient, who had two distinct streptococci in his first culture, had still a third strain on the second culture. The children with more numerous positive cultures were more likely to yield different strains of group A streptococci on serial cultures. Two or more streptococcal colonies were processed from 245 skin cultures (133 unselected and 112 selected be-

TABLE III

PERCENTAGE DISTRIBUTION OF ANTIBIOTIC SENSITIVITIES OF 478 STRAINS OF *STAPH. AUREUS* BASED ON INHIBITION ZONES AROUND ANTIBIOTIC DISCS

Antibiotic	Resistant	Inter-mediate	Sensitive
Penicillin	89.2% ($\geq$100 units/ml)	0	10.8% ($\leq$0.4 units/ml)
Streptomycin	7.5% ($\geq$200 γ/ml)	7.5%	85.0% ($\leq$6.3 γ/ml)
Tetracycline	11.5% ($\geq$25 γ/ml)	0	88.5% ($\leq$1.5 γ/ml)
Neomycin	6.9% ($\geq$200 γ/ml)	0.9%	92.2% ($\leq$6.3 γ/ml)

Numbers in parentheses indicate value or range of values of minimal inhibitory concentration by tube dilution tests performed on sample strains.

TABLE IV

MULTIPLICITY OF GROUP A STREPTOCOCCAL STRAINS IN RELATION TO NUMBER OF REPEATEDLY POSITIVE SKIN CULTURES IN INDIVIDUAL PATIENTS

Number of Positive Cultures for Group A Strep.	Number of Patients	Number of Distinct Streptococcal Strains				Period of Observation*
		1	2	3	4	
1	78	78	—	—	—	—
2	40	21	18	1	—	3 wk to 4 mo
3	14	7	6	1	—	6 wk to 6 mo
4	9	5	2	2	—	2 mo to 11 mo
5	7	1	2	4	—	3 mo to 9 mo
6	2	—	—	—	2	6 mo to 10 mo
7	6	—	1	4	1	3 mo to 8 mo
8	1	—	—	1	—	6 mo

* Period between first and last skin culture positive for group A streptococci

18

cause of differences in colony appearance) and in only eight of these cultures (3.3%) was more than one group A strain identified. Several patients had multiple lesions cultured simultaneously and, in all 10 instances where both skin cultures were positive for group A streptococci, the same serotype was present in both cultures. Hence, while multiple strains of group A organisms were commonly found on repeated skin cultures of the same patient, they were rarely detected in one lesion or in cultures of different lesions of one patient at one time.

Comparison of Respiratory Flora with that of Skin Lesions

In 214 of the 216 children whose initial skin cultures were positive for group A streptococci, nose and throat cultures were obtained at the same time. In 12 instances, both nose and throat cultures, as well as skin lesions, contained group A streptococci. In seven of these, nose, throat, and skin lesions contained the same strain; in two, the nose and skin strain were identical while the throat strains differed; in two cases, nose, throat, and lesions contained three different strains; and, in one, the skin and throat strains were identical while a different group A strain was present in the nose.

The nose and throat cultures are analyzed separately for the sake of simplicity (Fig. 5). In patients with skin lesions containing group A streptococci (mean age 7.7 years), the anterior nares also were positive in 42 (approximately 20%) and the streptococci in the two sites were identical in T-pattern or M-type in 37 of the 42 instances (88%). In contrast, only 7 (5%) of 145 children without skin lesions (mean age 7.7 years) had group A streptococci in nose cultures, a rate significantly less than in children with streptococci in their lesions (P value < .0001).

Fifty-one (24%) of the 214 children with group A streptococci in skin lesions had positive throat cultures (Fig. 5); in 23 the streptococci were identical and in 28 they

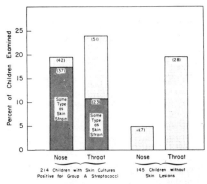

Fig. 5. Comparison of children with pyoderma and normal children with respect to presence of Group A streptococci in respiratory tract. (Figures in parenthesis refer to numbers of patients. "Type" refers to serological classification of M-protein or T-pattern.)

were different in the two sites. Throat cultures in the 145 normal children were positive for group A streptococci in 28 (19%), a rate not significantly different from the patients with positive skin lesions (P > 0.3).

The 185 children with skin lesions containing coagulase-positive staphylococci on initial culture were compared with 71 preschool and school children who had no skin lesions.|| Children with lesions containing staphylococci had positive nose cultures in 86 instances (46%) while the rate in the normal children was 26 of 71 (37%), a difference which is not statistically significant (P > 0.1). Staph. aureus was present in the throats of 58 of the 185 patients (31%) whose lesions contained staphylococci but in the throats of only 11 (15%) of the normal children (P = 0.01). In the case of children with staphylococci in nose and skin lesions, the strains were of identical phage types in 44% and different in 17%, while a determination was impossible in the remaining 38% because of non-typability. In the case of throat cultures, the

---

|| This includes the children from the 1965 survey but not those from the 1964 survey, since the staphylococci isolated in the earlier study were discarded without coagulase testing.

TABLE V

THE RELATIONSHIP OF GROUP A STREPTOCOCCI IN
INITIAL SKIN AND THROAT CULTURES TO INITIAL
STREPTOCOCCAL ANTIBODY TITERS

Group A Strep. in Cultures*		Number of Children	Geometric Mean of Titers†	
Skin	Throat		ASO	Anti-DNAse B
+	−	75	233	871
+	+	20	195	833
−	−	16	180	479

* Presence of group A streptococci is indicated by
+ and absence by −.
† ASO indicates antistreptolysin O and Anti-
DNAse B indicates antidesoxyribonuclease B.

skin and pharyngeal were identical in 31%,
different in 26%, and indeterminate in 43%.

Streptococcal Antibody Titers

Serial titers of antistreptolysin-O (ASO)
and anti-desoxyribonuclease B (anti-DNAse
B) were determined in 113 of the 165 children who completed the study, but two
children with positive throat but negative
skin cultures were excluded from this analysis. Examination of the initial 111 titers
(Table V) indicates that there was no appreciable difference (less than 0.1 log or 1
tube) in the geometric mean ASO titer between patients with group A streptococci in
skin lesions (line 1 and 2 of table) and those
without (line 3) while the mean anti-DNAse
B titer was higher (by more than 0.2 log or 2
tubes) in children with positive skin cultures than in the small group with negative
skin cultures. The presence of group A
streptococci in the throat as well as in skin
lesions, on the initial examination (line 2)
was not associated with an appreciably
different initial titer of either ASO or anti-
DNAse B than was the presence of these
organisms in skin lesions alone (line 1).

As shown in Table VI, the mean of the
maximum titers for ASO and anti-DNAse B
achieved by children with group A streptococci in both skin lesion and throat (line 2)
at some time during their enrollment was

not significantly different from that in children with pyoderma who had consistently
negative throat cultures (line 1). The five
patients who never had positive skin cultures for group A streptococci were excluded from this analysis.

Previous experience with antibody titers
in this population indicated that the usual
normal values for this laboratory were not
applicable. Therefore, it was considered
necessary to compare titers from children in
this study with those from children without
skin lesions in the same population. The sera
from a group of normal Minnesota Indian
children were collected in 1964 as part of
another study.[5] For the present analysis, a
serum from this group was included only if
the donor was known to be free of skin lesions. There were 57 such sera and comparison of these titers with the initial values in
the 108 patients whose lesions contained
group A streptococci at some time (Fig. 6)
indicates a modest elevation of ASO and a
more striking elevation of anti-DNAse B in
patients with skin lesions. Since the control
group was significantly older than the study
group (mean age 12.6 vs 8.7 years), this
could explain the difference in antibody titers. Therefore, children were blindly eliminated from both groups in order to obtain a
strictly age-matched comparison (Fig. 7).
Only study patients whose initial skin cul-

TABLE VI

THE RELATIONSHIP OF GROUP A STREPTOCOCCI IN ALL
SKIN AND THROAT CULTURES (INITIAL AND FOLLOW-
UP) TO MAXIMUM STREPTOCOCCAL ANTIBODY TITERS
ATTAINED BY EACH PATIENT

Group A Strep. in Cultures*		Number of Children	Geometric Mean of Titers†	
Skin	Throat		ASO	Anti-DNAse B
+	−	61	263	1,060
+	+	47	254	970

* Presence of group A streptococci is indicated by
+ and absence by −.
† ASO indicates antistreptolysin O and Anti-DNAse
B indicates antidesoxyribonuclease B.

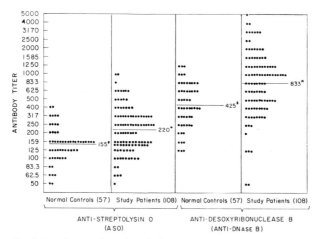

FIG. 6. Distribution of initial antibody titers in children with skin lesions and in normal Indian children. (Geometric mean is indicated by °.)

tures contained group A streptococci were included. The geometric mean of the initial ASO titers in children with skin lesions exceeded the mean of control titers by less than 1 tube (0.1 log). Although this difference was of borderline significance (P = 0.046), only 11 (26%) of the titers in the 43 study patients were above 250 Todd

units, compared with 6 (14%) of the titers in the 43 normal children, an insignificant difference (P = 0.2). On the other hand, the geometric mean of anti-DNAse B titers exceeded the mean of control titers by almost two tubes (0.2 log), a significant difference (P < 0.004), and 21 (49%) of the patients with lesions had initial titers above 833

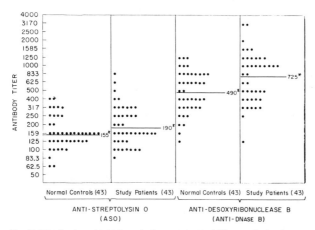

FIG. 7. Distribution of initial antibody titers in 43 children with skin lesions and in an age-matched group of normal children. (Geometric mean is indicated by °.)

21

units, as compared with 6 (14%) of the normal children (P < 0.001).

A significant serial increase in titer was defined as a rise of two tubes or more occurring in 9 weeks or less. By this definition, 14 of 58 (24%) of the children with group A streptococci in their initial skin cultures showed a response in ASO titer and 14 of 55 (25%) in anti-DNAse B. Twenty-one of 60 (35%) of these children manifested a response in one or both antibodies. No significant difference in frequency of response of either antibody was found between patients with frankly pustular lesions and those with crusted, non-purulent lesions.

Occurrence of Acute Nephritis

During the period covered in this report, there were seven instances of acute proliferative glomerulonephritis proven by renal biopsy. The diagnostic histopathological findings included enlargement of the glomeruli and definite endothelial cell proliferation, with or without polymorphonuclear exudation and bloodless loops in the glomerular capillaries, and without interstitial and tubular abnormalities.

Patient 1 was a 12-year-old female who served as a normal control for the nephritis follow-up study of 1964; her only manifestation was asymptomatic proteinuria. Patient 2, a 5-year-old girl with pyoderma, edema, and hypertension, received intensive antibiotic therapy before referral to the study.

Bacteriological data are available for the remaining five patients (Table VII). Patient 3 was enrolled in the study on August 2, 1965, at which time he had pyoderma lesions containing group A streptococci, with a T-pattern 5/27/44, and a normal urinalysis. Three weeks later, he and two siblings (patients 4 and 5) were found to have microscopic hematuria and type 12 (M and T antigen) streptococci in skin lesions and respiratory tract. Patient 6 was seen for the first time on August 2, 1965, with pyoderma and clinical signs of acute nephritis; his lesions contained group A streptococci with a

type 11-T antigen. Patient 7 had a group A streptococcus with a 4-T reaction in her eczematous lesions and in her nose, and she had a normal urinalysis on July 13, 1965. Three weeks later, microscopic hematuria appeared; at this time her lesions had cleared strikingly and the nose and throat cultures were unfortunately lost.

In only two of the seven patients (2 and 6) was nephritis clinically overt. Both of these children made a rapid recovery.

COMMENT

In one of the earliest descriptions of impetigo contagiosa, Fox distinguished between impetigo as a disease affecting the intact skin and the secondary "impetiginization" of other skin disorders.[17] While this distinction is still recognized,[18] in practice is it often a difficult one to make, especially if lesions are unavailable for observation at a sufficiently early stage. Except for the few children with obvious underlying eczema and second degree burns, it was usually impossible to determine the nature of the initial cutaneous insult in this study. However, factors which are known to predispose to secondary infection of the skin are extremely common in this population (scabies, lice, fleas, mosquitoes, minor trauma, and, perhaps most important, low standards of personal hygiene). For these reasons, we have avoided the term impetigo in describing our findings.

Both the relative frequency and the etiological significance of the β-hemolytic streptococcus and Staphylococcus aureus in superficial infections of the skin have been debated for many years. These questions have not been resolved by studies which have failed to reckon with the tendency of staphylococci to overgrow and conceal streptococci in mixed cultures on ordinary bacteriological media. Special precautions to offset this tendency may be taken, such as the use of appropriate inhibitory or selective media and the careful examination of primary culture plates with a hand lens or colony microscope. In studies where such measures have been used, convincing

TABLE VII

BACTERIOLOGICAL DATA ON FIVE INDIAN CHILDREN WITH BIOPSY-PROVEN ACUTE NEPHRITIS

Patient Number	Sex	Age (yr)	Serological Classification of Group A Streptococci* Isolated in Relation to Onset of Hematuria						Clinical Signs of Nephritis
			3 Weeks Before			Concomitant			
			Skin	Nose	Throat	Skin	Nose	Throat	
3	M	5	5/27/44	None	None	12	12	12	None
4	F	3	—	—	—	12	None	12	None
5	M	2	—	—	—	12	12	12	None
6	M	3	—	—	—	11	None	None	Edema, smoky urine, hypertension, oliguria
7	F	10	4	4	None	Healed	—	—	None

* Except for the type 12 strains, which contained both 12-M and T antigens, numbers refer to T-antigen (nontypable for M).

data have strongly implicated *Staph. aureus* alone in certain individual cases and in outbreaks of impetigo and other pyodermas.[19,20] Equally convincing bacteriological data indicate that β-hemolytic streptococci can play a dominant role in impetigo,[21] although this concept has not gained universal acceptance.[22] It appears that "streptococcal" and "staphylococcal" impetigo can sometimes be differentiated on clinical and epidemiological grounds.[21,23-26] As was often the case in other studies, β-hemolytic streptococci and coagulase-positive staphylococci were each recovered from skin lesions in this study with such frequency (80% and 70%, respectively) that it cannot be said, on this basis alone, whether the lesions represented streptococcal or staphylococcal pyoderma, although the clinical features were clearly not those of the classical bullous impetigo attributed to *Staph. aureus*. Moreover, the frequency of staphylococci and streptococci in follow-up cultures did not differ enough from the initial cultures to implicate either organism as a secondary invader.

The epidemiological observation that impetigo "breeds true," i.e., that secondary cases in an outbreak are expressed as fairly typical cases of impetigo rather than as other manifestations of staphylococcal disease (e.g., furunculosis) or of streptococcal infection (e.g., scarlet fever), prompted Simpson to predict that the responsible agent would prove not to be a typical member of either bacterial species.[27] The merit of this suggestion was borne out in 1955 when Parker, *et al.*[28] and Barrow[29] found that the coagulase-positive staphylococci and the group A streptococci isolated from skin lesions during outbreaks of pyoderma were indeed unusual strains. The staphylococci exhibited a characteristic phage susceptibility (usually type 71) and other unusual biological features, while the streptococci usually lacked detectable M-protein but fell into one of a few agglutination patterns which were much less prevalent in streptococcal infections at other sites. That the type 71 and related staphylococci are common in superficial skin lesions but infrequent in other staphylococcal lesions has since been confirmed in England[30,31] and in Europe.[32-34] In this country Dillon, *et al.*[35] have identified streptococci from skin lesions as predominantly of the T-patterns previously described by the British investigators, and Markowitz, *et al.*[36] have identified type 71 staphylococci in a significant proportion of impetigo cultures.

The findings in the present study are similar in that the most common agglutination T-pattern of group A streptococci isolated from skin lesions (3/13/B3264) and two of the other more frequent patterns (5/27/44 and 8/25/Impetigo 19) have been reported in earlier studies as being characteristic of strains encountered in superficial skin lesions. However, strains possessing the T-pattern 17/23/47, relatively common in skin lesions in this study, have not been previously identified with infections in this site. A second finding not reported previously is the presence of type 41-M protein in a significant proportion of the strains with the T-pattern 3/13/B3264. Special studies on some of these strains, including bactericidal tests, support the view that this reaction is a *bona fide* M-protein reaction and not a spurious observation.[37]

The staphylococcal strains identified in the skin lesions in this study differ from those isolated in earlier studies in that a relatively small proportion react with the group II phages (type 71, etc.), while the most common reaction is with concentrated phages of group III. In other studies, type 71 and related staphylococci have been common in cultures of lesions containing both staphylococci and β-hemolytic streptococci and have predominated in the pure cultures from "staphylococcal impetigo." If only specific "impetigo" staphylococci can produce superficial infections of the skin, the rarity of such strains in this report suggests that staphylococci may be secondary invaders in the lesions examined in this study.

The concept that pyoderma tends to be associated, clinically and epidemiologically, with streptococcal infection or colonization of the throat[26,38] is consistent with one recorded observation of the seasonal frequency of impetigo in Southampton, England, which resembled that of streptococcal respiratory infections, increasing in the late fall to a maximum in the winter months and declining in the spring to a low level during the summer.[39] However, the seasonal variation of impetigo in another British study,[31] in Denmark,[40] and in the southern United States[41,42] is apparently one of high frequency in late summer and early fall and

low frequency during the winter months. A season of high prevalence of pyoderma was not apparent in the studies reported here, but the lack of a fully comprehensive case-finding procedure may have obscured true seasonal variations. Other studies of seasonal incidence may be susceptible to such artifacts, as the English study which was conducted in a school clinic.[39]

Cultures from the upper respiratory tract in this study do not support a relationship between streptococcal infections of the skin and of the throat. Throat cultures of children with streptococci in their skin lesions contained group A streptococci at a rate (24%) not significantly different from that in Indian children without skin lesions (19%). In addition, when group A streptococci were simultaneously present in the pharynx and in skin lesions, they were at least as likely to be different as to be the same in serological classification.

On the other hand, children with group A streptococci in skin lesions carried group A organisms in the anterior nares, usually serologically identical, with about the same frequency (20%) as in the throat, but in children without skin lesions, nasal streptococci were distinctly uncommon (5%). The close serological relationship of group A streptococci in the nose to those in skin lesions prompts consideration of the possibility that the skin is infected from the nose, particularly since nasal carriers of streptococci have been shown to heavily contaminate the immediate environment, including the skin.[43,44] However, in the studies cited, the nasal cultures were strongly positive and were accompanied by and presumably the result of group A streptococcal infection of the pharynx. In contrast, the pyoderma patients in the present study with positive nasal cultures usually carried small numbers of streptococci at this site (<10 colonies per culture) and had the same group A strain in the throat in only 7 of 42 instances. These observations suggest rather that nasal streptococci are derived from those in skin lesions.

An examination of the antibody titers to

streptococcal products might help clarify the question of the significance of group A streptococci in superficial skin lesions. Burnett[45] reported elevated titers of ASO in approximately 15% of patients with pyoderma, some of whose skin lesions contained group A streptococci. In a more detailed examination of ASO titers, Markowitz, et al.[36] found in a group of children with impetigo that titers in 28% were elevated, while in a control group only 14% were elevated. In the present study, 26% of the patients with pyoderma (all with group A streptococci in initial cultures) had elevated ASO titers, while 14% of the age-matched controls had titers in this range,¶ a distribution which resembles that reported by Markowitz and his associates.[36]

The titers for antibodies to another streptococcal product, desoxyribonuclease B (DNAse B), were more significantly increased in children with skin lesions containing group A streptococci. The geometric mean of initial titers in children with pyoderma was significantly higher (by almost 2 tubes) than the mean value in children without lesions and 49% of the titers in pyoderma patients were above the upper limit of normal.¶ The explanation for the significantly greater frequency of elevated titers of anti-DNAse B than of ASO is not immediately apparent, but the occurrence of a differential antibody response in certain kinds of streptococcal infection has been observed by Ayoub and Wannamaker[9] who found relatively higher titers of anti-nicotinamide adenine dinucleotidase (anti-NADase, formerly anti-DPNase) and lower titers of anti-DNAse B in patients with acute nephritis as opposed to those with acute rheumatic fever, presumably related to the production of relatively large amounts of NADase by nephritogenic streptococci.[46] The apparent disso-

¶ The "upper limit of normal" was the same whether defined as 2 tubes above the geometric mean titer in normal controls, as by Markowitz, et al.,[36] or as the level dividing the upper 20% from the remaining 80% of control titers, as was previously reported from this laboratory.[9]

ciation of titers for ASO and anti-DNAse B in patients with pyoderma warrants further confirmation and comparison with titers in uncomplicated streptococcal pharyngitis, preferably in a population in which both skin and throat infections are prevalent.

A rather small proportion of patients in this study manifested a significant serial rise in streptococcal antibody titers. Only 24% showed a rising titer for ASO, 25% for anti-DNAse B, and 35% for at least one of the two antibodies. This may be a consequence of the relatively late stage of the infection at the time of examination. It is of interest that the presence of group A streptococci in the pharynx, as well as in skin lesions, was not associated with higher levels of either antibody. It has been suggested that because streptococcal skin infections are superficial, they are not usually associated with an immune response.[36] Despite the inability to demonstrate serial increases in antibody titers with regularity, the present study strongly suggests that a significant proportion of these patients had already developed an elevated antibody titer, particularly in response to streptococcal DNAse B.

The superficial nature of skin infections has also been related to the apparent lack of M-protein and hence relative avirulence of streptoccocci isolated from skin lesions.[36] That some of these skin strains may possess M-protein is clearly indicated by the fairly regular identification of type 41-M in strains of the agglutination pattern 3/13/B3264 isolated at the Cass Lake Reservation. Although systemic infections were not observed in this study, we have had occasion to observe a case of impetigo, bacteremia, and osteomyelitis caused by a group A streptococcus which was non-typable for M-protein but which was classified by the T-method as 3/13/B3264, a well-known "impetigo" strain. This clinical observation has stimulated investigations in this laboratory which indicate that certain of these strains which do not react as type 41-M nevertheless grow well in human blood and possess an M-protein not precipitated by any of the known typing sera.# Thus, both clinical and laboratory observations suggest that in at least some instances of impetigo or pyoderma there is the potential for invasive infection.

The long-recognized association between pyoderma and acute nephritis has been strengthened by a number of studies of concomitant pyoderma and nephritis in which β-hemolytic streptococci have been recovered from the skin lesions.[41,48] However, in one of the earlier reports of this nature, Futcher[49] isolated β-hemolytic streptococci with equal frequency in both skin and throat cultures of 11 patients with pyoderma and nephritis and pointed out the difficulty in assessing the relative significance, in the pathogenesis of nephritis, of streptococci in these two sites. In the other studies, throat cultures were not performed in a majority of patients. In the present study, in three nephritic patients (siblings), type 12 (M and T) streptococci were present in both skin and respiratory tract cultures. In another patient who was seen initially with nephritis and pyoderma, only the skin culture was positive for a group A strain agglutinating as an 11-T streptococcus, but this patient, like those in the reports cited, was not seen before developing nephritis and the possibility of a previous subclinical pharyngitis could not be excluded.

In the literature, the identification of nephritogenic types of group A streptococci has been largely based on studies of nephritis following pharyngitis, and it is conceivable that the strains responsible for pyoderma-associated nephritis may be quite different. Dillon, et al.[35] have identified the "impetigo" strains, 3/13/B3264 and 8/25/Impetigo 19, in the skin lesions of children with nephritis, as well as streptococci with type 14 T-protein, a strain previously recovered from cases of pharyngitis accompanying nephritis.[50,51] This occur-

rence of the 14-T strain is of additional interest because of its possible relationship to type 49-M,[52] the original "Red Lake" strain of 1953, as discussed in a recent review.[53] Enigmatically, type 49 apparently has virtually disappeared from the Red Lake Indian Reservation. In the current study, the patient with 11-T streptococci in his skin lesions is the only nephritic child who did not yield a recognized nephritogenic strain. Types 12 and 4 were recovered from the other nephritic children.

In recent studies of an extensive outbreak of pyoderma and nephritis in Trinidad, the strain most frequently recovered from the skin lesions and throats of patients with nephritis and also from individuals in areas where nephritis was epidemic was reported to be "type 41" by precipitation reaction.[54] In light of this finding, it is interesting that type 41-M strains, almost invariably accompanied in our experience by the T-pattern 3/13/B3264, were among the most common streptococci in skin lesions at one of the reservations under study (Cass Lake) but were not associated with nephritis. Subsequent studies, including bactericidal tests, suggest that the Trinidad strains are not true type 41-M strain[37,55] but that some are similar to the 3/13/B3264 strains in this study which react as a new M-type.[47]

Observations in this report of multiple strains of group A streptococci identified in repeated cultures of persisting skin lesions may be pertinent to a consideration of the nephritogenic role of streptococci in this study and perhaps in others. The isolation of different streptococcal types from serial cultures of a single patient's skin lesions may be a reflection of several types coexisting at one time or may indicate genuine shifts in the flora of skin lesions. Our limited studies to date would suggest that the latter is perhaps more common in this population. Regardless of the explanation, this finding indicates that, in this population at least, the identification of a particular strain in the skin lesions of a child with endemic acute nephritis does not exclude the possibility that other preexistent or coexistent

Approximately 50% of the 3/13/B3264 strains from initial skin cultures at Red Lake and 16% of the corresponding strains from Cass Lake appear to fall in this new M-type.[47]

streptococci may indeed be responsible for acute nephritis. On the other hand, the isolation of a group A strain from nephritic patients in an epidemic, as at Red Lake in 1953 when type 49 was the predominant type in children with nephritis,[3] is probably a more convincing indication that the strain played a significant role in the pathogenesis of nephritis.

In several of the children in this study and in almost all such cases reported in the literature, pyoderma first came under observation when evidence of nephritis was present. Under these circumstances, there is no reliable means of determining the possible occurrence or significance of preceding clinical or subclinical pharyngitis. Neither can one ascertain the role in the pathogenesis of acute nephritis of a group A streptococcus identified in skin lesions when nephritis appears, if rapid and multiple changes of streptococcal strains are characteristic of pyoderma in other populations, as they seem to be in this study. One approach which might cast some light on such questions is the performance of frequent, prospective observations of a normal population known to have endemic superficial infections of the skin. Such a study is now underway at the Red Lake Reservation.

SUMMARY

Serial observations were obtained over an 18-month period of 270 Indian children with pyoderma. Beta-hemolytic streptococci, predominantly group A, and coagulase-positive staphylococci were recovered from the majority of lesions (80% and 70%, respectively), both on the initial and on subsequent cultures. The predominant agglutination patterns of streptococcal strains were similar to those described in other studies of superficial skin infections. Another agglutination pattern, 17/23/47, not previously observed to be prevalent in streptococci from skin lesions, was identified in a significant number of skin cultures. In addition, the hitherto undescribed association of M-types, including type 41 and a new M-type, with strains of T-agglu-

tination pattern 3/13/B3264 was found. In striking contrast to the streptococcal strains, established "impetigo" strains of *Staph. aureus* (type 71 or other group II strains) were in the minority. Throat cultures of children with pyoderma suggested a limited relationship between infection or colonization of the pharynx and infection of the skin, while nasal streptococci were more closely correlated with and possibly derived from the flora of the skin lesions. Titers of ASO were not often elevated over control values in children with pyoderma, while anti-DNAse B titers were more commonly increased.

Group A streptococci isolated from skin lesions prior to or at the time acute nephritis was recognized included type 12 (M and T) and strains classified by T-agglutination as 5/27/44, 11 and 4. The role of infection or colonization of the upper respiratory tract in the relationship of pyoderma to nephritis was not clarified in these studies. Moreover, in view of the frequency of change of group A streptococcal strains in skin lesions, as shown in serial observations in this study, the nephritogenic significance of streptococci recovered from skin lesions at the time of recognition of nephritis must remain in some doubt. Questions concerning the pathogenesis of endemic nephritis associated with pyoderma can probably be most reliably answered by frequent, prospective observations of a normal population with significant occurrence of streptococcal skin infections.

REFERENCES

1. Kleinman, H.: Epidemic acute glomerulonephritis at Red Lake. Minnesota Med., 37: 479, 1954.
2. Reinstein, C. R.: Epidemic nephritis at Red Lake, Minnesota. J. Pediat., 47:25, 1955.
3. Updyke, E. L., Moore, M. S., and Conroy, E.: Provisional new type of group A streptococci associated with nephritis. Science, 121:171, 1955.
4. Wannamaker, L. W., and Pierce, H. C.: Family outbreak of acute nephritis associated with type 49 streptococcal infection. J. Lancet, 81:561, 1961.

5. Perlman, L. V., Herdman, R. C., Kleinman, H., and Vernier, R. L.: Poststreptococcal glomerulonephritis. J.A.M.A., 194:63, 1965.
6. Stetson, C. A., Rammelkamp, C. H., Jr., Krause, R. M., Kohen, R. J., and Perry, W. D.: Epidemic acute nephritis: studies on etiology, natural history and prevention. Medicine, 34:431, 1955.
7. Rantz, L. A., and Randall, E.: A modification of the technique for determination of the antistreptolysin titer. Proc. Soc. Exp. Biol. Med., 59:22, 1945.
8. McCarty, M.: The inhibition of streptococcal desoxyribonuclease by rabbit and human antisera. J. Exp. Med., 90:543, 1949.
9. Ayoub, E. M., and Wannamaker, L. W.: Evaluation of the streptococcal desoxyribonuclease B and diphosphopyridine nucleotidase antibody tests in acute rheumatic fever and acute glomerulonephritis. PEDIATRICS, 29:527, 1962.
10. Lancefield, R. C.: A serological differentiation of human and other groups of hemolytic streptococci. J. Exp. Med., 57:571, 1933.
11. Swift, H. F., Wilson, A. T., and Lancefield, R. C.: Typing group A hemolytic streptococci by M precipitin reactions in capillary pipettes. J. Exp. Med., 78:127, 1943.
12. Williams, R. E. O.: Laboratory diagnosis of streptococcal infections. Bull. WHO, 19:153, 1958.
13. Parker, M. T.: The definition of Str. pyogenes serotypes by agglutination and precipitation. Zbl. Bakt. I. Ref., 196:64, 1964.
14. Blair, J. E., and Williams, R. E. O.: Phage typing of staphylococci. Bull. WHO, 24:771, 1961.
15. Petersdorf, R. G., and Sherris, J. C.: Methods and significance of in vitro testing of bacterial sensitivity to drugs. Amer. J. Med., 39:766, 1965.
16. Rammelkamp, C. H., Jr., and Maxon, T.: Resistance of Staphylococcus aureus to the action of penicillin. Proc. Soc. Exp. Biol. Med., 51:386, 1942.
17. Fox, W. T.: On impetigo contagiosa, or porrigo. Brit. Med. J., 1:607, 1864.
18. Pillsbury, D. M., Shelley, W. B., and Kligman, A. M.: Dermatology. Philadelphia: W. B. Saunders Co., 1956.
19. Bigger, J. W., and Hodgson, G. A.: Impetigo contagiosa: its cause and treatment. Lancet, 1:544, 1943.
20. Sheehan, H. L., and Ferguson, A. G.: Impetigo: aetiology and treatment. Lancet, 1:547, 1943.
21. Davies, J. H. T., Dixon, K., and Stuart-Harris, C. H.: A therapeutic trial of penicillin in infective conditions of the skin. Quart. J. Med., 14:183, 1945.
22. Maibach, H. I.: Experimentally-induced infections in the skin of man. In Maibach, H. I., and Hildick-Smith, G., ed.: Skin Bacteria and Their Role in Infection. New York: McGraw-Hill, p. 85, 1965.
23. Tachau, P.: The bacteriology of impetigo contagiosa. Brit. J. Derm. Syph., 50:113, 1938.
24. Epstein, S.: Staphylococci impetigo contagiosa. Arch. Derm. Syph., 42:840, 1940.
25. Friedberg, R.: Bacteriological studies on impetigo, especially the streptogenic form. Acta Dermatovener., 23:297, 1942.
26. Cruickshank, R.: The epidemiology of some skin infections. Brit. Med. J., 1:55, 1953.
27. Simpson, R. E. H.: The impetigococcus. Lancet, 1:683, 1941.
28. Parker, M. T., Tomlinson, A. J. H., and Williams, R. E. O.: Impetigo contagiosa: the association of certain types of Staphylococcus aureus and of Streptococcus pyogenes with superficial skin infections. J. Hyg. (Camb.), 53:458, 1955.
29. Barrow, G. I.: Clinical and bacteriological aspects of impetigo contagiosa. J. Hyg. (Camb.), 53:495, 1955.
30. Spittlehouse, K. E.: Phage-types of Staphylococcus pyogenes isolated from impetigo and sycosis barbae. Lancet, 2:378, 1955.
31. Parker, M. T., and Williams, R. E. O.: Further observations on the bacteriology of impetigo and pemphigus neonatorum. Acta Paediat. Scand., 50:101, 1961.
32. Jessen, O., Faber, V., Rosendal, K., and Eriksen, K. R.: Some properties of Staphylococcus aureus, possibly related to pathogenicity. Acta Path. Microbiol. Scand., 47:316, 1959.
33. Van Toorn, M. J.: On the staphylococci and streptococcal etiology of impetigo. Dermatologica, 123:391, 1961.
34. Brundin, G., and Laurell, G.: Phage-typing in staphylodermia. Acta Dermatovener., 43:25, 1963.
35. Dillon, H. C., Moody, M. W., and Maxted, W. R.: Epidemiologic and bacteriologic aspects of impetigo and its complications: specificity of streptococcal types. Southern Med. J., 58:1578, 1965.
36. Markowitz, M., Bruton, H. D., Kuttner, A. G., and Cluff, L. E.: The bacteriologic findings, streptococcal immune response, and renal complications in children with impetigo. PEDIATRICS, 35:393, 1965.
37. Top, F. H., Jr., and Maxted, W. R.: Unpublished observations.
38. Mortimer, E. A., Jr., and Boxerbaum, B.: Diagnosis and treatment: group A streptococcal infections. PEDIATRICS, 36:930, 1965.
39. Newman, J. L.: Impetigo contagiosa, its

epidemiology and control. J. Hyg. (Camb.), 35:150, 1935.

40. Madsen, T.: Lectures on the Epidemiology and Control of Syphilis, Turberculosis, and Whooping Cough, and Other Aspects of Infectious Disease. Baltimore: Williams and Wilkins Co., 1937.

41. Blumberg, R. W., and Feldman, D. B.: Observations on acute glomerulonephritic associated with impetigo. J. Pediat., 60:677, 1962.

42. Dillon, H. C.: Personal communication.

43. Hare, R.: Haemolytic streptococci in normal people and carriers. Lancet, 1:85, 1941.

44. Hamburger, M., Jr., Green, M. J., and Hamburger, V. G.: The problem of the "dangerous carrier" of hemolytic streptococci. J. Infect. Dis., 77:96, 1945.

45. Burnett, J. W.: Management of pyogenic cutaneous infections. New Eng. J. Med., 266:164, 1962.

46. Bernheimer, A. W., Lazarides, P. D., Wilson, A. T.: Diphosphopyridine nucleotidase as an extracellular product of streptococcal growth and its possible relationship to leukotoxicity. J. Exp. Med., 106:27, 1957.

47. Top, F. H., Jr.: Unpublished observations.

48. Callaway, J. L., and O'Rear, H. B.: Pyogenic infections of skin: etiologic factor in acute glomerulonephritis of children. Arch. Derm. Syph., 64:159, 1951.

49. Futcher, P. H.: Glomerular nephritis following infections of the skin. Arch. Int. Med., 65:1192, 1940.

50. Feasby, W. R.: Survey of hemolytic streptococcus infections at Camp Borden, Ontario, 1943. War Med., 5:216, 1944.

51. Šramek, J.: A contribution to the epidemiology of acute glomerulonephritis associated with group A streptococci different from type 12. Zbl. Bakt. I. Ref., 196:56, 1964.

52. Köhler, W.: A common T-antigen of Str. pyogenes types 14–35–49–(51). Zbl. Bakt. I. Ref., 196:70, 1964.

53. Wannamaker, L. W.: The epidemiology of acute glomerulonephritis. In Metcoff, J., ed.: Proceedings of the 17th Annual Conference on the Kidney. National Kidney Foundation, in press.

54. Simon, N. S., Potter, E. V., Siegel, A. C., McAninch, J., Poon-King, T., Humair, L., and Earle, D. P.: Epidemic nephritis in Trinidad. J. Lab. Clin. Med., 66:1022, 1965.

55. Potter, E. V.: Personal communication.

Acknowledgment

The authors gratefully acknowledge the encouragement and advice of Dr. Robert L. Vernier and Dr. Dean S. Fleming, the logistical support of Dr. Sidney Finkelstein and the cooperation of Drs. Ronald D. Brown, Richard Bell, H. Bernie Orr, and their associates in the Cass Lake and Red Lake Public Health Service Hospitals. The study was conducted with the cooperation of the Indian Health Division of the U.S. Public Health Service. The following physicians participated in a number of field trips: Dr. Elia M. Ayoub, Dr. John M. Burns, Dr. Roger C. Herdman, Dr. Edward L. Isenberg, Dr. Edward L. Kaplan, Dr. Paul G. Quie, Dr. Franklin H. Top, Jr., Dr. Harold E. Windschitl. Technical proficiency was provided in the streptococcal identification, grouping, and typing by Mrs. Joyce Preston, Miss Carolyn McKay, and Mr. Howard Pierce, in staphylococcal identification and phage-typing by Mrs. JoAnn Watson, in performance of antibiotic sensitivities by Mr. Scott Giebink, in the antibody determinations by Mrs. JoAnn Nelson, Mrs. Jane Hall, and Mrs. Enid Thompson, and in other laboratory work by Mr. Steven Skjold. Mrs. James Kelley assisted in the field work. Dr. M. T. Parker and Mr. W. R. Maxted kindly reviewed the manuscript.

Anthropological and Physiological Observations on Tarahumara Endurance Runners

BRUNO BALKE AND CLYDE SNOW

In the fall of 1963, a party of American "river runners" attempted to conquer the twisting, boulder-strewn Barranca del Cobre, a gigantic canyon of the Sierra Madre Occidentale of North-Central Mexico. Unable to cover more than a few miles a day — at the cost of back-breaking effort — they ran dangerously low on food and were forced to abandon most of their equipment and to attempt climbing out of this gorge, which attains a depth of 1,500 meters in places. Their lives may have been saved only because of the help and guidance they received from some Indians chancing to cross their path. In describing the climb up the canyon wall one of the party stated: "Each one of us carried a canteen, but nothing else. For five miles we climbed that trail, which seemed designed only for goats. At one point, as we toiled upwards, the Indians passed us, each carrying a 60 pound pack of our gear. Suddenly, I realized it was their third trip of the day." (Sports Illustrated October 21, 1963, p. 33).

The Indians helping them were Tarahumara. This incident is recounted here because it is typical of hundreds of such casual observations made by travelers, missionaries and explorers of the region who, since the earliest days of Spanish contact, have marveled at Tarahumara feats of physical endurance. Well-documented accounts of such feats are also recorded in the anthropological literature of this tribe (Lumholtz, 1894, '02; Basauri, '29, '40; Bennett and Zingg, '35; Gajdusek, '53; Pennington, '63). Lumholtz, for example, mentioned a young Tarahumara who carried a 100-pound burden for a distance of 110 miles in 70 hours ('02: p. 241). Bennett and Zingg ('35: p. 160) stated that the Tarahumara competed successfully with mules as *cargadores*: Indians could be hired for 25 centavos a day to carry 50-pound loads at least twice as far as mules which carried 300 pounds and rented for 75 centavos a day. The latter authors also described the Tarahumara practice of hunting deer by following them at a steady pace for one or two days until the animal drops from exhaustion ('35: p. 113).

While such remarkable displays of physical endurance are common in the Tarahumara's day-to-day activities, they are best demonstrated in their popular sport of kick-ball racing. Kick-ball races have been described in detail by Lumholtz ('02: p. 281–294), Bennett and Zingg ('35: p. 335–341) and Pennington ('63: p. 167–172). These races vary considerably in length — depending on the age and sex of participants and the occasion. A very informal race, organized on a Sunday afternoon with boys 6 to 12 years old as runners, may last a little more than an hour and may cover a distance of ten kilometers. Elaborate inter-community events, on the other hand, involving men with great reputations as runners, may require several days or even weeks of organization and entail special "curing" ceremonies for the runners. Such big races may cover distances of 150–300 kilometers and attract crowds of several hundred spectators who bet heavily on the outcome. Similar races, only of shorter distance, are organized for women and older men (Lumholtz, '02: p. 293–294; Bennett and Zingg, '35: p. 339–340; Pennington, '63: p. 173). In the course of these events, the runners display capacities of physical endurance which equal or exceed the capabilities of well-trained athletes of our own culture. Such performances appear even more remarkable when it is considered that the race courses are laid out over extremely difficult terrain at altitudes of 1,800–2,500 meters, that the runners undergo little, if any, special training prior to a race and, finally, that their normal diet, in many ways, would be considered deficient by western standards.

Up to the present time, no functional data have been gathered on Tarahumara runners, although such information might contribute considerably to our understanding of the physiology of work, training and fatigue. In an effort to tap this source of potentially valuable information, two 10-day trips — in Fall 1963 and Spring 1964 — were made into the Tarahumara country with the purpose of establishing essential contacts and of collecting a preliminary set of physiological and performance measurements.

Geographic and ethnographic background

The 50,000 Tarahumara living today occupy some of the most rugged and remote terrain in North America. It is roughly coterminous with the Southern third of the Mexican State of Chihuahua (fig. 1). This area of about 300 × 500 kilometers straddles the north-central segment of the Sierra Madre Occidentale and embraces the watershed and tributaries of two large rivers — the Rio Concho, which drains the eastern aspect and the Rio Fuerte which flows to the Pacific.

The available archaeological evidence indicates that the Tarahumara have lived in their present habitat for a considerable period of time — perhaps as long as 2,000 years (Pennington, '63; Zingg, '33, '40; Ascher and Clune, '60). Physiographically, the area may be divided into two regions; uplands and canyon country (Pennington, '63). The uplands are pine- and pasture-clad plateaus with elevations of 1,200–2,400 meters and occasional peaks measuring 3,000 meters. The canyon country is formed by the Rio Fuerte drainage system and consists of gigantic gorges, the *barrancas*, which may attain depths of 800–1,800 meters and whose floors support a subtropical biota.

The summer climate of the *barrancas* is torrid and unhealthy, while that of the uplands is relatively cool and pleasant. In the winter, on the other hand, the climate of the uplands is the coldest in Mexico while the canyons offer warmth and shelter. Rainfall is scanty in both areas and tends to be concentrated in late summer and early fall.

The Tarahumara, whose rude technology poorly equips him for either upland winters or *barranca* summers (Zingg, '42), has responded to this environmental challenge by developing a seminomadic living pattern. In the spring, he moves to the highlands where he plants, tends and harvests his crops. In the fall, he retreats to the canyons where he overwinters in comparative comfort.

Tarahumara diet consists primarily of various preparations of corn, beans and squash supplemented with wild plant and animal resources of the region. Several varieties of Indian corn are cultivated and, in one form or another probably constitute 70–80% of the total caloric intake. Most commonly it is prepared as *pinole*, a gruel of parched corn meal and water. Bennett and Zingg ('35) estimated that pinole alone made up about 50% of the diet. *Esquiate*, various *atoles*, tortillas and tamales are also common. Beans, principally the true kidney bean (*Phaseolus vulgaris*) are a chief source of proteins. Although

31

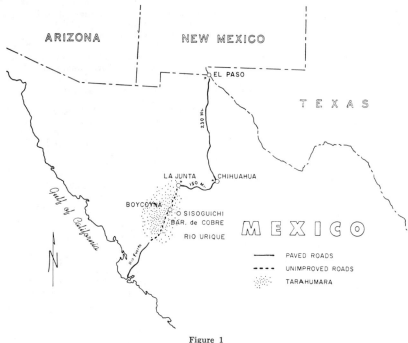

ARIZONA   NEW MEXICO

EL PASO

T E X A S

230 Mi.

LA JUNTA   CHIHUAHUA

150 Mi.

BOYCOYNA

O SISOGUICHI

BAR. de COBRE

RIO URIQUE   M E X I C O

Gulf of California

Rio Fuerte

N

— PAVED ROADS

- - - UNIMPROVED ROADS

⋯ TARAHUMARA

Figure 1

the Tarahumara have cattle, sheep and goats, these animals are kept principally as sources of fertilizer and wool. Only on rare occasions is a domestic animal slaughtered for food.

Background for the physical working capacity of the Tarahumara

The names that primitive peoples choose for themselves are often somewhat ethnocentric. Tarahumara is a Spanish corruption of Raramuri which means, literally "Fleet Foot." Historical and ethnographic evidence (Bancroft, 1884; Lumholtz, '02; Sauer, '35), indicates that the Tarahumara called themselves by this name from earliest contact times. From this, we may infer that for some centuries these people have prided themselves for their running abilities. With this in mind, let us examine some of the features of Tarahumara life and culture which have a bearing on their physical capabilities.

Arable land in the Sierra is scattered in widely separated patches along water courses. This situation has probably had some influence in determining the Tarahumara settlement pattern which, in contrast to the compact villages typical of most primitive agriculturists, consists of widely-scattered *rancherias* composed of one to several, usually related, families (Kennedy, '63). A *rancheria* may be separated from its neighbors by 2 to 10 kilometers of rugged terrain. The *rancherias* of a local area form a larger social unit, the *Pueblo*, governed by elected officials. Centrally located in the Pueblo area is a meeting place, the *Communidad*, where the members gather weekly to trade, gossip, hear mass, and to conduct Pueblo affairs. The typical Tarahumara covers a great deal of distance during the course of his daily activities. In addition to the weekly trek to the Communidad, a round trip of perhaps 10–30 kilometers, he must frequently visit his neighbors to trade, engage in communal labor projects, and perform other social tasks and duties. Also, he must herd his ranging flocks of sheep and goats and tend his fields which, because of peculiarities of the Tarahumara system of inheritance (Bennett and Zingg, '35), may be separated by many miles. Tarahumara hunting practices have already been mentioned.

In addition to such local activities, a considerable amount of inter-pueblo contact occurs, generally for the purpose of trade, to socialize or to attend religious fiestas. During Holy Week in Sisoguichi, for example, we encountered families who had traveled on foot from Pueblos as far away as Norogachic, some 150 kilometers to the south. In the modern Mexican city of Chihuahua, nearly 250 kilometers away, it is common to see whole families of Tarahumara *"turistas"* have trekked the entire distance with no other purpose than spending a few days wandering the streets and seeing the sights.

Mestizo settlers and the missions of the area commonly employ Tarahumara as messengers and it is generally conceded that a good runner can cover up to a hundred miles a day and sustain this pace for several days. Lumholtz ('02), for example, cites the case of a Tarahumara who carried a letter from Guazpares to Chihuahua and made the round trip, a journey of nearly 500 miles, in five days. Bennett and Zingg ('35) refer to the practice of Mexican ranchers hiring Tarahumara to chase and capture wild horses.

Thus, we see that in the course of his normal subsistence and social activities, the Tarahumara must spend a great deal of time traveling on foot, often carrying heavy loads. Here again we must emphasize the difficulty of the terrain: A journey of any distance on the map may actually amount to twice that distance on the circuitous trails of the region and may be interrupted by several steep ascents and descents. Whether to save time on an urgent affair or to simply break the mono-

tony of more casual errands is difficult to determine, but the Tarahumara often run while on such journeys. We, as well as others (Bennett and Zingg, '35; Pennington, '63), have been struck by the frequency with which one encounters the solitary Tarahumara jogging along the trail in a graceful and practiced trot.

While the day-to-day activities of the Tarahumara require a great deal of running, it is in their famous kick-ball races that their powers of endurance are most severely tested. These races, well-documented in the historical and ethnographic literature, follow cross-country circuits ranging from 10 to 40 kilometers in length. The number of laps to be run is pre-arranged for any given race. The usual distance covered ranges from 150 to 300 kilometers. The total time required to complete such a contest is 24 to 48 hours.

However simple or elaborate the contest, a special feature is the use of crudely carved wooden balls of about baseball size. The leading runners of the two teams propel these balls along the course using only their feet. An impressive feature of this performance is the precision with which the direction and distance of the ball travel is controlled. The runners — frequently barefoot — approach the ball with the dorsal-lateral side of either one of their feet and — with a kicking motion from the hips — send the ball in the desired direction. They are so skillful in this practice that turns and twists in the trail can be precisely short-cut by the ball flight, the ball landing on or close to the trail. The role of the "kicker" is the most strenuous one since proper and accurate control of the ball requires frequent changes of pace and direction. The other members of the team, by staying behind the kicking runner, are able to more evenly pace themselves. When the kicker becomes fatigued, he drops behind the rest of the runners and his place is taken by another, comparatively fresh, teammate. Touching the ball with the hands is only allowed when it inadvertently lodges in some otherwise inaccessible place. Often, the runner carries a stick along which he may use for placing the ball more favorably for his kick. He also may use it to assist his negotiations of steep slopes.

Throughout the race, the runners are usually accompanied by non-contestants as "active spectators." At night, the race goes on. Both — competitors and spectators — are then carrying torches — these being replaced as needed until dawn (Lumholtz, '02). Thus, the runners are under a more or less constant and impartial surveillance which tends to discourage either lagging or cheating. The fact that each participant usually bets upon himself also serves as a stimulus for good performance (Bennett, '35). The striving for maximum effort is indicated by reports that deaths from exhaustion have occurred.

Physiological aspect of the kick-ball races

The extraordinary physical accomplishments of these runners can only be assessed by an attempt to estimate the energy expenditure during such feats of prolonged effort. Although the average velocity is rather slow, judged by the standards of modern track and cross-country events, it is considerably above the speed a well-conditioned normal man of our culture can maintain for only 3 to 6 miles on a smooth course. One has to keep in mind that the course of the kick-ball race follows roads and trails over rocky terrain, climbs and descends frequently, and crosses many water passages. The many deviations and detours of the runners from a straight line, caused by the ball bouncing off-course, result in energy expenditures greater than would be calculated from the average velocity over the total distance. The frequent breaking of the running rhythm for picking up the ball, as well as the forceful swings of the ball-kicking legs also slow the average velocity down without, however, lowering the energy expenditures. Good runners cover steadily for many hours distances of 10–13 km per hour or, on the average, about 190 meters per minute. The physiological demands for such performance are best expressed in oxygen requirements which amount to approximately 43 ml/min per kilogram of the runner's weight — or to about 12 times his resting metabolic rate. At such a working rate, the total oxygen consumption of an individual weighing 60 kg would average about 2.5 liters per minute

which is nearly equal to an energy expenditure of 12 kcal per minute, or 720 kcal per hour. Thus, the total energy costs for a 100-mile race are well beyond 10,000 kcal. So far, physiological evaluations of feats of strenuous mountaineering or of long distance skiing or bicycling competitions — the most strenuous activities in man's voluntary physical efforts over many hours of duration — have yielded a limit of 10,000 kcal of energy expenditure within 24 hours. Thus, the reported performances of the Tarahumara require a revision of our physiological concepts of maximum work tolerance.

Actual observations on the Tarahumara's physical performance capacity

During our visit to Panalachi (2,100 m) in October 1963, a kick-ball race was organized with four boys as participants, two of them six years old, the other two of age nine and ten. The circuit measured approximately 2,500 meters and had to be run four times. All four runners finished within 70 to 80 minutes. The heart rate of the ten-year-old winner was 176 beats per minute immediately after the run, 154 at three and 132 at five minutes after the race. The nine-year-old's heart rate five minutes after the run was 108 beats per minute.

An attempt was made to evaluate the physical fitness level of a number of Mestizo and Tarahumara boys and to explore the possible existence of hereditary differences. The boys had lived for several years under the same conditions in a Mission School at Sisoguichi (2,000 m). Physical work capacity was assessed by a 15-minute run in which the boys were required to cover the greatest possible distance. The average velocity attained was converted into its physiological equivalent of oxygen requirements, a procedure justified because of the nearly linear relationship between running speeds and energy expenditures. Experimental comparison of this test procedure with a treadmill test of aerobic work capacity had indicated that the values of maximum oxygen intake during the treadmill test were closely approached by the estimated values of oxygen requirements for the average velocities attained during the 15-minute run (Balke, '63).

Results of this field test in Sisoguichi are presented in table 1. There was practically no difference in performance capacity between the boys of Indian or of Mestizo descent, the former averaging a mean velocity of 181 m/min, the latter 179 m/min. A few of the boys were apparently not turning out their best effort as can be concluded from the pulse rates counted immediately after termination of the run. Their average pace of 153, 176 and 160 m/min ellicited heart rates of only 78, 106 and 126 beats per minute, respectively. Such response is indicative of only light to moderate physical efforts.

American boys of comparable age, tested during a YMCA Summer Camp (Balke, '62), definitely did not perform as well. There, the *best* 17 out of a group of 80 boys attained an average velocity of 171 meters per minute, another group of 25 boys averaged only 155 m/min. Their pulse rates after termination of the run were all between 160–180 beats per minute.

The same test procedure was applied to six other male subjects of Tarahumara origin who had lived for several years in or around the Sisoguichi Mission. Their performances (table 2) were indicative of "very good" levels of work capacity (Balke and Ware, '59). The estimated metabolic equivalents for the average velocities were close to 14 times the resting metabolic rate. In comparison, nine medical officers of the U. S. Air Force, after eight weeks of physical conditioning, attained only a maximum energy expenditure of about 11 times the resting rate (Balke, '59).

During the Easter Holidays of 1964 a kick-ball race was organized at Sisoguichi. The four participants were Tarahumara Indians who had become permanent dwellers of this village, and hence, have become somewhat acculturated in diet and work habits. It is doubtful that they could match the physical efforts of less acculturated normal Tarahumara males. Since the race was a "short" one — only two circuits of 32 kilometers each — the runners

TABLE 1

		Age	Weight	Mean velocity	Oxygen requirement (estimated)	Heart rate 15-min run	
						Pre	Post
		years	kg	m/min	ml/kg/min		
Mestizo boys		13	38	204	45.5	93	152
		12	34	185	42.3	84	150
		12	36	176	40.7	72	106
		12	35	170	39.6	80	136
		12	36	160	38.0	64	126
	Mean:	12	36	179	41.2	79	134
Tarahumara boys		13	38	203	45.3	67	152
		12	36	189	42.9	62	140
		12	34	182	41.7	81	150
		12	36	176	40.7	86	158
		12	35	153	36.7	68	78
	Mean:	12	36	181	41.5	73	136

TABLE 2

Subject	Age	Weight	Blood pressure at rest	Heart rate		Mean velocity	Oxygen requirement (estimated)
				Pre	Post		
	years	kg	mm Hg			m/min	ml/kg/min
A.M.	14	45	115/80	80	156	235	50.8
D.C.	14	49	115/90	80	160	204	45.6
H.A.	16	52	125/92	68	148	197	44.2
V.	20	—	—	52	96	201	45.0
D.M.	21	65	135/80	64	160	251	53.5
R.	30	—	—	74	154	203	45.4

had made no special preparations and had not gone through the "curing" ceremonies described in detail by Bennett and Zingg, ('35). One of the runners — when asked — stated that "curing" was not considered necessary for such a short race.

This race was won by the oldest of the competitors, a man 43 years of age, who ran the distance of 64 kilometers in 6 hours and 18 minutes. The youngest (20 years), of Tarahumara-Mestizo descent, looked strongest and did very well initially but came in last in a total time of 6 hours and 52 minutes.

The winner's running velocities for consecutive segments of the race, his estimated accumulative energy expenditure, and the approximate course profile are presented in figure 2. The lower average velocities on the second circuit were less the result of fatigue than of a neglect on part of the organizers to provide for food supply at the half-way mark. Hence, after the runners had completed the first circuit of 32 kilometers in less than three hours they were somewhat discouraged when they found out that there were no refreshments available. Only the promise that food would be awaiting them after completion of the next 10 km urged them to go on — but at a reduced speed. The eventual rest period of several minutes

during which pinole and water was handed to them was included in the over-all running time and consequently affected the average velocity.

Several interesting physiological observations were made on all four runners (see table 3 and 4). The weight/height relationship indicated that all were on the lean side. Considering the relatively high temperature of about 27°C during the race, the average weight loss of 3 kg appeared not alarmingly high. The average performance during the nearly seven hour effort exceeded the maximum work capacity of the "normal" American male who can maintain not quite the same pace for only about 15 minutes.

The pre-race resting heart rates were of an order compatible with pre-race anxiety. Immediately after finishing the 64-km run, however, the heart rates were slower than expected, while the lower blood pressures were in line with the observations on people in a state of physical fatigue after extended periods of exercise. The serum cholesterol values were very low compared with the value of 180 mg% considered to be about "normal." The approximately 23% rise in cholesterol values after the run is consistent with the usual findings in trained men after physical exertion (Balke, '60) and must be explained as

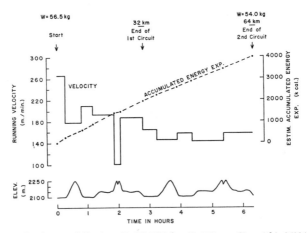

Fig. 2   Tarahumara L.D.; Age, 43; W, 56.5 kg; H. 169 cm; Sisoguichi, 3/29/64.

TABLE 3

Subject	Age	Weight		Height	Mean velocity	Oxygen requirement	Energy expenditure total kcal
		Pre	Post				
	years	kg	kg	cm	m/min	ml/kg/min	
L.D.	43	56.5	54.0	169	168	39.8	3960
L.V.	37	51.0	47.5	156	166	39.0	3350
J.D.V.	31	54.5	52.0	159	158	37.6	3890
R.B.	20	60.5	57.0	167	155	37.1	4180
Mean:	33	55.6	52.6	163	162	38.2	3845

TABLE 4

Subject	Heart rate per min		Blood pressure		Cholesterol		Hemoglobin		Hematocrit	
	Pre	Post	Pre	Post	Pre	Post	Pre	Post	Pre	Post
			mm Hg	mm Hg	mg %	mg %				
L.D.	80	102	110/75	130/80	114	135	17.0	18.8	51	56
L.V.	84	102	130/85	105/80	75	99	15.8	—	48	—
J.D.V.	87	112	135/85	105/80	63	81	17.3	17.8	53	56
R.B.	80	112	110/80	100/70	66	75	18.6	19.0	51	—
Mean:	83	107	121/81	110/77	79	97	17.2	—	51	—

mobilization of fat from the body reserves as an energy source. Hemoglobin and hematocrit values appear in line with those one can expect at elevation about 2,000 meters.

DISCUSSION

The principal objective of the present study was to scientifically confirm the hitherto largely anecdotal accounts of Tarahumara physical endurance. The physiological data presented are limited to the few simple procedures possible under the rigorous field condition of the region. They are sufficient, however, to establish guidelines for future research which should include not only more detailed and refined physiological assessments but anthropological studies to establish the role of diet, work habits, and other factors in adapting the Tarahumara to his environment.

Since the Tarahumara have inhabited the Sierra region for a considerable period and are exposed to environmental extremes which could act as selective agents, it is tempting to hypothesize that natural selection has played a role in adapting them to their arduous habitat. While such adaptations may be present, they were not detectable by the comparative techniques employed in this study: After 15 minutes of running, there was no significant difference in response between Tarahumara and Mestizo youngsters raised in a more or less uniform mission environment. Unfortunately, it was not possible to directly compare Mission students of Tarahumara origin with the performance of non-acculturated Tarahumara boys, but it was our impression, based on the 15-minute runs of the Tarahumara students, that they would not be able to sustain the pace set by the 6-10-year-old unacculturated Tarahumara youngsters in their 72-minute race at Panalachi. Thus, the evidence gathered so far indicates that Tarahumara endurance is predominately a matter of conditioning rather than primary genetic adaptation.

In this regard, however, it should be remembered that "conditioning," "endurance," and "physiological work capacity" are complex concepts involving the interplay of many physiological and morphological variables and it is unlikely that any genetic factors involved would be so simple and obvious that they would be revealed by the relatively crude field assessments employed in the present study. It should also be mentioned that certain features of generalized American Indian physiology and physique may represent preadaptations which may facilitate the development of Tarahumara physical capabilities. Thus, in general, Mongoloids display a somewhat larger thorax in relation to total body size than do other racial groups. Such a morphological feature might give the Tarahumara some slight advantage in the rate with which he can condition himself to endurance running. Another "pre-adaptive" feature may be the relatively slow heart which characterizes the American Indian. Hrdlička ('08), who gathered data on the resting heart rate of many hundred American Indians of several dozen tribes, found the mean resting rate is about ten beats per minute slower than the accepted normal of 72/minute for Caucasoids. On the other hand, regular strenuous physical activity lowers the resting heart rate of most any man to values between 50 and 60 beats per minute.

There is also the matter of how well the individuals we studied represented the total Tarahumara population. Only the school children in the 15-minute run tests were selected in a random manner. The remaining individuals, the various adults and the four children who raced at Panalachi, were volunteers who raced for the small inducements we offered. It is likely that they tend to be individuals who more or less regularly participate in kick-ball races and hence are somewhat better-conditioned than the average Tarahumara male. On the other hand, it should be noted that most of our subjects were to some degree acculturated and may actually under-represent the potentialities of their more primitive co-tribesmen.

LITERATURE CITED

Ascher, R., and F. J. Clune 1960 Waterfall cave, southern Chihuahua. American Antiquity, 26: 270–274.

Balke, B., and R. W. Ware 1959 An experimental study of "physical fitness" of Air Force personnel. U. S. Armed Forces Medical Journal, 10: 675.

Balke, B. 1959 Unpublished data.
——— 1960 The effect of physical exercise on the metabolic potential, a crucial measure of physical fitness. Colloqium on Exercise and Fitness. The University of Illinois College of Physical Education and the Athletic Institute Champaign-Urbana, Illinois.
——— 1960 Work capacity at altitude. In: Symposium of Exercise and Sports Science. Warren R. Johnson, ed., Harper Publishing Co., New York.
——— 1962 Unpublished data.
——— 1963 A simple field test for the assessment of physical fitness. Civil Aeromedical Research Institute Report 63-6, April 1963.

Bancroft, H. H. 1884 History of the North Mexican states and Texas. Vol. I, 1531–1800. A. L. Bancroft, San Francisco.

Basauri, C. 1929 Monografía de los Tarahumara. Talleres Graficas de la Nacion. Mexico, D.F.
——— 1940 La población indígena de Mexico. Vol. I, pp. 299–352. Secretaría de Educaión Publica, Mexico, D.F.

Bennett, W. C., and R. M. Zingg 1935 The Tarahumara, An Indian tribe of northern Mexico. University of Chicago Press, Chicago.

Dunne, P. J. S. 1948 Early Jesuit missions in Tarahumara. University of California Press, Berkeley.

Gajdusek, D. C. 1953 The Sierra Tarahumara. Geographical Review, 43: 15–38.

Hrdlička, A. 1908 Physiological and medical observations among the Indians of the southwestern United States and northern Mexico. Bureau of American Ethnology Bulletin 34, Smithsonian Institution, Washington, D. C.

Kennedy, J. G. 1963 Tesguino complex: The role of beer in Tarahumar culture. American Anthropologist, 65: 620–640.

Lumholtz, C. 1894 Tarahumara life and customs. Scribner's Magazine, 16: 296–311.
——— 1902 Unknown Mexico. Charles Scribner's Sons, New York.

Pennington, C. 1963 The Tarahumara of Mexico. University of Utah Press. Salt Lake City, Utah.

Sauer, C. 1935 Aboriginal populations of northwestern Mexico. Ibero-Americana 10. University of California Press, Berkeley.

Zingg, R. M. 1940 Report on the archaeology of southern Chihuahua, III. Contributions, University of Denver.
——— 1942 The genuine and spurious values in Tarahumara culture. American Anthropologist, 44: 78–92.

NORRIE'S DISEASE IN NORTH AMERICA

by

FREDERICK C. BLODI & WILLIAM S. HUNTER

In 1927 NORRIE described several families in whom the male members were born blind or became blind soon after birth. He also noticed at that time that many of these affected children had defective hearing or were deaf. In some of them there was also mental retardation. He clearly recognized this entity as a sex-linked recessive trait and subsequent reports have verified this assumption.

The eye disease, in general, resembles that of Coats' disease. In both retinas there appear numerous hemorrhages and later on an organized white mass is visible behind the lens. The eyes become atrophic and a cataract and degenerative corneal changes develop.

Histologic examination of enucleated globes have only rarely been done. In general they show a hemorrhagic retinal detachment with secondary degenerative changes, rubeosis of the iris, posterior synechiae and ectropium uveae.

In a recent monograph WARBURG (1966) has accumulated all available material on this condition. The first sibship in the United States was described only a year ago by HANSEN (1968).

The relationship to Coats' disease is an obvious one. Coats' disease is also a vascular retinal lesion occurring usually in young male patients but it affects only one eye in the majority of the cases. It is also characterized by exudation and hemorrhage into and beneath the retina. The primary lesion is here a congenital retinal teleangiectasia. Leber's disease of the retinal vessels is probably only an early or minimal phase of Coats' disease. The primary lesion of Norrie's disease is unknown, though it may very well also

39

be a retinal angioma. Coats' disease has recently been reviewed and delineated by MANSCHOT & DE BRUIJN (1967) and by GOMEZ MORALES (1965). Some variations in the clinical picture and course have been described. While most cases are unilateral (WOODS & DUKE, 1963) bilateral cases do occur (GREEN, 1967). The disease may become manifest or be detected in patients who have reached middle or old age (HENKIND & MORGAN, 1966).

The congenital nature of the condition could lead one to suspect that this is a genetically determined disease. However, familial Coats' disease has been observed only extremely rarely. In one family, reported by SMALL (1968), the children also suffered from muscular dystrophy, deafness and mental retardation. This family is somewhat of a link to Norrie's disease.

We would like to describe two families with Norrie's disease, in which the condition was present in several generations. In a number of instances enucleated eyes became available for histologic examination.

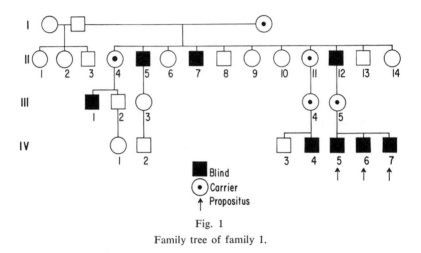

Fig. 1

Family tree of family 1.

Family 1 (fig. 1):

Our attention was drawn to this family because we saw in our clinic three brothers (IV-5, IV-6, IV-7) who were all blind since early infancy and who had defective hearing. Two of the eyes are available for histologic examination. The first eye was enucleated in 1957 and at that time the suspicion was

40

high that this could be a retinoblastoma. The other eye was enucleated because of painful, degenerative changes.

1) J.A.K. (48–4929 [IV/5]) was born on December 27, 1947. His birth weight was 9 lbs and 1 oz. Pregnancy and delivery had been normal. Soon after birth a white reflex was noticed by the mother in each eye. The child behaved like a blind infant.

He was first seen at the University Hospital in Iowa City on April 28, 1948. There was a searching nystagmus in both eyes. In the right eye the cornea was clear, but there was no anterior chamber, the brown iris being plastered against the cornea. Through the dilated pupil a white-yellow mass was seen behind the clear lens. Numerous blood vessels and few fresh hemorrhages were seen in that mass. A red reflex was seen in the periphery of the fundus. The left eye also had no anterior chamber. The pupil was irregular because of posterior synechiae and partly occluded by a membrane. Back of the lens was a similar hemorrhagic mass. No red fundus reflex could be obtained.

The child's hearing was definitely decreased. X-rays of the orbits did not show any calcifications within the globes. The child was examined under anesthesia, but nothing additional was found.

The patient was followed for several years. He attended the Iowa Braille and Sight Saving School. In 1952 both eyes became atrophic. In 1963 a band keratopathy developed in both eyes.

He graduated from high school and is gainfully employed.

2) R.H.K. (58–3124 [IV/6]) was born on February 20, 1949. His birth weight was 6 lbs and 1 oz. Pregnancy and delivery had been normal. The termination of pregnancy was on term and no supplemental oxygen was given. It soon became apparent that the child was blind. As of the age of one year he had a few tonic-clonic seizures. He was slow in growth and development. His hearing was diminished, but he spoke his first word when he was one. He did not walk until he was two. His psychomotor deficit became more apparent and his attacks more frequent. The EEG was grossly abnormal showing widespread cerebral involvement and a probable deep, midline disturbance. Skull films were negative. The cerebrospinal fluid was negative.

He was first seen in our clinic on May 1958. Both eyes were atrophic and deeply set in the orbit. Neither eye had light perception and both showed a searching nystagmus. The right conjunctiva was slightly injected. There was a band keratopathy on that side and the cornea was too cloudy to see the interior of the eye. The left cornea also had a band keratopathy and a degenerative pannus. The anterior chamber was here shallow with many peripheral anterior synechiae. The left pupil was occluded by a membrane.

The right eye became progressively painful and was enucleated on April 10, 1959.

The patient developed fairly well. He was put on medication because of chronic epilepsy with infrequent grand mal seizures. Though his hearing was defective

41

he could attend the Iowa Braille and Sight Saving School. He died by drowning in the summer of 1963.

The histologic examination of the enucleated right globe (Path. 3791) reveals an atrophic globe (18 × 19 × 20 mm) with a flattened, opaque cornea, which is markedly thickened. Its epithelium is irregular and basophilic deposits are found beneath it. The stroma is thick and vascularized. The anterior chamber is nearly absent because of extensive anterior synechiae. The iris is thick and the pupil is occluded. The lens is partly calcified.

The retina is completely detached showing numerous old and recent hemorrhages. The retina is drawn anteriorly by a cyclitic membrane on the temporal side (fig. 2). Nummerous cysts and cholesterol clefts are seen in the atrophic

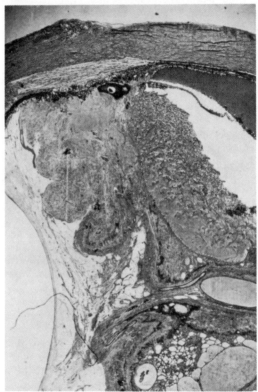

Fig. 2

Complete, hemorrhagic detachment of the right retina in case 2 (IV/6). Vascularized membrane in front of the retina and blood beneath it. Bone formation at the ora serrata. (Hematoxylin and Eosin, x15).

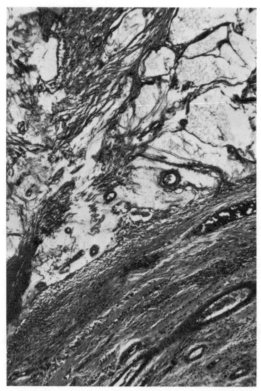

Fig. 3

Higher magnification of figure 2. Dilated blood vessels and hemorrhages in the retina; vascularized membrane on it. (Hematoxylin and Eosin, x100).

retina. On its anterior surface lies a fibrous, vascularized layer of connective tissue extending from one part of the ciliary body to the other (fig. 3). The choroid shows bone deposition and many calcified drusen.

3) M.K.K. (57–15979 [IV/7]) was born on August 30, 1957. His birth weight was 7 lbs and 5 ozs. Pregnancy and delivery had been normal. When he was two months old he was seen by his local ophthalmologist because of persistent tearing on the right side. The lacrimal duct was irrigated and at the same time a large fundus hemorrhage was noted on this side. Two weeks later a retinal hemorrhage was found in the left eye.

He was first seen in the Eye Clinic on December 5, 1957. The right eye was larger than normal, the cornea hazy and the pupil large and nasally displaced. It did not react to light. A white, elevated mass was seen in the fundus. Tension was normal to fingers. The left cornea was clear and the pupil reacted to light. A white mass was seen in the temporal periphery of the fundus. Tension was normal to fingers.

Four days later the child was examined under general anesthesia. The right eye was enucleated because a retinoblastoma could not be excluded. With the pupil dilated, the left fundus showed a marked dilatation of the temporal retinal vessels. The disc was blurred. Temporally a smooth, elevated white mass was seen with small vessels on it. A few hemorrhages were spattered over the fundus.

Three months later (2/27/68) the left anterior chamber was shallow, the pupil measured 3 mm in diameter and was fixed. A huge yellow detachment was seen in the fundus. On May 6, 1958 the left retinal detachment had become complete and hemorrhages were found behind the retina nasally. A hyphema appeared in September.

When examined in February, 1960 cholesterol crystals filled the anterior chamber and the eye was soft. He was last seen in 1964 with an atrophic left globe. At the present time he is still a student of the Iowa Braille and Sight Saving School.

The enucleated right globe (Path. 3493) is of normal size. The anterior chamber is shallow and the lens shows beginning cataractous changes. The retina is totally detached and shows severe pigmentary and glial degeneration. Numerous old, organizing and fresh hemorrhages are in and on the retina (fig. 4). The detached retina is covered by a layer of newformed blood vessels (fig. 5). In the choroid are a few inflammatory foci.

The first eye was enucleated because of the strong possibilty that it harbored a retinoblastoma. When it became evident that we were dealing with a familial hemorrhagic retinal disease we attempted to construct the family tree (fig. 1). The three brothers, who are the propositi, are IV/5, IV/6 and IV/7. All the members with the exception of II/4 and her offspring, live or had lived within the State of Iowa.

It turned out that the grandfather (II/12) of the three brothers had also been seen in the Eye Clinic.

4) Mr. L. A. (62–22577 and 44–4003) was born in 1894. He was first seen in the Eye Clinic on September 23, 1948 at the age of 54. He stated that he had been practically blind and poor of hearing since childhood.

At that time the left eye was atrophic and had no light perception. The cornea was milky white and showed a marked band keratopathy. The right eye had a visual acuity of 3/60. The cornea showed a beginning band keratopathy. The lens was completely opaque. Both eyes showed a rotatory nystagmus.

On September 29, 1948 the right cataract was extracted. The fundus could later on be seen. There was diffuse chorioretinal atrophy, gliosis and large elevated

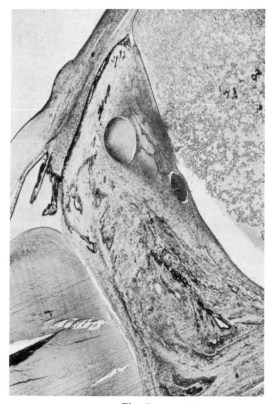

Fig. 4

Complete, hemorrhagic retinal detachment in the right eye of case 3 (IV/7).
(Hemotoxylin and Eosin, x15).

scars were seen in the temporal periphery. Vision with aphakic correction was
6/60.

The patient died in 1962 because of a bronchogenic carcinoma.

5) The cousin of the propositi, (IV/4), was examined by another ophthalmologist. He too was blind since birth and hard of hearing. Both eyes were atrophic
and the corneas opaque.

6) A similar eye report was obtained from a cousin of the mother of the propositi
(III/1).

No eye report is available on II/5 and II/7. The mother of the propositi had.

45

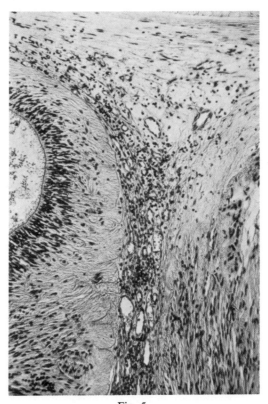

Fig. 5

Higher magnification of figure 2. A dense vascularized membrane lies on the
retina. (Hematoxylin and Eosin, x 150)

however, known them and was sure that they had been blind and nearly deaf
since childhood.

Family 2 (fig. 6):

The second family was originally reported 20 years ago by WILSON (1949).
It is a family of Indians from the Manitoulin Island in Ontario and most of
the affected males could be examined at the Hospital for Sick Children in
Toronto. We could extend this family tree by one more generation. Three

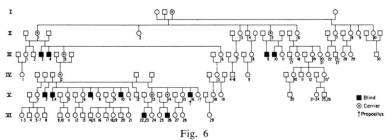

Fig. 6

Family tree of family 2.

more affected males were detected and more pathologic material could be studied.

The family tree (fig. 6) shows again that only males are affected. The defect is transmitted through the females. This is especially apparent in the offspring of IV/2 where six blind males have three different fathers but the same mother.

1) The patient who first drew the attention of the ophthalmologists to this family was W. McM (V/16). He was admitted September 9, 1947 at the age of 18 days. The eyes had been red from birth. The pregnancy was normal and delivery was on term. The birth weight was 6 lbs and 8 ozs.

On physical examination the right pupil appeared large with a green-white reflex in it. Behind the lens were blood vessels and blotches of blood in a whitish mass. Behind it smooth, dark folds were visible, apparently representing the retina. Cornea, sclera, conjunctiva and iris appeared normal. There was no light perception in this eye.

The left eye appeared essentially the same but there seems to have been some light perception.

Intraocular pressure was 21 in both eyes.

The right eye was enucleated on October 2, 1947.

The child remained mentally retarded and was brought up in an institution.

The enucleated right eye (147–47) is smaller than normal. The cornea is clear. The anterior chamber is shallow and filled with an eosinophilic, homogeneous fluid. There are peripheral anterior synechiae. The lens shows beginning cataractous changes. The retina is completely detached. The subretinal fluid contains blood and there are fresh hemorrhages in the retina. On the retina is a thin, vascularized membrane (fig. 7).

2) The oldest halfbrother (V/2) of the propositus was only seen once. The right eye showed posterior synechiae and a soft, greyish-yellow lens. The left iris was atrophic and the pupil dilated. The lens was small and the vitreous filled with a pinkish mass.

47

3) The second oldest halfbrother of the propositus is L.T. (V/3). He was admitted in August 1928 at the age of five years. At birth his eyes appeared normal. At the age of two months they became greyish and the child had never been able to see.

On psysical examination the right eye showed a dilated pupil and a small atrophic lens which was dislocated backward. The anterior chamber was deep. The eye itself was small and a large opaque mass was seen behind the lens.

The left eye showed a dense opacity of the cornea. The lens was cataractous and the pupil well dilated but did not react to light. The eye itself was small and soft.

The right eye was enucleated August 28, 1928.

The left eye became atrophic and was covered by a shell for cosmetic porposes.

The child developed with normal intelligence, but was deaf. He was well known among his tribe as a witch-doctor ('Bear walker').

Histologic examination of the enucleated right eye (2833-28) shows a phthisical globe with a deep anterior chamber and extensive peripheral anterior synechiae. An extension of Descemet's membrane and proliferating pigment epithelium cover the anterior surface of the iris. Calcium and bone are deposited at the posterior pole. The interior of the eye is filled with an organized hemorrhage, fresh blood, old blood pigment and cholesterol crystals (fig. 8).

4) The boy A.T. (V/4) is a brother of the previous patient. He was admitted to the hospital in August 1928 at the age of seven years. At that time his mother said that his eyes had been normal at birth and for the first two months of life. pregnancy had been normal and delivery on term. Later a greyish reflex appeared in the pupillary area of both eyes. Since then he has never been able to see, but could only appreciate bright light. His health was otherwise normal.

On examination the right eye appeared smaller than the left one. In the right eye numerous posterior synechiae were seen in a greyish yellow reflex in back of the lens. The left pupil was dilated and did not react to light. The lens was small and opaque and the vitreous behind it was filled with a pinkish mass. The iris was somewhat atrophic.

The child was definitely of normal intelligence, but completely deaf. He died three years later in an institution for the blind.

5) A younger brother is W.T. (V/7). He was admitted in July 1935 at the age of 2½ months, his mother stated that at birth his eyes seemed to be normal. He could follow movements during the first few days. The pregnancy had been normal and the delivery was on term. At the age of ten days the colored part of the eye became cloudy and smoky. This condition got worse in the next two weeks.

On examination the child appeared to be blind, though there was a slight indication of some light perception. Both pupils were dilated showing an ectropion uveae and they did not react to light. The lenses were clear. A yellow, partly

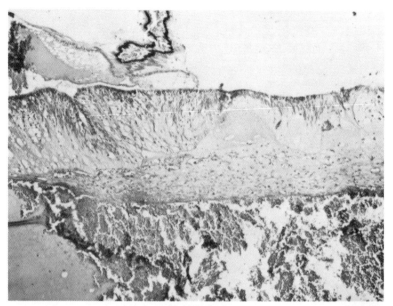

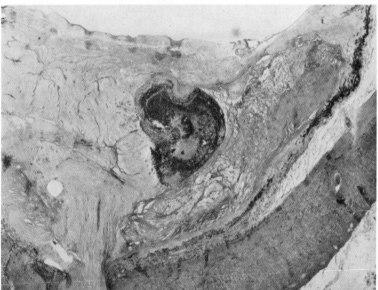

Fig. 7 and 8

Hemorrhagic detachment in the right eye of case 1 (V/16). The retina is hemorrhagic and edematous. (Hematoxylin and Eosin, x 125).

Fresh blood (center) and organized old blood fill the right eye of case 3 (V/3). (Hematoxylin and Eosin, x 15).

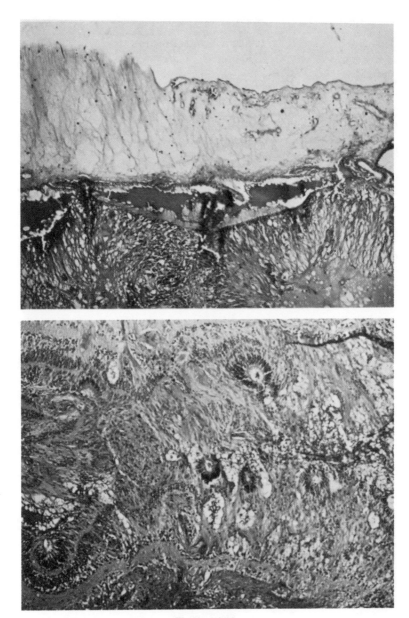

Fig. 9 and 10

Detached retina with a vascularized, preretinal membrane. Left eye of case 5
(V/7). (Hematoxylin and Eosin, x 125).

Completely disorganized detached retina filled with edema and blood in the same
eye as figure 9. A few rosettes are present. (Hematoxylin and Eosin, x 125).

vascularized mass lay behind each lens. The intraocular pressure was increased in both eyes.

The left eye was enucleated on July 24, 1935.

The boy has developed with normal intelligence but has been completely deaf.

Histologic examination of the left eye (3218-35) shows extensive peripheral anterior synechiae. An extension of Descemet's membrane and proliferating pigment epithelium cover the anterior surface of the iris. There is a moderate ectropium uveae. The retina is completely detached and blood is found in the retina and beneath it. A vascularized preretinal membrane is present (fig. 9). A few small, rosette-like structures are seen in the retina (fig. 10).

6) The youngest affected halfbrother of the propositus was W. T. (V/10). He was admitted in August 1928 at the age of 2½ years.

His mother stated that his eyes appeared normal at birth but at the age of two months they became greyish. He has not been able to see since then but he could perceive bright light.

On examination both corneas were clear and the pupils dilated. They did not react to light. Numerous posterior synechiae had developed in both eyes and the lenses were opaque bilaterally. The fundus could not be seen.

The patient died at the age of six of an unknown cause.

7) The oldest affected male in the sixth generation is K.B. (VI/22), born May 31, 1961. He was admitted July 10, 1961 at the age of 41 days. The mother had noticed a white reflex in the left pupil from birth. The child was born on term and the birth weight was 7 lbs and 3 ozs.

On physical examination both eyes showed a wandering, uncoordinated nystagmus. The right retina appeared detached with a mass visible on the temporal side behind the lens.

In the left eye a white retrolental mass was seen against the posterior lens surface. This mass was infiltrated with blood vessels and had a definite concave anterior surface.

The child was examined under general anesthesia and no definite lens changes were noted, nor could any elongated ciliary processes be found at the periphery of the lens.

The left eye was enucleated on August 8, 1961.

In September, 1961 the right anterior chamber was flat. The iris appeared frayed and atrophic and was pressed against the cornea. The pupil was fixed.

In 1967 his hearing was tested and apparently he was not deaf.

Histologic examination of the left eye (AFIP Acc. 1014117) shows the iris bowing backwards with dense posterior synechiae. Newformed bloodvessels cover the anterior iris surfae. The retina is completely detached and lies in a funnel-shaped form behind the lens. In the atrophic retina are large vessels and hemorrhages (fig. 11). There is also blood in the subretinal fluid. A few rosette-like structures are seen in the retinal tissue (fig. 12).

51

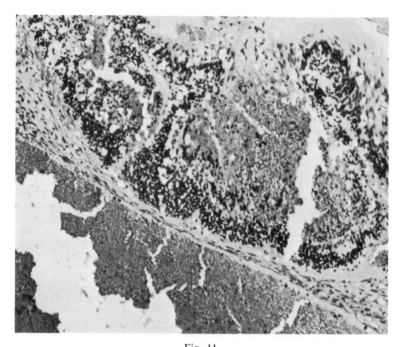

Fig. 11

Hemorrhagic retina with blood in the subretinal fluid in the left eye of case 7
(VI/22). (Hematoxylin and Eosin, x 75).

8) The younger brother of the previous patient is M.B. (VI/23). He was born on
April 10, 1962 on term after normal delivery. The mother noticed soon after
birth a whitish appearance of the pupils similar to the one seen in his brother.

The patient was examined May 4, 1962. Both fundi showed large vitreous strands
and opacities. In the left eye a hyaloid artery was present.

The patient was re-examined in November 1962. At that time the right anterior
chamber was absent and a white opaque mass was seen behind the lens. In the left
eye a similar white mass was seen nasally behind the lens. A red reflex was
obtainable temporally and the anterior chamber on that side was shallow.

The child developed with some mental retardation.

9) A cousin of the preceding two patients is K.A. (VI/26). He was born November
29, 1965 on term and after normal delivery. Soon after birth the mother had
noticed a whitish reflex in the pupils.

He was seen in the clinic in June, 1967. Both eyes showed a band keratopathy
and microphthalmos (fig. 13).

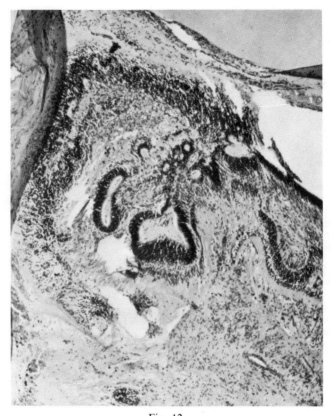

Fig. 12

Rosette-like structures in the disorganized retina. Same eye as figure 11. (Hematoxylin and Eosin, x 75).

The patient was examined under general anesthesia on October 6, 1967. The right cornea measured 8.5 x 7 and the left 9 x 8 mm. Both corneas were moderately hazy. The intraocular pressure was 2/10 gm with Schiøtz. The iris appeared dark brown in both eyes and there was an extropion uveae with posterior synechiae present bilaterally. The pupils were irregular and did not react to light. Anterior chambers were shallow and the lenses almost touched the cornea. A whitish mass was visible behind the lens in both eyes.

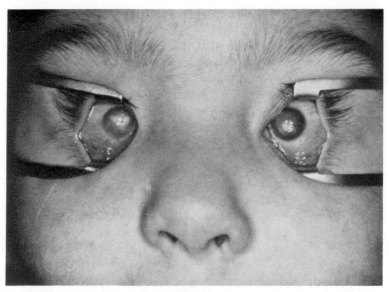

Fig. 13
Clinical appearance of the eyes in case 9 (VI/26).

CONCLUSION & SUMMARY

NORRIE's disease is a congenital or infantile, bilateral, hemorrhagic retinal detachment which is transmitted as a sex-linked recessive. Many of the affected children are poor of hearing, some are mentally retarded.

Two affected families are reported from North America. They encompass three and four generations respectively. Nineteen affected males are described clinically and six eyes could be studied histologically. The salient features of the histologic picture are: A complete retinal detachment, retinal hemorrhages and edema, a vascularized preretinal membrane and secondary degenerative change. These features are identical with those found in the usual Coats' disease.

REFERENCES

GOMEZ MORALES, A. Coats' disease. *Amer. J. Ophthal.* 60, *855–865* (1965).

GREEN, W. R. Bilateral Coats' disease. *Arch. Ophthal.* 77, *378–383* (1967).

HANSEN, A. C. Norrie's disease. *Amer. J. Ophthal.* 66, *328–332* (1968).

HENKIND, P. & G. MORGAN Peripheral retinal angioma with exudative retinopathy in adults (Coats' lesion). *Brit. J. Ophthal.* 50, *2–11* (1966).

MANSCHOT, W. A. & W. C. DE BRUIJN Coats' disease. *Brit. J. Ophthal.* 51, *145–157* (1967).

SMALL, R. G. Coats' disease and muscular dystrophy. *Trans. amer. Acad. Ophthal. Otolaryng.* 72, *225 231* (1968).

WARBURG, M. Norrie's disease. *Acta. ophthal.*, Suppl. 89 (1966).

WILSON, W. M. G. Congenital blindness (pseudoglioma) occurring as a sex-linked developmental anomaly. *Canad. med. Assoc. J.* 60, *580–585* (1949).

WOODS, A. C. & J. R. DUKE Coats' disease. *Brit. J. Ophthal.* 44, *385–412* (1963).

Alloalbuminemia

Albumin Naskapi in Indians of the Ungava

Baruch S. Blumberg, MD, John R. Martin, MD,
and Liisa Melartin, MD

Physicians usually associate inherited biochemical traits with "inborn errors of metabolism" and disease. The relatively rare but important inherited conditions, such as galactosemia and phenylketonuria, have received considerable attention in the past few years because of the success achieved in deter..ining the basic inherited biochemical defect and the steps that have been taken to ameliorate the dread effects of these genes. However, not all inherited biochemical variation is directly associated with disease. There are many systems in which several common inherited forms of a protein, carbohydrate, or other biochemical not directly associated with disease have been detected. Included among these are the red blood cell groups, the serum haptoglobins, transferrins, group-specific components (Gc groups), and the glucose-6-phosphate dehydrogenase and other enzyme variants. In these systems, two or more of the variants are common in many human populations, and none is directly associated with abnormalities. These systems are termed polymorphisms (after E. B. Ford) and, according to current genetic theory, are maintained in the population by a balance of selective forces acting on the different forms. Other genetic mechanisms may also be involved in maintaining the polymorphism. In some instances, interaction of an external agent with a variant can lead to illness. For example, individuals with an inherited deficiency of glucose-6-phosphate dehydrogenase are, under ordinary circumstances, unaffected by this "abnormality." However, if they ingest fava beans or a variety of drugs including antimalarials and salicylates, a hemolytic anemia, which can be severe, may develop. When persons with an inherited variant of serum pseudocholinesterase are given succinylcholine (suxamethonium) chloride or related muscle relaxants, apnea may develop; whereas such persons are quite normal under other circumstances.

One of the most interesting features of the polymorphic traits is the striking differences in gene frequency in different human populations. For example, the frequency of the gene which determines the haptoglobin type 1.1 protein (Hp¹ gene) may vary from less than 25% (India) to more than 85% (West Africa) in different human populations. The glucose-6-phosphate dehydrogenase deficiency gene is extremely rare in northern European populations but may occur in 30% or more of males in some Greek and Kurdish communities. Hence, if clinical conditions are associated with the trait, they would be of far greater consequence in the populations, native or immigrant, in which the variant is common than those in which it is absent or rare.

Variants of serum albumin have been found rarely in European and American populations. Recently, we described an albumin variant (albumin Naskapi) common in North American Indians and Eskimos but absent in the other populations tested. A clinical study was made of Indians who have only the albumin variant (albumin Naskapi homozygotes) and of those who have albumin Naskapi and common albumin (heterozygotes).

During the past ten years, there have been several reports of albumin variants detected in routine paper or cellulose acetate electrophoresis. In most of the reported cases, the albumin variant has been shown to be inherited as a simple autosomal codominant trait. In the early cases, only the heterozygotes

56

were detected. The presence of two albumin bands led to the use of the term "bisalbuminemia" for this condition. Bisalbuminemia was found to be extremely rare in the populations in which it was found, ie, one in 4,750 in Sweden,[1] and one in 1,015 in Norway.[2] The heterozygotes (ie, patients with bisalbuminemia) did not have any clear evidence of disease, although slightly elevated cholesterol levels were reported in two studies.[3,4] However, these findings were not statistically significant. Generally speaking, the bisalbuminemia was persistent although its transient occurrence has been reported.[5,6] There has been very little study in the isolation or biochemical characterization of the variant albumins. Gitlin et al[7] separated albumin A from the slow variant albumin B. Hydrolysis with chymotrypsin released one anomalous peptide from the slow albumin, while hydrolysis with trypsin yielded two anomalous peptides. The data indicate that an anomalous lysine residue is present in albumin B, replacing a residue in albumin A which most probably contains a free carboxyl group.

In the early cases, the variant albumin (albumin B) was reported to be slower moving than the common albumin (albumin A). Additional rare variants had been reported before 1966, which were both slower moving (albumin B) and faster moving (albumin Reading[4]; albumin Ra[8]) than common albumin A.

Despite the large number of heterozygotes reported in these studies, no variant homozygote was described until 1966. In that year, Melartin and Blumberg[9] reported a fast-moving variant of serum albumin (subsequently shown to be different from albumin Reading and albumin Ra) which was quite common in the populations in which it was found. The original discovery was made in the Naskapi Indians of Labrador and the variant was given the name albumin Naskapi. Several individuals homozygous for the Naskapi were found in the Naskapi Indians and in the closely related Montagnais Indians. Subsequently, homozygotes were also found among the Sioux and Athabascan Indians who also have this gene in relatively high frequency. Bell et al[10] have reported homozygotes for a fast-moving albumin found in Cree Indians. Although this variant has not been compared to albumin Naskapi it is likely to be the same variant.

The term "alloalbuminemia" (from the Greek *allo* meaning different) is recommended for the condition in which the individual has an albumin variant different from common albumin A. Individuals can be either heterozygous or homozygous for the variant; theoretically an individual heterozygous for two uncommon variants may be found. The specific variant could be designated by the second word in a binomial, eg, alloalbuminemia Naskapi, alloalbuminemia B, or alloalbuminemia Mexico. The albumin variants which have been compared in our studies are shown in Fig 1 along with the nomenclature.[11]

Tribal History.—Prior to the arrival of the Euro-

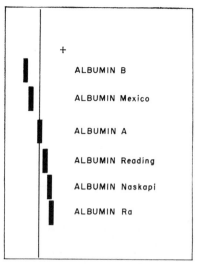

1. Inherited albumin variants which have been compared to albumin Naskapi, Symbols A1 B, A1 Naskapi, etc, re used for albumin phenotypes. Symbols A1^B, A1^{Na}, A1^{Me}, etc, are used for genes. (Adapted from Melartin[11].) The term "Gent" has recently been substituted for Ra (Weime, personal communication).

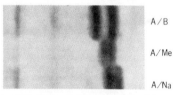

2. Starch gel electrophoresis experiment in which mobility of albumin Naskapi is compared to that of albumin A, albumin B and albumin Mexico.[14,15] The origin is at left and positive pole to right.

peans, the hunting grounds of the Naskapi and Montagnais ranged over a large part of the Labrador peninsula. With the establishment of the fur trade, the two groups polarized; the Montagnais becoming tributary to trading posts along the north shore of the St. Lawrence River, and the Naskapi eventually focusing on posts in the northern part of the peninsula. With the establishment of an iron mine in Schefferville (nearly midway between these points), a railroad line was constructed from Seven Island on the north shore of the St. Lawrence to the mining area. Approximately 30 Montagnais families traveled

Table 1.—Clinical Features in Homozygous, Heterozygous and Normal Subjects

Table 1.—Clinical Features in Homozygous, Heterozygous and Normal Subjects

Patient No.	Albumin Type	Age (yr)	Sex	Height cm (in)	Weight kg (lb)	BP Right Arm (mm Hg)	Peripheral Pulses	Fundi	Miscellanea	Tribe
C12728	Na/Na	46	M	171.5 (67.5)	85.3 (188)	110/78	Strong	Normal	...	Naskapi
C12765	Na/Na	28	F	177.8 (70)	64.4 (142)	90/0	Strong	Normal	Eight months pregnant	Montagnais
C12727	A/Na	13	M	142.2 (56)	32.2 (71)	100/60	Strong	Normal	...	Naskapi
C12730	A/Na	19	M	168.9 (66.5)	49.9 (110)	110/64	Strong	Normal	...	Naskapi
C12731	A/Na	65	M	157.5 (62)	58.5 (129)	140/80	Strong	Early copper wire changes	Arcus senilis	Naskapi
C12732	A/Na	66	M	163.9 (64.5)	68 (150)	150/96	Strong	Normal	...	Naskapi
C12733	A/Na	68	F	... ...	... ...	150/80	Strong	...	Bilateral cataracts; arcus senilis, and bilateral pterygia	Naskapi
C12761	A/Na	29	F	... ...	... ...	130/70	Strong	Normal	...	Montagnais
C12763	A/Na	32	F	160 (63)	42.2 (93)	100/60	Strong	Normal	...	Naskapi
C12726	A/A	10	F	139.7 (55)	35.4 (78)	100/60	Strong	Normal	...	Naskapi
C12729	A/A	13	M	149.8 (59)	38.1 (84)	90/58	Absent dorsalis pedis pulses	Normal	...	Naskapi
C12762	A/A	63	F	163.9 (64.5)	70.8 (156)	180/90	Strong	Early copper wire changes	...	Montagnais
C12764	A/A	62	M	165.1 (65)	57.2 (126)	120/78	Absent right dorsalis pedis pulse	Normal	Arcus senilis	Montagnais

to Schefferville and established residence in a village adjacent to the mining town. Shortly afterwards, the Naskapi, who had centered on the Fort Chimo area of Ungava Bay, traveled to the Schefferville area and established themselves in a village near the Montagnais constructed by the Canadian government for their use. The Naskapi are nearly all Anglicans in religion, and only a few of them speak English. Most are literate in their own language. The Montagnais, who are nearly all Roman Catholics, speak French and are literate in that language. Until recently, there has been relatively little intermarriage between these two groups despite their proximity in the Schefferville area.[12]

The Naskapi and Montagnais are part of the large Indian Algonquian language family which is spread throughout southern Canada from the West Coast of Hudson Bay to the eastern provinces of Canada, and through the midwestern United States.

Material and Methods

A total of 203 blood specimens was collected

from among the Naskapi. The population of the tribes in 1963 was 224. Hence, more than 90% of the entire Naskapi population of Schefferville was tested during the course of this study. A total of 128 blood specimens was collected from the Montagnais residents of Schefferville. This represented somewhat more than 50% of the population in the village at the time that the study was done. Clinical studies were performed on two Naskapi/Naskapi homozygotes, seven Naskapi/A heterozygotes, and four A/A homozygotes (ie, individuals with the usual kind of albumin), selected from Naskapi and Montagnais residents in Schefferville. Because of the previous reports of elevated cholesterol levels associated with albumin heterozygotes,[3,4] serum lipid studies and clinical evaluations of conditions associated with hypercholesterolemia were included. The studies included, for some or all of the subjects, a complete physical examination; an abbreviated medical history; roentgenograms of the chest; electrocardiogram; hemogram; urinalysis; and deter-

Table 2.—Laboratory Results in Homozygous, Heterozygous, and Normal Subjects

Patient No.	Albumin Type	Hemoglobin, gm/100 ml	WBC/cu mm	Urinalysis	Cholesterol, mg/100 ml (160-260)*	Triglycerides, mg/100 ml (50-150)*	Lipase, cc (0.1-1)*	Amylase, Units/ml (5-23)*
C12728	Na/Na	...	7,200	Normal	230	84	0.25	14
C12765	Na/Na	...	12,150	Normal	239	223	...	...
C12727	A/Na	...	...	...	159	106	...	...
C12730	A/Na	14.0	7,100	Normal	180	42	0.6	20
C12731	A/Na	14.3	6,600	Normal	160	139	0.6	12
C12732	A/Na	...	...	...	210	107	0	18
C12733	A/Na	11.2	5,650	Normal	245	123	0.5	20
C12761	A/Na	...	...	...	152	81	...	...
C12763	A/Na	...	...	...	144	56	0.45	16
C12726	A/A	...	...	...	244	195	...	...
C12729	A/A	...	...	...	244	230	0.15	18
C12762	A/A	...	...	...	282	125	...	...
C12764	A/A	...	...	...	209	63	0.5	16

*Normal value.

58

mination of serum cholesterol, triglyceride, lipase, amylase, calcium, alkaline phosphatase and uric acid levels; and a thymol turbidity test. The hematologic examinations, ECG's, and roentgenographic studies were performed in Schefferville. The cholesterol and triglyceride levels were determined at the Hospital of the University of Pennsylvania, and the remainder of the studies were done at the clinical laboratory of Jeanes Hospital, Philadelphia. Routine clinical techniques were used for these determinations. The medical examinations were performed primarily by one of us (J.R.M.), with the assistance of the other authors.

The albumin phenotype was determined using the starch gel electrophoresis technique with the discontinuous buffer system of Ashton and Braden[13] at pH 8.6. This buffer system contains lithium hydroxide, boric acid, citric acid, and tromethamine. Details of the procedure are given in the original paper by Ashton and Braden,[13] and in the paper by Melartin and Blumberg.[9]

Results

A picture of results of a starch gel electrophoresis experiment is shown in Fig 2. In this, albumin Naskapi is compared to albumin A (common albumin), albumin B (the slow-moving rare albumin) and albumin Mexico (a slow-moving albumin). In Fig 1, albumin variants which have been studied in our laboratory are shown in a diagram in which their relative mobilities are compared. From these it is clear that albumin variants can be readily distinguished on the basis of differences in their electrophoretic mobilities.

Report of Cases

CASE 1 (C12728).—A 46-year-old Naskapi Indian man born in Fort Chimo, Quebec, who was homozygous for albumin Naskapi, felt well at the time of examination. Results of the system review of the head, eyes, ears, nose, and throat (HEENT), cardiorespiratory system, gastrointestinal system, genitourinary system and neuromuscular system were all normal. On physical examination, the patient's height was 171.5 cm (5 ft 7½ inches); weight, 85.3 kg (188 lb); blood pressure (sitting), right arm, 110/78 mm Hg; and

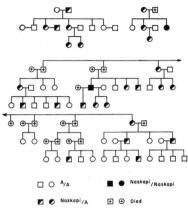

3. Typical pedigrees showing segregation of albumin Naskapi in Naskapi and Montagnais Indian families. (Adapted from Melartin and Blumberg.[9])

pulse, 68 beats per minute. His dentition was good. The pupils reacted equally to light. His fundi were pale, and the disks and fundal vessels appeared normal. There were no abnormal findings in the heart and lungs, nor were there masses in his abdomen. There was no evidence of hernia, and the genitalia were normal. Deep tendon reflexes (DTR) were not elicited at the knees, and were diminished at the ankles. The Babinski reaction was normal, and results of the remainder of the neurologic examination were within normal limits. Laboratory studies showed that the white blood cell count (WBC) was 7,200/cu mm; urine was pH 6 and contained no protein or sugar. Other values were as follows: cholesterol 230 mg/100 ml; triglycerides, 84 mg/ 100 ml; serum amylase, 14 units/ml; serum calcium, 10.5 mg/100 ml; lipase, 0.25 cc; alkaline phosphatase, 3.7 Bodansky units; thymol turbidity, 1.6 units; and serum uric acid, 6.1 mg/100 ml.

The chest roentgenogram was within normal limits, except that the left ventricle was minimally enlarged. The ECG showed intraventricular conduction delay and clockwise rotation.

CASE 2 (C12765).—A 28-year-old Montagnais Indian woman was eight months pregnant at the time of examination. She had no complaints referable to her pregnancy, nor to any other system. Results of review of HEENT, cardiorespiratory system, gastrointestinal system, genitourinary system, and neuromuscular system were all normal. On physical examination, the patient's height was 177.8 cm (5 ft 10 inches); weight, 64.4 kg (142 lb); blood pressure (sitting), right arm, 90/0 mm Hg, left arm, 110/0 mm Hg. Her pulse rate was 92 beats per minute and regular. On ophthalmoscopic examination, the fundi were pale, and the vessels and disks were normal. There were no abnormal findings in the heart and lungs. The liver and spleen were not palpated. The fetus was palpable at the umbilicus, and the genitals were normal. The peripheral pulses were normal with the exception of an absent left post-tibial pulse. The DTR and Babinski reactions were normal, and results of the remainder of the neurologic examination were within normal limits. Laboratory studies showed that the WBC was 12,150/cu mm, and that the urine was pH 8 and contained no sugar or protein.

Calcium, Units/ml (9-11)*	Thymol Turbidity, Units (0-5)*	Alkaline Phosphatase, Units (1.5-4)*	Serum Uric Acid, mg/100 ml (2-6)*
10.5	1.6	3.7	6.1
...	...	...	...
...	...	...	...
12.0	4.2	6.1	5.1
9.5	3.5	1.6	5.1
12.0	3.9	2.8	5.8
11.5	3.2	3.1	4.2
...	...	...	...
10.5	1.8	3.0	5.6
...	...	...	...
11.0	5.1	9.1	3.6
...	...	...	...
10.5	2.0	3.5	6.2

Table 3.—Roentgenographic and ECG Results

Patient No.	Albumin Type	Roentgenogram	ECG
C12728	Na/Na	Minimal enlargement of left ventricle	Intraventricular conduction delay. Clockwise rotation
C12765	Na/Na	Bilateral pleural thickening at bases	Normal
C12730	A/Na	Normal	Peaked T waves. Elevated ST segment
C12731	A/Na	Pleural thickening, tenting diaphram, calcified nodes, concentric left ventricular hypertrophy	Minimum left ventricular hypertrophy
C12733	A/Na	Normal	Normal

Because of the patient's pregnancy, the roentgenogram and ECG were deferred until after delivery. At that time the chest roentgenogram showed minimal pleural thickening at the bases of both lungs. Her ECG was within normal limits and showed a vertical electrical position of the heart.

The results of these examinations and those of the A/NA heterozygotes and of the A/A homozygotes are given in Tables 1 to 3. One of the heterozygotes (patient C12730) had a slightly elevated alkaline phosphatase level, and an elevated alkaline phosphatase level was also found in an individual (C12729) with albumin A. The same individual had a slightly elevated thymol turbidity value.

In summary, none of the individuals with albumin Naskapi appeared to have clinical or laboratory findings which could be ascribed to alloalbuminemia.

Comment

Previous studies have shown that albumin Naskapi is inherited as a simple autosomal codominant trait. Several of the pedigrees are shown in Fig 3, and an analysis of the family studies is given in Table 4 (taken from Melartin and Blumberg[9]). From this, it can be seen that the number and phenotypes of offspring of A/A × Na/Na and the A/A × A/Na families are very close to those expected on the basis of autosomal codominant inheritance. No exception to the genetic hypothesis has been found. The distribution of albumin Naskapi in various

American Indians and other populations is shown in Table 3. From the studies completed to date, we can conclude that albumin Naskapi occurs in a restricted range. It is found in several northern North American Indians but not in American Indians from southern North America and South America, nor in Europeans, white Americans, Africans, Indians, and others who have been tested. The studies in the southwestern United States are fragmentary, but albumin Naskapi has been reported in Navajo Indians from Idaho (J. L. Robbins, MD, unpublished data). The distribution of the trait crosses several Indian linguistic and cultural divisions. In addition, the trait has been found in Eskimo groups in north Labrador and in west Alaska as well as in a single Aleut (B. S. Blumberg et al, unpublished data).

Recently we found another polymorphic variant of serum albumin termed albumin Mexico[14,15] which is relatively common in the Uto-Aztecan Indians of Mexico and the southwestern United States. This trait has not been found in the northern American Indians in which albumin Naskapi is common, nor in any non-Indian populations tested.

A particularly interesting feature of the albumin variants is the finding that the albumin locus is closely linked to the locus for the genes determining the Gc serum protein variants, ie, the loci for these two traits are located on the same chromosome.[16-18] (The Gc proteins are inherited α-protein variants first described by Hirschfeld.[19]) Prior to the discovery of this linkage, there were some five well-documented examples of autosomal linkage (ie, on non-sex chromosomes) known in man. These are characterized by the rarity of families in which the linkage could be studied. Since the albumin Naskapi polymorphism is relatively common in the populations in which it is found, and the Gc trait is polymorphic in all of these populations (polymorphic implies that two or more of the inherited forms of the trait occur fairly commonly in the populations), the discovery of this linkage system should make possible extended studies on the biology of linkage.

The clinical studies reported here suggest that there are no striking abnormalities associated with the presence of albumin Naskapi either in heterozygote or homozygote form.

This does not mean that other forms of alloalbuminemia would be without clinical findings. It would not be surprising if homozygotes for the rare albumins (ie, albumin B, albumin Reading) were severely ill.

Despite these negative findings, there are certain considerations

Table 4.—Segregation of Albumin Types in Families*

Albumin Type of Parents	No. of Families	Albumin Type of Children						Children, Total
		A/A		A/Na		Na/Na		
		Observed	Expected	Observed	Expected	Observed	Expected	
A/A-Na/Na	1	0	0	2	2	0	0	2
A/A-A/Na	10	17	16	15	16	0	0	32

*Adapted from Melartin and Blumberg.[9]

Table 5.—Distribution of Albumin Naskapi in Different Populations*

Population	No. Tested	Na/Na	A/Na	A/A	Gene Frequency A1
Naskapi, Canada	203	1	54	148	0.138
Montagnais, Canada	128	2	19	107	0.090
Sioux, US	160	0	2	158	0.007
Athabascan, US and Canada	230	1	11	218	0.028
Eskimos, Labrador, Canada	124	0	3	121	0.012
Eskimos, Alaska and continental US	262	0	4	258	0.008
Various Indians, Mexico†	687	0	0	687	0
Haida, Canada	365	0	0	365	0
Cashinahua, Peru	92	0	0	92	0
Quechua, Peru	100	0	0	100	0
White and Negro, US	353	0	0	353	0
Asian and Oceanic population	1,252	0	0	1,252	0
Other non-Indian populations	3,100	0	0	3,100	0

*Adapted from Melartin.[11]
†Albumin Mexico[14,15] was present in this population.

which may prove to be of impórtance in relation to the health of American Indians. Serum albumin is the major plasma protein involved in blood transport of cations, anions, dyes, drugs, and various physiological substances. Several substances bind almost exclusively to albumin (ie, bromophenol blue, fatty acid, bilirubin), and several other substances which bind to other serum protein also bind to serum albumin. Examples of substances which bind to a serum protein in addition to albumin are thyroxine, which binds mainly to α-globulin, and hemoglobin, which binds mainly to haptoglobin. Both of these will bind to albumin when they are present in sufficiently high concentrations. The biochemical differences between albumin variants which result in differences in electrophoretic mobility might also have an effect on their binding properties for particular substances. For example, it has been shown that only the variant band of albumin in some heterozygote sera (albumin B in A/B heterozygotes and albumin Reading in A/Reading heterozygotes) binds thyroxine when a small amount of thyroxine is added. Also, in A/Reading heterozygotes only albumin Reading binds bromophenol blue and the albumin A component remains unstained, while in an A/B heterozygote the dye binding capacity of the albumin component appears to be equal. In our experience, bromophenol blue binds more readily to albumin Naskapi than to albumin A, and in other studies it was shown to bind more readily to albumin A than to the slow-moving albumin Mexico. There does not appear to be any differential binding of thyroxine and hemoglobin to albumin Naskapi in the amounts that have been used so far. Many antibiotics and other drugs such as barbiturates bind to albumin. It has been shown that penicillin in large amounts distorts the appearance of all the albumin variants with which it has been associated (D. Arvan et al, unpublished data). It is not known, however, if this would have any effect on the antibiotic action of the drug. In summary, there is differential binding between variants for certain substances; an investigation of these may yield information of clinical importance.

The albumin variants are also of considerable interest in the study of the physical anthropology of American Indians. Albumin Naskapi appears to be associated with northern North American aboriginal tribes. The second common albumin variant we have found, albumin Mexico,[15] is common in some southern tribes. This may, therefore, provide a powerful tool for the study of the interrelation of these tribes in North America and their affinities with Old World people still living in eastern and northern Asia. It also brings up the very interesting question of why these traits should have persisted and increased to relatively high frequency in these particular tribes while it is not found in other North American aborigines. This could be due to the major differences in environment to which these populations have been subjected over the generations, as well as to their tribal interrelations.

This investigation was supported by Public Health Service research grants CA-06551 and CA-08069 from the National Cancer Institute.

M. Gelinas, MD, performed the electrocardiographic and roentgenographic studies. Cholesterol and triglyceride levels were determined by P. T. Kuo, MD.

J. MacEachen, minister of national health and welfare, government of Canada, granted permission to undertake this study.

Generic and Trade Names of Drug

Succinylcholine chloride—*Anectine Chloride, Quelicin Chloride, Sucostrin Chloride, Sux-Cert, Suxinyl.*

References

1. Laurell, C.B., and Niléhn, J.E.: A New Type of Inherited Serum Albumin Anomaly, *J Clin Invest* 45:1935-1945 (Dec) 1966.
2. Efremov, G., and Braend, M.: Serum Albumin: Polymorphism in Man, *Science* 146:1679-1680 (Dec 25) 1964.
3. Earle, D.P., et al: Observations on Double Albumin: A Genetically Transmitted Serum Protein Anomaly, *J Clin Invest* 38:1412-1420 (Sept) 1959.
4. Tárnoky, A.L., and Lestas, A.N.: A New Type of Bisalbuminemia, *Clin Chim Acta* 9:551-558, 1964.
5. Scheurlen, P.G.: Ueber Serumeiweissveränderungen beim Diabetes Mellitus, *Klin Wschr* 33:198-205 (March) 1955.
6. Gabl, F., and Huber, E.G.: Passagere, nicht Hereditäre Doppelalbuminämie, *Ann Paediat* 202:81-91, 1964.
7. Gitlin, D., et al: Observations on Double Albumin: II. A Peptide Difference Between Two Genetically Determined Human Serum Albumis, *J Clin Invest* 40:820-827 (May) 1961.
8. Wieme, R.J.: On the Presence of Two Albumins in Certain Normal Human Sera and Its Genetic Determination, *Clin Chim Acta* 5:443-445, 1960.
9. Melartin, L., and Blumberg, B.S.: Albumin Naskapi, a New Variant of Serum Albumin, *Science* 153:1664-1666 (Sept 30) 1966.
10. Bell, H.E., et al: Bisalbuminemia of the Fast Type With a Homozygote, *Clin Chim Acta* 15:247-252, 1967.

11. Melartin, L.: Albumin Polymorphism in Man: Studies on Albumin Variants in North American Native Populations, *Acta Path Microbiol Scand*, to be published.
12. Blumberg, B.S., et al: Blood Groups of the Naskapi and Montagnais Indians of Schefferville, Quebec, *Hum Biol* 36:263-272 (Sept) 1964.
13. Ashton, G.C., and Braden, A.W.H.: Serum β-globulin Polymorphism in Mice, *Aust J Biol Sci* 14:248-253 (April) 1961.
14. Melartin, L., and Blumberg, B.S.: Inherited Variants of Human Serum Albumin, *Clin Res* 14, Dec 13, 1966, adv p 48.
15. Melartin, L.; Blumberg, B.S.; and Lisker, R.: Albumin Mexico: A New Variant of Serum Albumin, *Nature* 115:1288-1289 (Sept 16) 1967.
16. Weitkamp, L.R., et al: Genetic Linkage Between Structural Loci for Albumin and Group Specific Component (Gc), *Amer J Hum Genet*, July 1967, pp 559-571.
17. Blumberg, B.S.; Kaarsalo, E.: and Melartin, L.: Autosomal Linkage Between Albumin and Gc Loci, *Clin Res* 14:481 (Dec 13) 1966.
18. Kaarsalo, E.; Melartin, L.; and Blumberg, B.S.: Autosomal Linkage Between the Albumin and Gc Loci in Humans, *Science*, 158:123-125 (Oct 6) 1967.
19. Hirschfeld, J.: The Gc-system, *Progr Allerg* 6:155-186, 1962.

Measles Vaccine Field Trials in Alaska

II. Vaccination on St. Paul Island, Pribilofs, Where Measles Had Been Absent for 21 Years

Jacob A. Brody, MD, Irvin Emanuel, MD, Robert McAlister, MD, and E. Russell Alexander, MD

Since the development of measles vaccines, several studies of clinical reactions to vaccines among older individuals have been done.[1,2] The present investigation deals with clinical and serologic responses in an island population where measles had not occurred for 21 years. Almost all residents received vaccine regardless of previous exposure to measles. Live attenuated measles virus vaccine (LV) plus γ-globulin was given to those under age 21, while LV with or without γ-globulin was administered to older people who had not been exposed to measles virus for over 20 years.

Background

St. Paul, one of the Pribilof Islands, lies in the Bering Sea off the coast of Alaska. Home of the fur seal industry, the islands by international treaty (Great Britain, Canada, the Union of Soviet Socialist Republics, Japan, and the United States) are under the direct administration of the United States government through the Bureau of Commercial Fisheries, Department of Interior. The resident Aleut population of St. Paul was 350 during the period of measles vaccination. Other island residents included a Coast Guard contingent of 30 men, about 50 Department of Interior employees, a nurse with the US Public Health Service, Alaska Native Health Program, and several practical nurses.

e standard of living on the Pribilofs compares favorably with urban Alaskan communities, and is far above that encountered in most other Aleut, Indian, and Eskimo villages. This is reflected in the high level of general health. A pediatric consultant for the Alaska Department of Health and Welfare who examined all preschool and school children on St. Paul in June, 1963, reported that, except for tooth decay, the health of St. Paul children and their growth and development was similar to that which she observes in private practice in Anchorage.[3]

Measles occurred among Pribilof residents in 1942 when they were moved from their islands to the mainland following the Japanese occupation of the Island of Attu. Prior to 1942, a very severe epidemic occurred in 1910 during which the older residents recall many fatalities. It is possible that measles appeared again in 1933 or 1938. This, however, is somewhat doubtful since during the 1942 epidemic there were numerous cases among adults.[4] Since 1942 there had been no clinical cases of measles on St. Paul Island and prevaccination serology reveals the virtual absence of immunity among those under age 20 (Table 1).

In late May and early June, a rubella epidemic occurred on St. Paul.[5] Two physicians, one from the Arctic Health Research Center, Public Health Service, and the other from Headquarters, Medical Battalion, Fort Richardson, USA, were on the island investigating the outbreak. On June 15, an 8-month-old infant was seen at the clinic with a rash and cough which in the opinion of the two physicians was compatible with rubeola. The child had arrived on St. Paul Island five days previously in apparent good health from the mainland village of Bethel. A radio message to the Public Health Service Alaska Native Hospital in Bethel revealed that a rubeola epidemic was in progress, and that rubella had not been seen. In the face of this apparent medical emergency, the Public Health Service Alaska Native Health Area Office purchased measles vaccine and γ-globulin which arrived on St. Paul on June 19. Serum specimens from this infant drawn two weeks and three months following the onset of illness, when subsequently tested,

Table 1.—Population and Vaccination Data of St. Paul Island and Prevaccination Serologic Status

Age Years	Resident Population	No. Receiving LV		No. Bled		Geometric Mean Titer (Prevaccination Bleeding)
		With γ-Globulin	Without γ-Globulin	Pre-Vaccination	Post-Vaccination	
0-1	10	10		8	7	
1-2	12	12		12	10	
2-3	11	11		11	10	
3-4	10	10		10	10	
4-5	12	12		12	11	
Total 0.5	55	55		53	48	1.6
5-9	42	42		41	40	1.8
10-14	43	43		41	41	1.5
15-19	44	33	16	36	20	3.2
20-29	48	31	20	36	30	12.0
30-39	41	13	20	23	19	24.7
40-49	40	18	20	28	20	18.3
50+	37	6	26	26	17	17.4
Total	350	241	82	284	235	

failed to reveal the presence of measles antibodies. It must therefore be concluded that in spite of the clinical appearance, it is doubtful that the child had rubeola.

Materials and Methods

Measles vaccine was administered to 323 of 350 residents on June 19 and 20. Sufficient quantities of specific γ-globulin were not available so 92 adults received vaccine with sodium chloride injection. Age distribution of the entire population and of the vaccinees is listed in Table 1, along with the distribution of those from whom blood samples were collected. During the two weeks prior to vaccination, blood samples were drawn from a total of 284 individuals (primarily in connection with rubella studies, and new samples were obtained on 235 of these four months later.

Live attenuated measles vaccine (LV) was administered according to the manufacturer's dosage schedule: LV, ½ ml, subcutaneously in one arm, and γ-globulin intramuscularly in the other arm, 0.01 ml per pound body weight (40 units per pound). Surveillance for vaccine reactions was conducted for 14 days following vaccination. Women volunteers instructed in temperature taking made

daily home visits, recorded the oral or rectal temperatures of each household member, and examined them for rashes. Anyone with an oral temperature over 99.4 F (37.4 C), or a rectal temperature over 100.4 F (38 C), or with a rash was seen by one of two physicians who were in continuous residence. (In the text, all temperatures recorded are oral, unless otherwise indicated.)

Serologic determinations were conducted at the Arctic Health Research Center using methods previously described.[6,7] Hemagglutination inhibition (HI) tests were done on sera extracted to an initial dilution of 1:3.

Results

Clinical Reactions.—Since this was not a controlled study, it was difficult to delineate those reactions which were associated with vaccine. Febrile responses during the 14-day surveillance period among 164 individuals who were seronegative for measles antibody and who received LV plus γ-globulin are presented in Table 2. An accumulation of temperature elevations occurred between days 8 and 13 following vaccination. For purposes of subsequent analysis, reactions occurring between days 5 and 14 will be considered as probably related to the vaccine. Febrile responses of eight seronegative individuals have been deleted because clear diagnosis of another illness was established as the more likely cause of temperature elevation (one tooth abscess, one herpes stomatitis, and six rubella cases).

The maximum temperature recorded for these susceptible individuals is shown by age in Table 3. Of these 27% had a temperature of 100 F (37.8 C) or greater. The highest temperature recorded was 105.2 F (40.7 C) rectally in a 3-year-old child. Temperature elevations were more frequent in children under age 5; in this group 47.1% had temperatures of 100 F (37.8 C) or more, and 15.7% had temperatures of 102 F (38.9 C) or more. Within age group 0 to 4 years, there was no tendency for febrile responses to be higher among infants less than 2 years of age. Two of six susceptibles, ages 20 to 29, had low-grade fevers with

Table 2.—Daily Rectal and Oral Temperatures of Seronegative Individuals Receiving LV Plus γ-Globulin Following Measles Vaccination

Temperature F*	Day 1	2	3	4	5	6	7	8	9	10	11	12	13	14
R 105-105.9 / O 104-104.9							1							
R 104-104.9 / O 103-103.9									1	1	1		1	
R 103-103.9 / O 102-102.9		1	2	2	1	1				3	3		2	
R 102-102.9 / O 101-101.9		2		1				3	2	5	1	3	1	
R 101-101.9 / O 100-100.9	3	1	7	1	1	3	3	5	10	14	7	5	2	2
R 100.4-100.9 / O 99.4-99.9	4	9	5	2	4	9	3	6	11	7	8	4	6	6
R <100.4 / O <99.4	157	151	150	158	158	151	157	150	140	134	144	152	152	156
Totals	164	164	164	164	164	164	164	164	164	164	164	164	164	164

*Centigrade equivalents appear in the text.

Table 3.—Age and Maximum Temperature Among Seronegative Individuals 5-14 Days Following Measles Vaccination With LV plus γ-Globulin

Temperature F	Age, Years					Total 0-4	Age, Years				Total
	<1	1	2	3	4		5-9	10-14	15-19	20-29	
R 105-105.9 O 104-104.9					1	1					1
R 104-104.9 O 103-103.9			1		1	2	1	1			4
R 103-103.9 O 102-102.9	1	1		2	1	5	2				7
R 102-102.9 O 101-101.9				1	1	2	3	1			6
R 101-101.9 O 100-100.9	3	1	5	2	3	14	3	7	2		26
R 100.4-100.9 O 99.4- 99.9			3		2	8	10	4	4	2	28
R <100.4 O <99.4	4	7	5	2	1	19	22	26	21	4	92
Total	8	12	11	10	10	51	39	41	27	6	164

temperatures of 99.4 to 99.8 F (37.4 to 37.7 C) and were not ill.

Rash probably associated with measles vaccine occurred in 10 individuals. In five instances, exanthem appeared in the absence of fever. Rashes tended to occur about equally in all age groups (one 20-year-old, two 15-19, two 10 to 14, two 5 to 9, and three 0 to 4 years of age).

LV without γ-globulin was given to five individuals who did not have preexisting antibody to measles. All were over age 30 and had remained on the Pribilofs during the evacuation in 1942. None recalled having had measles at any time in his life. Only one had a temperature of 100.4 F (38 C) for one day, and complained of very slight fatigue. Others remained afebrile.

A total of 115 individuals with preexisting measles antibodies were vaccinated. Temperatures of 99.4 to 99.8 F (37.4 to 37.7 C) of one day's duration occurred in eight of these individuals, all between days 5 and 14 following vaccination. No other signs of illness were noted in these eight cases, and there was no antibody rise above preexisting levels. Ages ranged from 29 to 73 years. Four received γ-globulin with vaccine and four did not.

Serologic Responses.—The geometric mean HI titer of 150 susceptible individuals who received LV plus γ-globulin was 15.4 four months after vaccination (Table 4). Eight of 150 susceptible individuals

remained seronegative at 1:3 initial dilution for a failure rate of 5.3%. There was no strong pattern of variation by age although titers were somewhat higher in the very young and lower among six individuals, aged 20 to 29 years. The geometric mean HI titer of five susceptible individuals over age 30 who received LV without γ-globulin was 8.5.

The degree of maximum temperature did not appear to be related to the height of antibody response. The geometric mean titer of those with oral temperatures of 100 F (37.8 C) or more was 17.0, while for those whose maximum temperature was below 100 F (37.8 C), it was 14.8.

The titers before vaccination of individuals in whom preexisting antibody was demonstrated revealed little variation by age among those 20 and over (Table 5). The geometric mean titer of 13 individuals younger than 20 years of age was 31.3. Of these, ten had had measles within the previous eight months, one while hospitalized in Anchorage, and nine while in residence at a boarding school in Sitka. There was essentially no difference between geometric mean titers of prevaccination and postvaccination blood specimens regardless of the age of the individual, or whether LV with or without γ-globulin was given (Table 5). Clinical and inapparent rubella infection as measured by antibody response occurred among persons undergoing successful measles vaccination. These simultaneous cases will be presented more fully in a subsequent report.[16]

Comment

With widespread use of measles vaccines, a situation analogous to that of smallpox may soon exist

Table 4.—Age and Titer of 164 Individuals Initially Seroimmune 4 Months After Vaccination With LV plus γ-Globulin

Age	HI Titer							Total	Geometric Mean HI Titer
	0	3	6	12	24	48	96		
<1		1	1	3	1	1		7	24.0
1-2		2	1	5	2			10	19.5
2-3			2	3	4			10	14.8
3-4	1		1	3	2	2	1	10	17.0
4-5		1	2	2	3		1	9	14.0
Total 0-5	1	1	8	10	18	5	3	46	17.2
5-9		3		10	13	8	4	38	11.4
10-14	1	1	3	12	11	10	3	41	20.6
15-19	2		2	4	4	6	1	19	17.9
20-29	1	1	2	2				6	5.3
Total	8	3	25	41	41	25	7	150*	15.4

*Excludes 14 individuals for whom no postvaccination specimen was available.

Table 5.—Geometric Mean HI Titers of Those With Preexisting HI Antibodies Prior to and Following Vaccination

	Paired Sera of Vaccinated Individuals							
	Prebleeding		With γ-globulin			No γ-globulin		
Age	No.	Geometric Mean	No.	Pre-vaccination	Post-vaccination	No.	Pre-vaccination	Post-vaccination
0-19	13	31.3	5	31.6	41.8	....		
20-29	30	18.2	9	13.0	17.6	15	24.0	20.9
30-39	22	28.1	9	24.0	22.2	9	25.9	28.0
40-49	25	24.7	9	25.9	25.9	9	24.0	25.9
50+	25	19.2	1	24.0	24.0	15	20.9	18.2
Total	115	22.7	33	21.6	24.0	48	23.3	22.0

in which measles disappears from more highly developed areas. As is the case with smallpox,[14,15] a substantial proportion of the population may not be vaccinated against measles. In addition, the duration of protection afforded by measles vaccine is not yet known. It is not inconceivable that mass measles vaccination of all age groups would suddenly become a necessity.

The measles vaccine study on St. Paul Island provided an opportunity to document clinical and serologic reactions to commercial vaccine among susceptible individuals up to age 20 and in a smaller group of older individuals. In addition, the older residents, who in all probability had been exposed to measles only once within their lives and not for the past 21 years, were studied to determine persistence of antibody under these unusual circumstances and also the response of these individuals to live attenuated measles vaccine with or without simultaneous administration of γ-globulin.

Among susceptible individuals, reactions to measles vaccine were mild. Febrile response over 102 F (38.9 C) orally occurred in 7% of the susceptible population. Temperatures were somewhat higher in the 0 to 4 years age group, and were quite low in the small group of older individuals studied. Rash appeared in 6% of the vaccinees, and was not appreciably more common at any age group.

There were eight vaccine failures in a population of 150. This is a somewhat higher rate than previously reported for LV with γ-globulin.[8,10] Antibody responses were highest among those less than one year of age and lowest in the group over age 20, although in general, antibody titers did not seem strongly related to the age of the vaccinee.

Reactions tended to be milder than those reported by Black and Gudnadottir in Iceland[1] for similar age groups in spite of the fact that these authors used twice the dose of γ-globulin (80 units per pound of body weight) that we employed. In a study in Chevak, Alaska,[6] where we used 20 units per pound of body weight, the maximum febrile response and geometric mean antibody response were similar to those in St. Paul, although fevers were more prolonged and rashes were considerably more frequent. This may, in part, be due to the fact that basic health standards and living conditions were considerably higher in St. Paul than in Chevak.

In previous studies[1,3,6] children under two had significantly higher maximum temperature responses than older individuals. In St. Paul, temperatures were higher in the entire group, age 0 to 4 years, but there was no concentration of high temperatures in those under age 2. Relationship between maximum temperature and height of antibody response has also been noted in the past[6,11] but was not demonstrated in St. Paul.

No individual with preexisting antibody to measles had a febrile response of 100 F (37.8 C) or more between the 5th and 14th day following vaccination in spite of the fact that the majority of these individuals had been exposed to measles only once in their lives, and not within the past 21 years. Geometric mean titer before vaccination did not vary appreciably in older age groups, which is in agreement with the observation by Black and Rosen[13] that naturally acquired measles antibodies persist at high levels in the absence of reexposure to measles. The geometric mean titer of seroimmune individuals did not rise following vaccination. This was equally true for those who received LV with γ-globulin and those who received LV without γ-globulin, further testifying to the solidity of immunity following natural measles infection.

Participation by the University of Washington, Seattle, was supported in part by US Public Health Service grants CC36-02 and 5TIA1206.

Members of the Sisterhood of the Russian Orthodox Church, St. Paul helped in the collection of data. Major contributions to the field study were made by Major Robert Cutting, USA, Alaska, and Eliza Bridenbaugh, RN, and her staff. William J. L. Sladen, MD, permitted the use of his field laboratory on St. Paul Island.

Generic and Trade Names of Drug

Measles Virus Vaccine, Live, Attenuated—*Lyovac Rubeovax, Gammagee.*

References

1. Black, F.L., and Gudnadottir, M.: Measles Vaccination of Adults in Iceland, *Lancet* 1:418-420 (Feb) 1963.

2. Hoekenga, M.T., et al: Experimental Vaccination Against Measles. II. Tests of Live Measles and Live Distemper Vaccine in Human Volunteers During Measles Epidemic in Panama, *JAMA* 173:868-872 (June 25) 1960.

3. Whaley, H.S.: Personal communication to author.

4. Around Alaska, *Alaska's Health*, vol 2, 1944.

5. Brody, J.A., and Sever, J.L.: Unpublished data.

6. Brody, J.A., et al: Measles Vaccine Field Trials in Alaska.

I. Use of Killed Vaccine Followed by Attenuated Vaccine and γ-Globulin With Live Attenuated Vaccine, *JAMA* 189:339-342 (Aug 3) 1964.

7. Brody, J.A., et al: Use of Dried Whole Blood Collected on Filter Paper Discs in Adenovirus Complement Fixation and Measles Hemagglutination Inhibition Tests, *J Immun* 92:854-857 (June) 1964.

8. Terry, L.L.: Status of Measles Vaccines. Technical Report, US Department of Health, Education, and Welfare, 1963.

9. Stokes, J., et al: Efficacy of Live, Attenuated Measles-Virus

Vaccine Given With Human Immune Globulin, *New Eng J Med* **265**:507-513, 1961.

10. Fulginiti, V.A.; Leland, O.S.; and Kempe, C.H.: Evaluation of Measles Immunization Methods. Clinical and Serologic Evaluation of Three Different Methods, *Amer J Dis Child* **105**:5-11, 1963.

11. Weibel, R., et al: Administration of Enders' Live Measles Virus Vaccine With Human Immune Globulin, *JAMA* **180**:1086-1094 (June 30) 1962.

12. Krugman, S., et al: Studies With Live Attenuated Measles-Virus Vaccine, Comparative Clinical Antigenic and Prophylactic Effects After Inoculation With and Without γ-Globulin, *Amer J Dis Child* **103**:366-372, 1962.

13. Glack, F.L., and Rosen, L.: Patterns of Measles Antibodies in Residents of Tahiti and Their Stability in Absence of Reexposure, *J Immun* **88**:725-731 (June) 1962.

14. Collins, S.D., and Councell, C.: Extent of Immunization and Case Histories for Diphtheria, Smallpox, Scarlet Fever, and Typhoid Fever in 200,000 Surveyed Families in 28 Large Cities, *Public Health Rep* **58**:1121-1151, 1943.

15. Beneson, A.S.: Continuing Threat of Smallpox, *Arch Environ Health* **96**-1000, 1963.

16. Brody, J.A.: To be published

Draining Ears and Deafness
Among Alaskan Eskimos

JACOB A. BRODY, MD; THERESA OVERFIELD, RN, MPH; AND ROBERT McALISTER, MD

Middle ear pathology in Alaska is a problem of considerable magnitude. Various studies [1-3] reported hearing loss in 14% of Caucasians and 34% of Eskimos and evidence of chronic otitis media in about one third of Alaskan natives. An infant morbidity and mortality study conducted by the Arctic Health Research Center in Eskimo villages revealed that of 323 infants, 38% had at least one episode of draining ears during their first year of life.[4]

To combat acute and chronic otitis media, routine medical and surgical treatment is dispensed within the limits of available personnel, and an aggressive tonsillectomy and adenoidectomy campaign is in progress.[5] The present study was undertaken to investigate the natural history and epidemiology of ear disease and also the relationship between hearing loss and otitis media.

Material and Methods

The major portion of the study was conducted in the Bethel area in southwestern Alaska among Eskimos in the villages of Hooper Bay, Chevak, Nightmute, Akiachuk, Tuluksak, Kipnuk, Pilot Station, Mountain Village, and Tuntutuliak. For comparison, similar investigations were conducted on St. Paul Island in the Pribilofs, where the population is primarily Aleut, and in Wasilla where a majority of the people are Caucasians homesteading in Alaska. In addition, we conducted a small study of the children of school teachers who reside in native villages in Alaska and of the children of school teachers living in other states.

Reprint requests to 945 Sixth Ave, Anchorage, Alaska 99501 (Dr. Brody).

Our primary techniques were to make house-to-house visits in villages and ask mothers if their children had suffered a draining ear one or more times in their lives. In village schools, we conducted hearing tests using an Ambco portable otometer, model 600. In the Eskimo villages, our sample approached 100% of the population under 20, while in Wasilla and St. Paul, sampling was more limited (about 20%).

For purposes of analysis, the population was divided into three groups: those who never had a drainnig ear; those whose ear drained once; and those whose ear drained more than once. Otometer scores were graded as normal if there was no hearing loss of 20 db from frequencies of 500 to 6,000. Severe hearing loss was defined as hearing loss of 40 db or more from frenquencies of 1,000 to 3,000. All hearing losses 20 db or greater, but not 40 db, between frequencies of 1,000 and 3,000 were classified as moderate. Hearing tests and histories of illness were collected by physicians or nurses of the Arctic Health Research Center. Since physicians were able to perform otoscopic examinations on only a small percentage of the individuals, these data are not considered in this report.

The study of children of school teachers in Alaska and in other states was conducted entirely by mail. Alaskan school teachers were contacted and asked to complete a form, giving data on earaches and draining ears for their children, both while in residence in Alaska and previously. The Alaskan school teachers were asked to recommend a school teacher with approximately the same number of children living in any other state. A similar form was sent to the teachers thus recommended.

Results

1. *History of Draining Ears.*—Table 1 gives the number and per cent of children with a history of a draining ear at some time in their lives. More than one episode of draining ear had occurred in 23% of Alaskan Eskimos; while in Wasilla, 15% had more than one episode; and on St. Paul, 5% had

TABLE 1.—*History of Draining Ear in Alaskan and Non-Alaskan Populations*

Series	Ethnic Group	No.	History of Draining Ear		
			Never, %	Once, %	More Than Once, %
Wasilla	Caucasian	103	80	5	15
Alaskan teachers' children	Caucasian	162	93	4	4
Non-Alaskan teachers' children	Caucasian	99	85	10	5
St. Paul, Pribilof Islands	Aleut	95	89	6	5
7 Eskimo villages	Eskimo	1,003	69	8	23

more than one episode. Among Alaskan teachers' children, 4% had draining ear more than once as opposed to 5% of teachers' children from other states. Single episodes of draining ear were reported from approximately the same percentage of children in all groups studied, with the highest rate being 10% for non-Alaskan teachers' children. In

Moderate hearing loss ranged from 25% to 36% in the various groups.

3. *Further Analysis of Chronic Otitis Media and Hearing Loss Among Alaskan Eskimos.*—Hearing loss as determined by otometry correlated with history of draining ear (Table 3). Only 3% of those with no history of draining ear had severe hearing

TABLE 2.—*Hearing Loss in Various Alaskan Populations*

Series	Ethnic Group	Total	Otomerer Reading		
			Normal Hearing,* %	Moderate Loss,† %	Severe Loss,‡ %
Wasilla	Caucasian	244	63	36	1
St. Paul, Pribilof Islands	Aleut	87	74	25	1
Eskimo villages	Eskimo	327	61	26	13

* No loss of 20 db from frequency of 500-6,000.
† Loss of 20 db or more at any tone from frequency of 500-6,000 but not in severe category.
‡ Loss of 40 db or more from 1,000-3,000.

Eskimo villages, 69% of children had no history of draining ear at any time.

2. *Hearing Loss Determined by Otometer.*

The results of the hearing tests are recorded in Table 2. In St. Paul and Wasilla, 1% of children tested had severe hearing loss. In the Bethel villages, 13% of the Alaskan Eskimos had severe hearing loss.

loss, while 32% of those having more than one episode of draining ear had severe hearing loss. Of all those with severe hearing loss (Table 4), 23 of 35 had a history of draining ear more than once, and seven had one episode of draining ear (ie, 86% of all those with severe hearing loss had a history of draining ear). The age of individuals with a

TABLE 3.—*Correlation Between History of Draining Ear and Hearing Loss Among Alaskan Eskimos*

Otometer Rating	Total Tested	History of Draining Ear					
		Never		Once		More Than Once	
		No.	%	No.	%	No.	%
Normal	189	150	80	14	48	25	35
Moderate loss	65	33	17	8	28	24	33
Severe loss	35	5	3	7	24	23	32
Total	289	188	100	29	100	72	100

68

TABLE 4.—*Correlation Between Hearing Loss and History of Draining Ear Among Alaskan Eskimos*

History of Draining Ear	Total	Otometer Rating					
		Normal Hearing		Moderate Loss		Severe Loss	
		No.	%	No.	%	No.	%
Never	188	150	80	33	50	5	14
Once	29	14	7	8	12	7	20
More than once	72	25	13	24	37	23	66
Total	289	189	100	65	99	35	100

history of draining at any time in their life is presented in Table 5. Approximately 69% of the people in each age group denied ever having a draining ear, while 8% claimed to have had a draining ear once in their life, and 23% suffered more than one draining ear at some time.

Households in which there were one or more children with a history of draining ear or moderate or severe hearing loss were studied to determine whether ear pathology was familial. The total number of children from whom complete household data were available was 656. Of these, 246, or 38%, had some degree of pathology. There were 118 households with 529 children in which hearing pathology existed. By subtracting the index case in these households, we have 408 children of whom 125, or 31%, had evidence of ear pathology. Thus, the siblings of index cases had a lower rate of ear pathology than the community at large (38% versus 31%).

Comment

In collecting and analyzing these data, we have attempted to utilize the simplest types

TABLE 5.—*Past History of Draining Ear Among Alaskan Eskimos by Age Group*

Age Group	Total	History of Draining Ear, %		
		Never	Once	More Than Once
0-3	246	66	9	25
4-8	273	67	9	24
9-13	229	69	7	24
14-18	136	72	7	21
19 & over	119	76	8	16
Totals	1,003	69	8	23

of information. Initially, we tried to analyze earaches as well as draining ears but found that data concerning earache were variable and dependent upon the informant. We, therefore, limited our investigation to draining ears which is a more objective and, apparently, a more memorable event. In our study population, only 3% of children with no history of draining ear at any time had severe hearing loss. Our definition of severe and moderate hearing loss was arbitrary. We adopted the standard of a 40 db loss between 1,000 and 3,000 cps for severe hearing loss, because we were certain that a loss of this magnitude in the speaking range indicated definite pathology which was likely to interfere with normal hearing and learning. Most of our analyses were based upon this group. The significance of a moderate hearing loss was not as clear-cut. We accepted in this group anyone with a loss of greater than 20 db who did not fall into the severe category. We did this to increase the significance of our normal and severe group. In many instances, we worked under less than optimum conditions where background noise, language barriers, and immaturity of the subject may have interfered with results. We doubt that anyone in the group with moderate hearing loss should be in the group with severe hearing loss. However, it is quite possible that under better conditions, some of these people would have normal hearing.

History of draining ear was strikingly more common among Alaskan Eskimos (31%) than among the other groups. Residents of St. Paul Island, primarily Aleuts, teachers' children, both living in Alaska and living in other states, had rather similar rates of draining ear, 11%, 8%, and 15%, respectively. We were surprised to find that a group in Wasilla comprised primarily of Caucasian children born in Alaska had a high rate (20%) of draining ear. It is the opinion of many Alaskan physicians [1] that acute and chronic ear conditions are unusually prevalent even among nonnative Alaskans. Unfortunately, we know of no comparable study of rate of draining ears in other areas. Crude incidence rate of acute otitis media was estimated at 2.8% in England with rates up to 20% in 6-year-olds.[6] Physicians with the Division of Indian Health, Public Health Service, now stationed in Alaska state that draining ears were unusually common on Indian reservations in other states. In a study of Swedish Lapps,[7] a high rate of chronic otitis media and hearing loss was reported.

Otometric tests revealed that approximately 1% of residents of St. Paul or Wasilla had severe hearing loss, while severe loss was encountered in 13% of Eskimos. In otometric testing of school children and preschool children in Reading, Pa,[8] New York,[9] and Erie County, New York,[10] hearing loss ranged from 2% to 8% on initial screening. These data are not comparable to ours, since different criteria and methods of testing were used.

A close correlation between history and otometric evaluation was noted among Alaskan Eskimos. Only 3% of children with no history of draining ear had severe hearing loss. On the other hand, in the group found to have severe hearing loss, 86% of children had a history of draining ear. With limited medical facilities available in Alaska, reliance on medical histories would seem a valid approach in selecting groups for study and therapeutic regimens.

Of the Eskimos, 31% gave history of draining ears at least once in their life, while 69% had never suffered a draining ear. Rates of draining ear were slightly higher among children under 36 months of age and slightly lower among those over 18, but there was no statistical difference between rates at any age.

In a one-year prospective study, it was shown that 38% of children had suffered at least one episode of draining ear by age 1. These data imply that chronic otitis media is established by age 1 or 2. There is no cumulative effect, since a similar percentage of older children gave history of having had a draining ear at some time in the past. Most intriguing is the fact that two thirds of the people at any age group deny ever having had a draining ear, and only 3% of this population had severe hearing loss. In the English study of acute otitis media, it was shown that the risk of subsequent attack increased with each successive attack.[6]

It is tempting to postulate that approximately 30% of Eskimos react to stimuli, either allergic or more probably infectious, in such a way as to set up an acute and then chronic otitis media. This is rather analogous to Jackson's and Dowling's findings with the common cold.[11,12] These authors have documented a group of people who react to stimuli by developing symptoms of a cold at a much higher rate than the remainder of the community. The factors leading to hyperresponsiveness are unclear, and it is far less clear what would lead to hyperresponsiveness of the middle ear.

No familial correlation was found for ear pathology in the Eskimo villages under study. Within individual villages, wide differences in sanitation and maternal care existed between households. It is the impression of Public Health Service physicians who frequently visit native villages that they did see families with a high prevalence of draining ears. While this is undoubtedly true, these families did not contribute measurably to the overall rate. These physicians also reported that variation exists between villages in respect to the number of chronically draining ears. This fact certainly bears investigation, although it was not demonstrated in the villages selected in this study.

Conclusions

The data presented in this study were collected over a six-month period. There seems little doubt that ear pathology among Alaskan Eskimos is unusually prevalent. Chronic otitis media was the major cause for hearing loss. As many as 69% of the people denied ever having a draining ear and only 3% of these had severe hearing loss. A total of 86% of the severe hearing loss occurred among individuals with a history of one or more episodes of draining ears. The observation that otitis media is established in a third of the population before age 2 and does not seem to affect two thirds of the population at any age strongly suggests that this specific subgroup reacts differently than the rest of the population to environmental stimuli by developing middle ear inflammation. In order to prove the concept of a predetermined chronic otitis media group, it will be necessary to follow those children in whom we have demonstrated draining ears until they are old enough to be tested for hearing loss and similarly to follow those whose ears have not drained to see if they have normal hearing.

Summary

Hearing loss and history of draining ears were analyzed for a large group of Alaskan Eskimos and smaller populations of Aleuts and Caucasian Alaskans. The rate of chronic otitis media and hearing loss was very much higher among Alaskan Eskimos than other groups tested. A strong correlation was shown between history of draining ear and hearing loss. It was suggested that ear pathology is established in approximately one third of the Eskimo village population by about age 2, and that this group may comprise the population which goes on to have severe hearing loss, while those who by age 2 have not had draining ear are unlikely to develop ear pathology in subsequent years. No familial relationship was shown for ear pathology.

The nurses with the Bethel Field Unit of the Arctic Health Research Center (Catherine Haley, Mary Lou Heminghous, Earline Isabel, Nancy Wetmore) and Dr. Irvin Emanuel, Senior Fellow, Department of Preventive Medicine, University of Washington School of Medicine, aided in collecting the data.

REFERENCES

1. Eye, Ear, Nose and Throat Infections in Alaska, Anchorage, Alaska, Alaska Department of Health, 1956.
2. Hayman, C. R., and Kester, F. E.: Eye, Ear, Nose and Throat Infection in Natives of Alaska: Summary and Analysis Based on Report of Survey Conducted in 1956, Northwest Med 56:423 (April) 1957.
3. The McGrath Project: Documentation on Study and Prevention of Upper Respiratory Disease, Anchorage, Alaska, State of Alaska, Department of Health and Welfare, and Children's Bureau, DHEW, 1962.
4. Maynard, J., and Hammes, L.: Personal communication to the authors.
5. Fritz, M. H.: Tanana Revisited, Northwest Med 62:589 (Aug) 1963.
6. Acute Otitis Media in General Practice: Report of a Survey by Medical Research Council's Working-Party for Research in General Practice, Lancet 2:510 (Sept) 1957.
7. Mellbin, T.: Children of Swedish Nomad Lapps: Study of Their Health, Growth and Development, Acta Paediat (suppl 131) 51:1-97 (Jan) 1962.
8. Wishik, S. M.; Kramm, E. R.; and Koch, E. M.: Audiometric Testing of School Children, Public Health Rep 73:265 (March) 1958.
9. Belkin, M., et al: Evaluation of Hearing Testing Program in New York City Elementary Schools, Public Health Rep 78:681 (Aug) 1963.
10. Mosher, W. E., and Maines, A. E.: A Screening Program for Detection of Hearing Loss in Preschool Children, Amer J Public Health 45:1,101 (Sept) 1955.
11. Jackson, G. G.; Dowling, H. F.; and Muldoon, R. L.: Acute Respiratory Diseases of Viral Etiology: VII. Present Concepts of Common Cold, Amer J Public Health 52:940 (June) 1962.
12. Dowling, H. F.; Jackson, G. G.; and Inouye, T.: Transmission of Experimental Common Cold in Volunteers: II. Effect of Certain Host Factors Upon Susceptibility, J Lab Clin Med 50:516 (Oct) 1957.

Biliary Tract Disease
Among the Navajos

James E. Brown, MD, and Chris Christensen, MD

WHILE MUCH has been written concerning the increased incidence of cholelithiasis and cholecystitis among the Southwestern Indians in general, there has been little data concerning the severity and natural history of biliary tract disease among them. The largest single nation of Indians in the Southwest is the Navajo nation, found predominantly in Arizona and New Mexico, with the majority of the people living on reservation and numbering about 100,000. The exact incidence of cholecystitis and cholelithiasis is unknown among the Navajos. Sievers and Marquis[1] reported that 32% of autopsied Southwestern Indians more than 15 years of age harbored biliary tract disease. However, Navajos constituted a small percentage of the patients autopsied. Also, Kravetz[2] stated that 54% of adult Southwestern Indians over 21 autopsied at the Phoenix Public Health Service Hospital between 1955 to 1960 had some form of biliary tract disease.

While the exact incidence of cholecystitis and cholelithiasis among Navajos is unknown at this time, due to geographical problems, cultural limitations, and other factors, some estimate of the severity and importance of biliary tract disease can be made from available data. The purpose of this communication is to present an analysis of 104 consecutive primary operations on the biliary tree, with an attempt to draw some conclusions on the natural history of the disease among the Navajos.

Results

There were 104 patients who received a primary operation for biliary tract disease, 19 of which were males and 85 of which were females. Thus 82% of all patients were females. The average age of the male patients was 56.8 years, while the average age of the female patients was 39.9 years. The average age of the total number of patients in the series was 43 years.

Methods

A review of all the operations done at the Shiprock Public Health Service Indian Hospital between July 1964 to December 1966 was undertaken. The hospital at Shiprock is a general hospital of 75 beds which services approximately 24,000 Navajos. One hundred and four cases of primary biliary tract surgery were found. The data gathered from each chart were age, sex, pathological diagnosis, operative procedure, serum bilirubin levels, presence or absence of cholelithiasis, and the presence or absence of choledocholithiasis. All charts were reviewed for follow-up visits to the outpatient clinic. Thus, all of the patients except one were seen at least one time after discharge from the hospital.

Reprint requests to 4612 S Clairborne Ave, New Orleans 70125 (Dr. Brown).

Cholecystectomy was done in all patients except one who had agenesis of the gallbladder. Of the 104 cases reviewed, 74 (72%; 9 males and 65 females) had chronic cholecystitis. Two males and two females in this group did not have associated cholelithiasis. There were 21 patients (20%) operated on for acute cholecystitis, seven males and 14 females. In this group of 21 there were two males without associated cholelithiasis. There were three patients (3%; two males and one female) who had carcinoma of the gallbladder. Four patients (3%; one male and three females) had diagnoses of subacute cholecystitis. With the exception of the single case of agenesis of the gallbladder, diagnoses were reached by review of the pathology report alone despite any conflicting clinical opinions.

Choledochostomy was performed in 34 (32.7%) of the patients who underwent cholecystectomy. Choledocholithiasis was found in 19 of 34 patients who underwent common bile duct exploration, giving a recovery rate of 56%. Of the patients with acute cholecystitis, eight of 21 (38%) were found to have choledocholithiasis. Of the 74 patients with chronic cholecystitis, 11 (15%) also had choledocholithiasis. The average age of patients with choledocholithiasis was 46 years. Females made up 84% of the patients with choledochoithiasis with an average age of 44 years. There were only three males with choledocholithiasis with an average age of 61 years.

The indications for common duct exploration were the commonly accepted criteria: dilated common duct, palpation of stone in the common duct, jaundice, cholangiographic evidence of choledocholithiasis, and a history of pancreatitis. The presence of small stones in the gallbladder was not used alone as an indication for exploration. Also, the use of cystic duct cholangiography varied from surgeon to surgeon. In this series, 56% of the patients with dilated common ducts (larger than 1 cm) had stones. Of those patients with elevated bilirubin levels (serum bilirubin value greater than 1.2 mg/100 cc) 39% had choledocholithiasis; however, 63% of the patients with choledocholithiasis had elevated bilirubin levels. Of those patients with elevated serum alkaline phosphatase levels (greater than 4 Bodansky units), 44% had choledocholithiasis; however, 82% of the patients with choledocholithiasis had elevated alkaline phosphatase levels.

There were no deaths in the series. Thus far there have been two cases of retained stones.

Comment

Since the purpose of this review is to reach some conclusions concerning the natural history of biliary tract disease among the Navajos, it seems necessary to compare the data from this review with other reviews from non-Navajo populations. It is of interest to note that no other similar study on Navajos was found in the literature.

Colcock and Perey[3] in a review ot 1,756 patients (operated on from 1954 to 1958) who underwent a cholecystectomy or cholecystostomy for cholecystitis found the average age for all patients to be 53.5 years; 53.4 years for women and 53.7 years for men. This was similar to findings of Adams and Stranahan[4] and of Colcock and McManus.[5] In the present review, the average age of patients who underwent cholecystectomy was 43.3 years, females being 39.9 years and males averaging 43 years. Also, in some series,[3-5] the male-to-female ratio is approximately two to one. In this series there were 82% females and only 18% males. Thus, it would seem that biliary tract disease not only occurs earlier in Navajos than in the general populations, but is less predominant in Navajo males than caucasian males.

It is also interesting to speculate on the actual incidence of biliary tract disease among the Navajos as compared to other populations. The actual incidence of biliary tract disease per unit popula-

tion at risk was not determined in this study. However, it must be noted that 50% of the entire Navajo populationis under the age of 15. Also, since biliary tract disease is one of the most common diseases seen on the surgical service at Shiprock Public Health Service Indian Hospital, it would appear that this condition is more common in Navajos than the usual populations around the country. However, this is speculation.

In a study by Smith et al,[6] the average age of all patients with choledocholithiasis was 57.8 years. This is in agreement with other large series. In the series reported here, the average age of patients with choledocholithiasis was 46, which is significantly lower. If one assumes that choledocholithiasis represents advanced biliary disease as compared to cholelithiasis,[7] then certainly it would appear that calculous biliary tract disease not only occurs earlier in Navajos but also has a more aggressive course.

Colcock and Perey[8] reported a choledochostomy rate of 28.6% in 1745 cholecystectomies. Hornfield and Albritten[9] reported that indications for choledochostomy were present in 40% of their 111 cholecystectomies. In this study choledochostomy was performed in 32.7% of the patients who underwent cholecystectomy. A choledocholithiasis recovery rate of 56% was found. This is in keeping with the recovery rate of 53% reported by Smith et al.[6] However, this recovery rate of 56% is definitely higher than that reported by Colcock and Perey[8] (27%) and by Hornfield and Albritten[9] (35%). This difference in rate probably represents the variation in criteria for exploration of the common duct.

Of the patients with chronic cholecystitis in this series, 15% were found to have choledocholithiasis. This is at variance with other series, which report a much lower rate. Of the patients with acute cholecystitis in this series, 38% were found to have choledocholithiasis. This is also higher than most series. These results would seem to point up again that calculous biliary tract disease in the Navajo is a more aggressive form of the disease than that found in the usual American non-Navajo population.

In this series there were seven internal biliary fistulas. Two occurred in carcinomatous gallbladders and five in benign biliary tract disease. Of the five benign internal biliary fistulas, three were cholecystoduodenal, one was cholecystocolic, and one was cholecystocholedochal. Of the two malignant fistulas, one was cholecystocolic and one was cholecystoduodenal. The biliary internal fistula rate in this series for benign disease is 5%. Puestow[10] discovered 16 instances of fistula in 500 operations for a rate of 3%. Dean[11] reported that, in his series, 1.2% of patients admitted with cholecystitis harbored fistulas. In a recent review of 12,152 cholecystectomies performed with or without exploration of the common duct (between July 1932 and June 1965 at the Columbia Presbyterian Hospital in New York[12]), there were 26 single spontaneous biliary enteric fistulas for an incidence of approximately .2%. Thus it would seem that the incidence of biliary fistulas is higher among the Navajos than the general population.

The operative incidence of carcinoma of the biliary tree in this series is 3%. This is higher than most series in the literature, most values being between .5% to 1.4%.[13-15] The youngest patient of the group was 59, the oldest 77.

Considering the age incidence of cholecystitis and cholelithiasis among the Navajos, the increased incidence of choledocholithiasis in the patients with cholecystitis, the increased incidence of carcinoma of the biliary tree, the increased incidence of internal benign biliary fistulas, and the early appearance of choledocholithiasis in the population, it would appear safe to state that biliary tract disease is more aggressive in Navajos than non-Navajo populations.

References

1. Sievers, M.L., and Marquis, J.R.: The Southwestern American Indian's Burden: Biliary Disease, *JAMA* **182**:570-572 (Nov 3) 1962.

2. Kravetz, R.E.: Etiology of Biliary Tract Disease in Southwestern American Indians: Analysis of 105 consecutive cholecystetomies, *Gastroenterology* **46**:392-398 (April) 1964.

3. Colcock, B.P., and Perey, B.: The Treatment of Cholelithiasis. *Surg Gynec Obstet* **117**:529-534 (Nov) 1963.

4. Adams, R., and Stranahan, A.: Cholecystitis and Cholelithiasis: An Analytical Report of 1,104 Operative Cases, *Surg Gynec Obstet* **85**:776-784 (Dec) 1947.

5. Colcock, B.P., and McManus, J.E.: Experiences With 1,356 Cases of Cholecystitis and Cholelithiasis, *Surg Gynec Obstet* **101**:161-172 (Aug) 1955.

6. Smith, R.F.; Conklin, E.F.; and Porter, M.R.: A Five Year Study of Choledocholithiasis, *Surg Gynec Obstet* **116**:731-740 (June) 1963.

7. Glenn, F., and Beil, A.R.: Choledocholithiasis Demonstrated at 586 Operations, *Surg Gynec Obstet* **118**:499-506 (March) 1964.

8. Colcock, B.P., and Perey, B.: Exploration of the Common Duct, *Surg Gynec Obstet* **118**:20-24 (Jan) 1964.

9. Hornfield, H.J., and Albritten, F.F.: The Roles of Choledochostomy and Antibiotics in Gall Bladder Surgery, *Surg Gynec Obstet* **113**:277-282 (Sept) 1961.

10. Puestow, C.B.: Spontaneous Internal Biliary Fistula, *Ann Surg* **115**:1043-1054 (June) 1942.

11. Dean, G.O.: Internal Biliary Fistulas: Discussion of Internal Biliary Fistulas Based on 29 Cases, *Surgery* **5**:857-864 (June) 1939.

12. Amoury, R.A., and Barker, H.G.: Multiple Biliary Enteric

Fistuals, *Amer J Surg* 111:180-185 (Feb) 1966.

13. Van Heerden, J.A.; Judd, E.S.; and Dockerty, M.B.: Carcinoma of the Extrahepatic Bile Ducts, *Amer J Surg* 113:49-55 (Jan) 1967.

14. Neibling, J.M.; Dockerty, M.B.; and Waugh, J.M.: Carcinoma of the Extrahepatic Bile Ducts, *Surg Gynec Obstet* 89: 429-438 (Oct) 1949.

15. Judd, E.S., and Gray, H.K.: Carcinoma of the Gall Bladder and Bile Ducts, *Proc Int Assembly Inter-State Post Grad Med Assoc North America*, 7:342-345, 1931.

Epidemiological Studies on Rheumatic Diseases

Thomas A. Burch

I͟T HAS BEEN suggested that by studying populations with different frequencies of a rheumatic disease it might be possible to detect the responsible environmental factor which may well throw light on causation.[1] Very few studies have been reported, however, in which the same investigators have conducted epidemiological studies on different populations using the same methods. Yet when this is not done it is very difficult to assess whether reported differences in prevalence of diseases or conditions are due to differences in the population or differences in the investigators.

The present report describes the findings of two surveys for arthritis and rheumatism conducted by the same team of investigators using the same methods and diagnostic criteria on population groups living under extremely different climatic conditions.

American Indians were selected for this study since within certain Indian reservations, many of the adults and almost all of the children have spent their lives within a few miles of the place of their birth. Many Indian reservations are located in the ancestral tribal home and hence the present inhabitants have lived there for generations. It would be very difficult to find a white population in the United States so identified with their home area. This is especially true of our southwest desert where there has been an extremely high immigration rate. For example, according to the 1960 census, only 6 per cent of the white population of Arizona of the ages that we surveyed were born in that state, yet all of the Arizona Indians included in this study were natives of that state.

The Blackfeet Indians (Fig. 1) were selected since their reservation in northern Montana is located in one of the coldest areas of the United States, while the Pima Indians of Arizona live in one of the hottest areas of the country. The warmest months on the Blackfeet Reservation have about the same mean temperature as the coldest months on the Pima Reservation (Fig. 2).

Material and Methods

An area survey was conducted on each reservation in which 86 per cent of the Indians of the specified tribe, aged 30 years or older, who actually lived on the reservation were examined.[2,3] All examinations and procedures were carried out in large vans equipped as mobile clinics which were located at various strategic locations about the reservations. Transportation to and from the clinics was furnished by local Indian chauffeurs who also served as translators. Many of those who either could not or would not attend the clinic were visited at their home using portable equipment. Approximately 1,000 Indians of each tribe were examined. Each respondent was questioned carefully and examined by a staff physician with special training in rheumatology. Radiographs of the hands, feet, cervical spine and pelvis were taken of all male respondents and the hands, feet and cervical spine of all female respondents. Radiographs

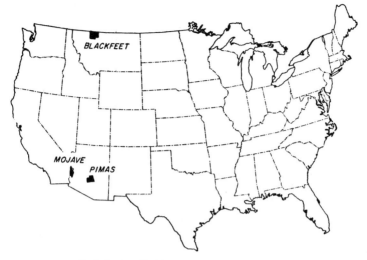

Fig. 1. Location of Indian Reservations Indicated in Studies.

of the pelvis were only taken on female respondents aged 45 years and older. Serum samples were collected and tested for rheumatoid factor by both the bentonite flocculation test (BFT)[4] and the sheep cell agglutination test (SCAT) done by the method of Ball.[5] Radiographs were graded for osteoarthrosis and erosive arthritis in accordance with the standards developed by the group at the University of Manchester[6,7] and rheumatoid arthritis was diagnosed in accordance with the criteria of the American Rheumatism Association[8] as well as the physician's clinical impression at the time of the examination.

In the following account age and sex adjusted rates have been calculated by applying

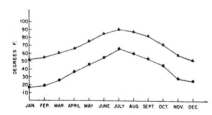

Fig. 2. Mean Monthly Temperature in Browning, Montana, and Phoenix, Arizona.

the age sex specific rates from each tribe to a standardized population consisting of the combined population of the two tribes. While in this instance there were but slight differences between these standardized rates and the crude rates, there can be considerable differences, if the populations being compared differ in their age and sex composition.[9]

Results and Discussion

There were but slight differences in the frequency of acknowledged arthritis or rheumatism, history of swollen joints or painful peripheral joints in the two populations (Table I). The women of both tribes complained of painful peripheral joints more frequently than the men. The difference in rates between the sexes was only significant, however, among the Blackfeet.

The Blackfeet reported pain in the hips, shoulders and back as well as pain with a segmental distribution much more frequently than the Pimas. The examining physicians made a clinical diagnosis of ankylosing spondylitis more than five times as frequently in the male Pima Indians as in the male Blackfeet. This would suggest that the frequent

TABLE I

AGE AND AGE-SEX ADJUSTED RATES PER HUNDRED OF RHEUMATIC COMPLAINTS AND
CONDITIONS IN TWO TRIBES OF AMERICAN INDIANS

Condition	Blackfeet			Pima		
	Total	Male	Female	Total	Male	Female
No. Examined	1101	622	479	969	483	486
History						
Arthritis	42	40	44	37	33	41
Joint swelling	18	14	22#	16	15	17
Pain: peripheral joints	35	29	41#	40	36	45#
Hips/shoulders	21*	20	21	9	9	10
Spine	27*	30	22	14	16	11
Segmental	23*	26	20	14	13	15
Physical Examination						
Joint swelling	6	5	6	6	5	6
Pain on motion	17	13	20#	13	10	16
Limitation of motion peripheral joints	22	26#	16	23	35#	8
Radiographs (hands & feet)						
OA gr 2	68	74#	61	65	74#	56
OA gr 3	24	26	21	23	30#	14
RA gr 2–4	3	4	2	3	2	5
RA gr 3–4	1	1	1	1	0	2
Rheumatoid Factor						
BFT ≥1:32	6	6	7	20*	22	18
≥1:64	5	4	5	13*	14	11
SCAT ≥1:32	6	6	5	9	7	11
Clinical Diagnosis						
Rheumatoid arthritis	5	4	6	4	3	6
Ankylosing spondylitis	0	1	0	3*	5#	0
Diagnosis by ARA criteria						
Probable or definite	4	3	5	5	5	5
Definite	1	1	1	1	0	2

* 95% confidence limits (11) did not overlap with those of other tribe.
# 95% confidence limits (11) did not overlap with those of other sex of same tribe.

back complaints of the latter were for the most part unrelated to spondylitis. It is tempting to attribute this difference to the fact that the Blackfeet are largely cattlemen and horsemen and hence it would seem likely that they have much more trauma to their shoulders, hips and spine than the Pimas who use but few horses.

The frequency of abnormal findings during physical examination of the joints was essentially the same in both tribes. The males of both tribes, however, had objective evidence of limitation of motion of one or more peripheral joints much more frequently than the females. This was especially marked in the Pimas where 35 per cent of the males but only 8 per cent of the females were affected. A similar, but less marked difference, between the sexes was also noted for radiological evidence of osteoarthrosis of the hands and feet.

The age-sex adjusted rate of probable plus definite rheumatoid arthritis was 4 and 5 per cent respectively in the Blackfeet and Pima Indians. This difference is not significant. In

TABLE II

PREVALENCE OF RHEUMATOID ARTHRITIS AND RHEUMATOID FACTOR IN BLACKFEET
AND PIMA TRIBES (Age Specific Rates)

| | Blackfeet | | | | Pima | | |
Age Groups	No.	R.A. (%)	Pos. BFT (%)	Pos. SCAT (%)	No.	R.A. (%)	Pos. BFT (%)	Pos. SCAT (%)
30–34	165	1.8	2.6	4.5	143	1.4	14.2	7.1
35–44	319	3.4	5.6	4.9	265	4.5	18.2	7.2
45–54	241	3.7	5.6	4.8	187	6.0	15.1	6.0
55–64	203	6.4	5.2	7.9	189	8.4	28.6	15.1
65–74	108	5.6	8.8	4.0	122	6.5	13.1	8.2
75+	66	4.5	9.8	4.8	62	4.8	25.8	12.9

both populations, RA was more prevalent among females than males. This difference, however, was slight and was not greater than could be expected from chance alone. The age distribution of RA was similar in both tribes (Table II) with the lowest frequency in the youngest and the highest in the 55-64 year age group, and then a gradual decline in prevalence.

The frequency of rheumatoid factor as shown by the bentonite flocculation test, was more than three times greater in the Pimas than in the Blackfeet and half again as great when tested by the sheep cell agglutination test.

The prevalence of rheumatoid factor as tested by the BFT was not significantly different in males and females. There was a definite age trend of positive BFTs in the Blackfeet with the lowest frequency in the youngest and the highest in the oldest age group examined (Table II). This trend is compatible with a constant incidence of the factor so that there is a steady accumulation with time of individuals in the population demonstrating a positive test. Another possible explanation is that whatever evokes rheumatoid factor became progressively less frequent since the older individuals were initially exposed.[10]

Among the Pima Indians all age groups had a high frequency of positive BFTs of about 15 per cent except for those aged 55-64 and 75 years and older, who had approximately twice the prevalence of other age groups (Table II).

It would appear that the entire population of the Pimas was exposed to some environmental factor that resulted in the production of an unusually high frequency of individuals with rheumatoid factor and that individuals age 55-64 and 75 and over were exposed to a far greater extent than the other age groups. This view is strengthened by similar findings on the Mojaves who are a culturally and genetically distinct group of Indians living on another reservation in Arizona.[3]

Summary and Conclusions

The frequency of arthritis and rheumatism in the Blackfeet Indians living in a cold climate and the Pima Indians living in a hot climate was similar, except that the Blackfeet had more complaints referable to shoulders, hips, spine and pain with a segmental distribution while the Pimas had a significantly higher frequency of clinical ankylosing spondylitis and positive tests for rheumatoid factor. There is no evidence that these differences are attributable to differences in climate *per se* but may be due to other environmental factors such as frequency and severity of infections and different occupations. Further studies on these aspects are in progress.

Acknowledgments

This work would have been impossible without the valuable help of the Division of Indian Health of the U. S. Public Health Service and the Tribal Councils of the Blackfeet and Pima Tribes. The other physicians who participated in the investigations were Dr. William M. O'Brien, Dr. John S. Lawrence and Dr. Peter H. Bennett. The serological tests for rheumatoid factor were performed by Mrs. Janie B. Taylor and Mrs. Anna M. Newell.

REFERENCES

[1] Lawrence, J. S., Methods of assessing rheumatoid arthritis in population studies and initial findings, Excerpta Medica, 53:15, 1960.

[2] Bunim, J. J., Burch, T. A., and O'Brien, W. M.: Influence of genetic and environmental factors on the occurrence of rheumatoid arthritis and rheumatoid factor in American Indians, Bull. Rheum. Dis., 15:349, 1964.

[3] Burch, T. A., O'Brien, W., Lawrence, J. S., Bennett, P. H., and Bunim, J. J., Prevalencia de artritis reumatoidea y factor reumatoide en Indios Americanos. Rev. Med. Chile, 92:183-186, 1964.

[4] Bozicevich, J., Bunim, J. J., Freund, J. and Ward, S. B., Bentonite flocculation test for rheumatoid arthritis. Proc. Soc. Exper. Biol. and Med., 97:180, 1958.

[5] Ball, J., Serum factors in rheumatoid arthritis agglutinating sensitized sheep red cells, Lancet, 2:520, 1950.

[6] Kellgren, J. H., and Lawrence, J. S., Radiological assessment of rheumatoid arthritis, Ann. Rheum. Dis., 16:485, 1957.

[7] Kellgren, J. H., and Lawrence, J. S., Radiological assessment of osteroarthrosis, Ann. Rheum. Dis., 16:494, 1957.

[8] Ropes, M. W., Bennett, G. A., Cobb, S., Jacox, R., and Jessar, R. A., 1958 revision of diagnostic criteria for rheumatoid arthritis. Bull. Rheum. Dis., 9:175, 1958.

[9] Swaroop, S., Introduction to Health Statistics, E & S Livingston Ltd., London, 182 pp., 1960.

[10] Ball, J. and Lawrence, J. S, Epidemiology of the sheep cell agglutination test. Ann. Rheum. Dis., 20:235, 1961.

[11] Mainland, D., Herrera, L. and Sutcliffe, M. I., Tables for use with binomial samples. N.Y. Univ. College of Medicine, 83 pp., 1956.

Northern Sylvatic Helminthiasis

Thomas W. M. Cameron, DSc

THE fundamental influence of the theory of evolution on medical thinking was to enforce the realization that man is an animal related to all other mammals. Physiologically he is a rather unspecialized mammal, and so experimental medicine became a valuable tool in medical research.

Later it became obvious for much the same reason that organisms infecting other animals could sometimes be transferred to him and quite frequently cause disease. Parasitic organisms like all other living things had evolved pari passu with their hosts, and usually had in consequence become physiologically specialized to these hosts. Sometimes however, the degree of specialization was insufficient to prevent their transference to man, and some could adapt themselves to the new human host. Propinquity and feeding habits favored this. Very few parasites came from the highly specialized herbivores, but the domestic carnivores were more generous donors. Specialization in parasites was often to an intermediate host, and the adult stages in the definitive hosts could live comfortably in many different animals. On the other hand, parasites sometimes had very specific final hosts, but could infect a great variety of intermediate hosts.

In spite of the general acceptance of the theory of evolution, progress in developing medical implications was slow. Comparative medicine in its true meaning did not take formal shape until the 1920's, but what we

Reprint requests to Department of Microbiology and Immunology, McGill University, Montreal (Dr. Cameron).

unfortunately now call zoonosis, began to attract medical attention as *Diseases of Animals Transmissible to Man.* (I wrote the first book on this in a series under the editorship of Prof Frazer Harris of Halifax, Nova Scotia, in 1926).

It later became obvious that often wild animals played a part similar to that of domestic ones in causing disease in human beings. Perhaps the most important environment in which to observe this is the Boreal countries where domestic animals—other than dogs—are absent, and where man is not only essentially a carnivore in his food habits, but is in close association with both terrestrial and marine wild animals. Here zoonosis is sylvatic zoonosis—even though the domestic dog often acts as an important link between wild animals and man.

Some of these sylvatic zoonoses in the north are of great medical significance, such as tapeworms, hydatid cysts, and trichinosis —all of which have been subjects of intensive research on the part of my colleagues and myself, during the past 30 years.

Fish Tapeworms.—"Fish tapeworms" are tapeworms transmitted to mammals and birds through the agency of uncooked fish flesh. They belong to the genus *Diphyllobothrium* (or *Dibothriocephalus*), but the actual species involved are still in doubt. They are widespread in northern America in man, dog, and bears, and they are usually ascribed to the species *D latum,* a common European species associated, because of its high vitamin B_{12} requirement, with pernicious anemia in man in Scandinavia and the USSR. However, we have no definite knowledge of this relationship in North America, although it may exist. We may have a different variety here because while in Europe dogs are good hosts, in Canada, the tapeworm eggs which they pass are mainly sterile.

The tapeworm is not only big—up to 60 feet long—but it has a potential life in man of ten years. It produces about two million eggs daily, and as all its food comes from the partly digested contents of the intestine, it must make considerable inroads into the food intake of the host.

Diphyllobothrium latum is the "broad tapeworm," in which segments are wider than long, but as G. A. Webster, PhD, and I have shown, after unsuccessful treatment with Quinacrine (Atabrine) hydrochloride the segments may become longer than broad, showing a superficial resemblance to *Taenia species* which are absent from man in the Northlands.

Trematodes.—Fish-borne trematodes are prevalent in the southern part of northern Canada. One is the *Metorchis conjunctus* closely related to the classical oriental liver flukes. It is carried in the flesh of the common sucker fish and probably other fish. It lives as an adult in the liver of a large variety of fish-eating mammals and causes chronic cirrhosis. Its severity depends on the number of parasites present. As it cannot multiply in the adult stage, the numbers present depend on the cysts swallowed in the infected fish. Chronic cirrhosis is not uncommon among the Indians of northern Saskatchewan.

A small intestinal species, *cryptocotyle,* has been identified in eggs found in the stool of men in Thule. It is a parasite of young terns carried by sea snails and originally in ballast imported from Europe and carried to northeastern America. It has now spread both north and south along the coast. Its cercaria invade shore fish, such as flounder and it has caused serious enteritis in foxes and other animals which have fed on raw fish. Its presence in man is still a curiosity.

Hydatid Cysts.—Hydatid disease is one of the most widespread and serious of the helminthic infections of man. It is still uncertain how many species exist. Taxonomy is still further complicated by the wide variety of intermediate hosts and the pleomorphic character of the larval stage (which is partly conditioned by the reaction of the host). There are certainly two species at least and a great variety of biological strains.

Echinococcus granulosus canadiensis.—Prior to 1950, only sporadic cases of human hydatidosis had been reported from North America, and although there were occasional reports of hydatid cysts occurring in domestic and wild herbivores, the incidence in both the human and animal population was of such a low degree that the disease was regarded as a curiosity. At about this time, the Indian Health Service discovered, as a result of studies made by their x-ray service, that hydatid infections were relatively common in the Indian population in northwest Canada. With the active collaboration of that service and the Laboratory of Hygiene of the Department of National Health and Welfare, surveys were made to determine the prevalence of the disease in the inhabitants of this area and the relationship between sylvatic hydatidosis and native customs which might influence the disease pattern. In addition, extensive research has been carried out on the biology of the parasite and the development of serological tests for diagnosis.

The causative agent of hydatid disease is a cestode belonging to the genus *Echinococcus*. These tapeworms have a life cycle involving two hosts. The definitive host is a member of the family Canidae, and the intermediate host is normally a herbivore. While the definitive host is quite specific and the tapeworm stage is found only in carnivores, the larval (hydatid cyst) stage is much less so and is found in man as well as a large variety of grass-eating animals. Because of the wide distribution of the Canidae and the presence of some suitable intermediate host in most parts of the world, the parasite has an almost cosmopolitan distribution. The intensity of this distribution varies from place to place, being greatest where domestic herbivores are kept in numbers in close association with dogs and related Canidae, and where food containing cysts is more accessible to the dogs.

Although domestic animals are the most important hosts of this tapeworm they are not the exclusive ones; it occurs in wild animals also, and there is, therefore, a sylvatic cycle. This sylvatic disease extends through the five western provinces of Canada and the adjacent states in the United States. The cyst occurs naturally in moose (*Alces americanus*), caribou (*Rangifer arcticus*), elk or wapiti (*Cervus canadiensis*), and occasionally other deer. It does not occur in rodents or domestic herbivores in northern North America, and repeated attempts to infect voles, sheep, cattle, and pigs have failed. The adult cysts are carried by wolves (*Canis lupus*) and occasionally coyotes (*Canis latrans*), but not by grey or red foxes; dogs are often infected (25% or more) from cervine sources and carry the infection into Indian and Eskimo villages.

The cyst is of the classical type, and ideally, is a univesicular sphere ranging in size from that of an egg to that of a large grapefruit. It is composed of a dead outer laminated layer and an inner germinal membrane. The cyst is filled with a clear, water fluid which is under intercystic pressure so that the vesicle is always turgid. A fully developed cyst contains numerous secondary cysts called brood capsules. Each brood capsule produces within itself numerous protoscolices which are really inverted tapeworm heads. Growth is slow and several years may be required for the cyst to become fertile. Dogs become infected by eating the cyst and each protoscolex in six weeks or so becomes an adult tapeworm.

In 1952, Max Miller, MD, made a survey of the incidence of hydatid cyst in British Columbia at Fort Rae, Northwest Territory. He used an Australian test antigen prepared from hydatid fluid from sheep. He tested 613 persons in British Columbia, with 15 positive results, and 229 at Fort Rae, with no positive results. These figures were obviously unsatisfactory because the incidence in dogs was high in most areas where dogs were examined, and they did not accord with clinical experience. It was suspected that the test antigen might be at fault, and in 1953, L. Chocquette, MD, visited Aklavik during the reindeer kill and secured a quantity of hydatid fluid (15% of the reindeer were infected) and from this an Aklavik antigen was prepared.

Using this antigen during 1954 to 1956, my colleagues, (Drs. Wolfgang, Poole, Chocquette, and Whitten) conducted a series of surveys on Indians and Eskimos in the Yukon and Northwest territories. The populations tested were unselected and were not clinically ill. The results are shown in the Table.

The technique used in all cases was the intradermal injection of filtered fluid, which had been mixed with thimerosal (Merthiolate), from hydatid cysts collected from reindeer slaughtered at Aklavik. In 1954, the amount injected was 0.25 ml. Later, this was reduced to 0.10 ml, experience having shown that the smaller dose was sufficient. With the smaller dose, the reaction lasted for about four hours only, necessitating a prompt reading. This was an advantage when accompanying a Treaty party where time was important. Even then, however, not all persons injected returned for the reading of the test. It was believed that 0.05 ml would be satisfactory for future work because subdermal edemas, which were noted with the largest doses, still had been seen occasionally with 0.10 ml doses.

The interpretation of the intradermal test is essentially arbitrary and subjective. The reaction is usually noted 20 minutes after intradermal injection. It is compared with a saline control; if it is similar, it is regarded as negative. If the wheal is 2 cm in diameter with pseudopodia and a zone of erythema, it is regarded as positive, while one between 1 and 2 cm is doubtfully so.

All antigens used are "crude" antigens and electrophoresis has shown that they contain at least a dozen antigenic components—some of them of host (ie, reindeer) origin.

The composition of hydatid fluid is notoriously variable and, although various techniques have been employed to determine the differences between Canadian and sheep hydatid fluids, the results were somewhat inconclusive. However, there was a difference in carbohydrates, polypeptides and protein fractions; polysaccharides could not be demonstrated in deer antigens although they were clearly seen in sheep antigens, while amino acids were much more evident in Canadian material. Hydatid fluid from different species of deer showed slight differences between themselves, although these differences were less than that shown by sheep fluid.

Fractionation of cyst components indicated that proteins from the fluid are effective test antigens in both complement fixation and the indirect passive hemagglutination reaction. This protein fraction gives two distinct bands of specific precipitation in double-diffusion precipitin analysis, indicating that this fraction has at least two well-defined antigenic components which are of considerable value in the passive indirect hemagglutination test. Lipid extracts had a high antigenic activity—those from protoscolices especially so—but were found to yield some nonspecific complement fixation reactions. The lack of polysaccharides in the fluid rendered the direct hemagglutination test valueless.

It seems unlikely except when the cyst is ruptured, which is not uncommon when cysts are located in the lungs, that high molecular weight substances are involved in the associated immunological reactions. Low-molecular weight material can lead to dermal diagnostic reactions, but do not necessarily yield positive in vitro tests, such as complement fixation, precipitation, or hemagglutination.

It is not known how accurate the intradermal test is. Elsewhere than in Canada, authors have claimed an accuracy of from 54% to 100%. The average is about 90%. The Camsell Hospital tested 22 patients with proven hydatid disease. Of these, 15 were positive and seven negative, but all seven patients with negative results had been tested with Australian antigen. The hospital has had only one negative result with the Aklavik antigen in a proven case. However a positive reaction is of much greater significance than a negative one. Children with unruptured living cysts often have a negative result.

It is believed that the intradermal test reaction is positive for the lifetime of an individual even after the cyst has been removed or has, in the case of pulmonary cysts, ruptured and spontaneous cure has taken place. It may be assumed, tentatively, that the test reveals only about 90% of all cases (past and present). Accordingly, it would seem that about 42% of the Indians in the Yukon and 28% in the Mackenzie Valley are harboring or have harbored cysts; about 23% of the Eskimos at Eskimo Point are also infected. These figures may be much too low, as all doubtful cases have been regarded as negative; they may be too high because there may be unknown reasons for hypersensitivity in the Indians. The natural history of the disease and the cultural habits of the Indians seem to make this somewhat improbable. Epidemiological investigations showed that the intensity of human infection was correlated with the customs of each particular tribe. Those groups which subsist mainly on a fish diet have a low incidence, whereas hunting tribes are often heavily infected. For economic reasons, it is standard practice to feed the dogs portions of animals not suitable for human consumption (chiefly the

District	No. Tested	No. Positive
Yukon, central	291*	129
Old Crow	42	16
Mackenzie, Lesser Slave Lake	145	46
Fort Vermillion	313	109
Fort Norman	413	162
Yellow Knife	584†	79
Total indians tested	1,433	432 (28%)
Keewatin Eskimo Point	186	31 (21%)
Franklin Igloolik	63†	4

* This represents about one fifth of the total Indian population, giving a crude infection rate of about 40%. Approximately one third more females than males reacted (74:53).

† About half of the Yellow Knife Indians inhabit the Lesser Slave Lake area and are mainly fishermen, while the Eskimo at Igloolik have little contact with deer.

lungs where 99% of the cysts occur). One hunting tribe hung the lungs of their kill in trees as a sort of pagan offering, and consequently were relatively free from infection.

Dogs are valuable possessions in the territories and are, therefore, tethered close to or inside the dwellings. The custom of feeding infected viscera insures that many will harbor the tapeworms and that the soil in the immediate vicinity of the dwellings will be heavily contaminated with the eggs which are the only source of human infection and can remain viable for at least two years. This is the main source of infection in women and children, but men may also swallow eggs adhering to pelts they remove from wolve or coyotes—the only other carnivores which harbor the tapeworm.

Echinococcus multilocularis.—The second species, probably originating in northern Eurasia and discovered by R. Rausch, MD, in Alaska, is quite different. It is generally agreed that its name is *E multilocularis,* and although essentially an arctic species, it shows a tendency to move southward. It has been reported in Germany, northern Switzerland, and presently in North America, and already has reached across the Canadian prairies into the Dakotas. The adult tapeworm's original host was the white fox, but it can live in dogs and red foxes and, unlike *E granulosus,* in cats.

The larval stage does not occur in domestic herbivores, but in a large variety of rodents, such as field voles or mice; and in these, it develops as a rapidly growing, multicystic microvesicular body in the liver, lungs, and other organs. Although the adult

stage in the carnivore is relatively benign, the larval stage is malignant and usually fatal.

Dévé and others many years ago showed that if protoscolices, the immature heads of the tapeworm, were removed from the mother cyst of *E granulosus,* they would become vesicular and form a new cyst identical in all respects with the mother cyst. Daughter cysts and even granddaughter cysts are formed in this way usually, but not always by the rupture of the mother cyst by trauma.

Echinococcus multilocularis spreads in a different way—not usually by the vacuolation of the protoscolices, but by peripheral exogenous budding. Each small vesicle is completely filled with protoscolices and the fast, luxuriant growth may completely fill the rodent's liver and kill the animal within two months.

G. Lubinsky, MD, has shown that a portion of cyst inoculated into the body cavity of a rodent can establish itself as a fertile cyst. He has actually performed over 50 successive passive transfers without the intervention of adult tapeworms.

The cyst is almost immortal, and the only limits imposed on it are those of the host organs. It can live in men in its larval stage as the result of swallowing the egg as fecal contamination. Fortunately, because it is one of the most dangerous of the parasites affecting him, it is still uncommon.

According to evolutionary theory, man is a relatively recent host and he is, therefore, not a particularly good one. Uncomplicated liver and lung cysts of *E granulosus* are usually the typical spherical structures associated with this species but, on occasion, multilocular cysts do develop. When the larva settles in an unnatural site, such as the central nervous system or long bones, it also grows abberrantly. *Echinococcus multilocularis* always develops abnormally in man, producing a condition known as alveolar hydatid in which there is a mass of minute vesicles of irregular shape with degenerated hyaline membrane and little or no fluid. The cavities are enclosed in a heavy avascular, more or less amorphic fibrous stroma and are nearly always sterile. The cavities extend peripherally, with necrosis and cavitation in the center of the lesion, growth which is histologically similar to a colloidal carcinoma.

Growth is slow but malignant, and there is a definite tendency to metastasize. While the primary cyst is in the liver, secondary lesions have been reported from the lungs, lymph glands, and brain.

Diagnosis of the cyst in man is difficult; *E granulosus* test antigen is not specific, and even antigen prepared from *E multilocularis* cysts is a complex of host and parasitic material. The first step is obviously the in vitro cultivation of the cyst in a purely synthetic medium (we have been partly successful in this), and fractionating the fluid in the cysts so obtained. The insiduous development of the cyst in the human liver makes clinical diagnosis difficult until the condition has reached a state where it may be inoperable.

Trichinosis.—Trichinosis is caused by the ingestion of larvae of the nematode *Trichinella spiralis* encysted in the voluntary musculature of a food animal. The larvae are released in the stomach by peptic digestion of the cysts; they then pass into the small intestine where they rapidly mature and the sexes mate. The female worm begins releasing her progeny alive about ten days after fertilization and these young parasites rapidly penetrate the circulatory system and are carried throughout the body by the bloodstream.

The symptomatology of the disease is seldom characteristic, and its severity depends on the number of infective larvae in the original meal. Probably about half of these are immature females which mature sexually in the intestine, and over a period of several weeks give birth to 500 or 600 immature embryos. These are distributed at random throughout the body. They reach the terminal capillaries in various organs and die and degenerate, releasing various toxic substances. Others, however, ultimately reach the sarcolemma of the skeletal muscles, which they enter, where they develop into immature adults. They do not and cannot reach sexual maturity without being swallowed by another animal, and they cannot, accordingly, multiply in the original host. They do however cause muscle destruction and release more foreign material into the bloodstream. The signs and symptoms produced depend on a variety of causes, but most important on the number of living larvae ingested in the infective meal. Conse-quently, there may be no symptoms at all, or, if a heavy meal of meat from a heavily infected animal is consumed, the symptoms may be sufficiently violent to cause death.

Trichinosis was first identified in Canada as a human infection by William Osler while he was a medical student in Toronto, and later, as a porcine infection when he was a lecturer in helminthology at McGill University. Since then, it has occurred sporadically in Canada and has been the subject of various surveys from coast to coast. It has, however, been found to be a very serious endemic disease in the Arctic where the parasite occurs in wild animals, and where man is very frequently seriously infected.

Essentially an infection of flesh-eating animals, it reaches its greatest frequency in wild mammals in the Arctic. I found it in a polar bear in the London Zoo in 1926 (the bear had been newly introduced from Canada) and in numerous others since then. It has long been known to occur in the black or brown bear and Dr. Rausch and his colleagues have demonstrated its presence not only in other bears, but in numerous flesh-eating animals.

The parasite is highly resistant to putrefaction and can exist in the same carcass as the *Bacillus* of botulism—a combination of causes which can rapidly prove fatal if the carcass is eaten uncooked, as it so often is in the Arctic. C. Dolman, MD, believes that many of the fatal epidemics which wiped out whole tribes of Eskimo were botulism, but evidence suggests that the Trichina worm may be equally culpable.

The worm in meat is easily killed by heat; our experiments with artificially infected pork showed that a temperature of 131 F (55 C) was lethal. Pork protein in sausages (in which we had placed thermocouples) coagulated between 137 F and 140 F. Pork which changed color by heating contained no living trichinae. This is equally true with bear flesh. It is, however, quite resistant to drying, and dried bear muscle (jerky) not only can contain living larvae, but if eaten uncooked can prove fatal.

Eskimo methods of cooking often do not reach this temperature, and the patients flown in to southern Canada—some of which died, nearly always had a history of eating undercooked or raw bear meat.

A few had walrus meat in their diet, and, as we have found, an infection rate of 4% in bull walrus; this also is a probable source of human infection.

It is difficult to see how marine carnivores other than walrus become infected. The few cases discovered are probably accidental; any mammal that eats flesh infected with trichinosis can become infected. The case of walrus may be different, and an important cycle in the Arctic may well be a polar bear-walrus one. Steffenson found that in the sea, a bull walrus would engage and kill a polar bear while the reverse took place on land. Not all bull walruses confine their diet to clams, and some are quite active carnivores or scavengers.

Dogs, arctic foxes, and wolves, of course, are easily and frequently infected, but do not normally form part of the human diet. Their infections come from small rodents or from scavenging.

The presence of the parasite in man is usually determined by sensitivity intradermal tests or by serology. The damage done to the muscles of the subject as well as the death and degeneration of the larvae in the solid organs releases antigenic substances which produce both humoral and skin-sensitive antibodies. Neither, of course, are produced immediately and the intradermal reaction is of minor importance in making a clinical diagnosis, although both are of value in confirming one. The humoral bodies disappear within a year or so, but the skin sensitivity remains for a long period of time—probably for life. The intradermal test, consequently, is of great value in establishing the incidence of the infection in a population. It is believed to have an accuracy of at least 90%; however the antigen used, prepared from Trichina larvae isolated in vitro from an experimentally infected animal, dried, and extracted in saline, contains about a dozen, more or less, antigenic substances.

We have no accurate figures of the incidence of human trichinosis in the North American Arctic and sub-Arctic although we know it occurs extensively from the Labrador Coast to Alaska.

In 1949, Dr. M. Brown, and his colleagues found 40% positive reactions of 265 individuals tested on Southampton Island. In 1957 and 1958, Dr. L. E. C. Davis of the Camsell Hospital in Edmonton, using a saline extract of trichinae larvae, tested 644 individuals along the Arctic coast and found 144 positive reactions with 27 doubtful.

Dr. Whitten tested Eskimos at Igloolik and at the Hamilton Sanitorium, and Indians at North Larea; 31 of 192 had positive reactions. No community in the North is completely free from infection and many clinical cases are transported south by the Royal Canadian Air Force for hospital treatment.

We estimate that among the meat-eating tribes in the American Arctic, both in the islands and on the mainland, the incidence of infection is about 90%.

Strongyloides.—The most recent probable addition to the list of nematodes possibly transmitted from animals to man is Strongyloides. This genus of small intestinal worms is worldwide in its distribution, and a large variety of animals act as hosts. Numerous species have been described, but the differences in morphology are slight and their biology is largely undetermined. There may be biological strains which have become adapted to specific hosts, but which can occasionally infect man. It has been suggested, for example, that the occasional finding of Strongyloides in human beings in northern Saskatchewan is such an example. However, the report by Dr. Miller, of a massive infection in an Eskimo seal hunter from the Arctic, who had suffered several years of severe abdominal pain associated with an eosinophilia, suggests that the species infecting humans may exist in the North. The dog, at least, among the domestic mammals can be infected with Strongyloides, but we have no information about its occurrence in seals and whales.

The parasite is a pernicious one and unique among the helminths. It can reproduce and multiply at body temperature within the human body and can even bring about the death of the host. Normally, however, it has a well-developed external life cycle. Only parthenogenetic females are parasites, living normally in the mucosa of the small bowel where they lay eggs which hatch in situ and from which emerges a minute, active, feeding larva. This is evacuated with the feces, and it grows and gives rise to free-feeding males and females which are quite unlike the parasitic female from which they descended. These mate; the female gives rise to eggs, half of which normally develop males and half (usually called infective larvae) which have no visible sex organs, but which will ultimately become parasitic females. They are really "pre-adults" which cannot reach maturity unless, and until they enter the human body: this they do by penetrating the skin or mucous membranes and making their way via the bloodstream to the small intestine. The males of this parasitic generation which are similar to the free-living males are not parasitic, but die without fertilizing eggs of the females.

The story is even more complicated, for if conditions for development of the external sexual generation are unsatisfactory the larvae which normally would become free-living females become instead infective larvae (the males of course die), and are ready to return to the body at once and become parasitic females. The conditions which cause this can occur outside of the body in fecal particles lodged in the rugae of the rectum or even inside the intestine. In this way, an initial infection can multiply almost indefinitely within the body, overrun the mucosa and submucosa of the bowel wall, and even invade other organs. They usually cause nausea, epigastric distress, abdominal pain, and severe diarrhea. There are humoral changes sometimes including anemia, and a high degree of eosinophilia is characteristic. Children often have signs suggesting involvement of the upper respiratory tract. Infections may be very chronic and exist for years, or they may be relatively acute and end fatally. Diagnosis is made by demonstrating the presence of the newly passed larva (about 0.25 mm long) in a freshly passed stool—possibly after a mild saline purge.

Conclusion

The distribution of these parasitic worms in man is conditioned by the cultures and food habits of northern people. Fish-carried parasites postulate the consumption of raw or undercooked fish, while trichinosis similarly requires raw or undercooked flesh of carnivorous mammals. *Diphyllobothrium* is consequently widespread throughout the Canadian shield with its innumerable freshwater lakes and streams. Trichinosis, on the other hand, reaches its maximum intensity in the Arctic islands and the shores of the Arctic ocean where polar bear and walrus are commonly eaten. It is only slightly associated with caribou- or other deer-hunting cultures, but in the maritime regions of the American Arctic, it probably has the highest intensity in the world. *Echinococcus granulosus,* however, is associated with these cultures and has essentially an inland distribution throughout the north west of North America from Hudson Bay to Alaska. *Echinococcus multilocularis,* originally a circumpolar parasite, is associated with white fox pelting. Its distribution as it is moving southward in America is more likely to be associated with rural conditions where cats and dogs are partly feral and where red foxes are infected. For the present however, its greatest incidence would appear to be in northern Asia.

Generic and Trade Names of Drugs

Quinacrine hydrochloride—*Atabrine Hydrochloride.*
Thimerosal—*Merthiolate.*

A CONTROLLED TRIAL OF COMMUNITY-WIDE ISONIAZID PROPHYLAXIS IN ALASKA [2]

GEORGE W. COMSTOCK, SHIRLEY H. FEREBEE, AND LAUREL M. HAMMES

INTRODUCTION

The history of tuberculosis among the Eskimos of Alaska could be documented only recently. No one knows whether or not the disease existed among them prior to their contacts with Europeans. Throughout the nineteenth century and the first half of the present century, the prevalence of tuberculosis could be assessed only from scattered reports by explorers, missionaries, or a handful of physicians struggling to supply the needs for medical care (1). The first systematic information on the extent of the problem came from a BCG campaign conducted from 1949 to 1952 (2). Tuberculin testing at that time showed fantastically high levels of tuberculous infection. The situation was worse among Eskimos in the Bethel Hospital service area in southwestern Alaska, where each year 25 per cent of the nonreactors became infected, a rate far exceeding any we have been able to find in the medical literature. Shortly thereafter, a crash program was instituted to bring modern tuberculosis control methods to Alaska. At its height in 1956, there was one tuberculosis hospital bed for every 30 Aleuts,

Eskimos, and Indians, backed up by a far-flung system of itinerant public health nurses and village chemotherapy aides to provide pre- and posthospital care (3). By 1957, the tuberculosis situation had shown distinct improvement but, even so, the annual rate of acquiring new infections in the Bethel area was 8 per cent, and newly reported active cases of tuberculosis equalled 1 per cent of the population for that year (4). Because the high tuberculosis rates made it likely that the effectiveness of isoniazid prophylaxis could be estimated even with a relatively small study population and because a previous program of ambulatory chemotherapy had established a field facility and good rapport with the population in the Bethel area (5), conditions there seemed well suited for a controlled trial of isoniazid prophylaxis on a community-wide basis.

MATERIALS AND METHODS

The trial was sponsored and conducted cooperatively by four agencies: the Tuberculosis Program, the Arctic Health Research Center, the Division of Indian Health of the U.S. Public Health Service, and the Alaska Department of Health and Welfare. The Bethel Hospital service area is shown by the broken line in figure 1. In size, it exceeds the ninth largest state of the United States, but its population in 1957 was only about 10,000 persons. The trial was restricted to 28 villages and two boarding schools in the western half of the area, with a total population of 7,333 persons, of whom 95 per cent were Eskimos.

The conduct of the trial has been described previously and will only be summarized here (6). The initial step was an explanation of the nature of the study to each communtiy. After approval by each council and by a village meeting, a house-to-house census was conducted. Half of the house-

[2] Supported in part by Public Health Service Research Career Award No. 1-K6-HE-21, 670 from the National Heart Institute, and Graduate Training Grant No. CD-1-01-1-T1 from the Bureau of State Services, Public Health Service, Department of Health, Education, and Welfare.

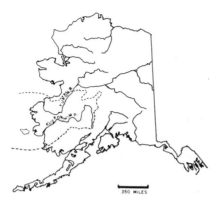

ALASKA

FIG. 1. Location of the Bethel Hospital service area, with boundaries indicated by the broken line.

holds, selected by using a table of random numbers, were furnished isoniazid tablets; the remaining half were given a placebo. Adults were asked to take three tablets (equivalent to 300 mg. of isoniazid) once each day for a year, whereas children were given smaller numbers of tablets according to their age. The recommended daily dosage furnished approximately 5 mg. of isoniazid per kilogram of body weight.

Because of difficulties with adverse weather, tuberculin testing was carried out in only a small proportion of the villages prior to the trial, and in some of these, testing was restricted to children. Chest film surveys were conducted in nearly every village before the trial started. Persons found to have active tuberculosis were removed from the study regimen and treated, almost always in a tuberculosis hospital. Persons already under treatment for tuberculosis were excluded from the trial, as were persons with a history of convulsions and children under two months of age.

Of the 7,333 persons in the study area, 3,017 took a placebo and 3,047 isoniazid. Another 211 took both products at some time during the medication year as the result of moving from one household to another. Most of the remaining 1,058 persons did not take prophylactic medication either because they were being treated for tuberculosis or because they came to the village too late to be included in the program. Less than 3 per cent of the population refused to participate.

The trial started in December 1957. Most of the communities entered the trial in the spring of 1958, but some started as late as the fall of 1959. The tuberculosis experience of these 30 communities has now been analyzed up to the date of

their examination during the winter of 1963 to 1964. For the purposes of this paper, a case may be either newly recognized disease or reactivation of previously known tuberculosis. Both types of tuberculosis cases were identified from the excellent case register maintained by the Alaska Department of Health and Welfare. To be included in this analysis, all cases must have had bacteriologic examinations positive for *Mycobacterium tuberculosis* either for the first time after the start of the trial, or if previously positive, their bacteriologic status must have changed from negative at the start of the trial to positive some time afterward. In addition, one of the following conditions was necessary for classification as a case: (1) death certified to be due to tuberculosis; (2) hospitalization for treatment of tuberculosis; or (3) roentgenographic evidence of active disease and outpatient chemotherapy for tuberculosis. As things turned out, all but 2 patients were hospitalized for treatment of their disease. Case records were considered to match population records only if a specified proportion of identifying information on the two records corresponded. Failing this, a field visit was made to obtain further information to allow a possible match to be verified or denied.

The trial was designed to be double-blind, with neither subjects nor observers at any level knowing who had received isoniazid or who had received the placebo. Records that identified subjects did not show the assigned medication, and cards used for analyses did not identify persons. Only one statistician in the office in Washington knew the products represented by the household serial number, and this person has never made any judgments related to classifying subjects as cases.

The amount of medication taken was ascertained in two ways. At each quarterly visit during the medication year, the field nurse asked a responsible person in the household how well each member was taking medication. From these answers, an individual medication index was derived, expressed as percent of the annual recommended dose. In addition, it was known how many tablets had been issued to each household during the year and how many were returned at the end. From these figures, an index of medication taking for the household was calculated. The two indices agreed reasonably well, but for this presentation only the individual medication index has been used.

RESULTS

Follow-up has been satisfactorily complete. The maximal possible length of observation for any village was 76 months, and for some was as short as 43 months because of delayed admission to the trial. The median length of observation for the total population was 69.3 months. Only 390 persons, or 5.3 per cent

90

of the initial population, were observed for less than 40 months. Most of those lost from observation prematurely were non-native families residing in the area temporarily or persons who died. A total of 284 deaths are known to have occurred during the period of observation, 85 among the 3,017 persons assigned a placebo, 79 among the 3,047 given isoniazid, 2 among 211 persons who received both the placebo and isoniazid because they changed households during the year, and 118 among 1,058 persons who were not assigned medication. Tuberculosis was the certified cause of death for 7 persons in the placebo group, 3 in the isoniazid group, and 16 in the nonparticipant group.

The magnitude of the tuberculosis problem in this population and some of its epidemiologic characteristics can be illustrated by the experience of the persons who took a placebo. To set the stage for this discussion, it is helpful to show the prevalence of positive reactors to 5 TU of PPD-S by age and sex among Eskimos in 1957, the year the trial was started. By the age of 15, nearly everyone had been infected with tubercle bacilli, the prevalence of infection being essentially the same for males and females. This is shown in figure 2.

Tuberculosis case rates in per cent for the entire study period are shown in figure 3 for persons who took the placebo.[3] Rates are low in childhood because a large proportion of young children did not become infected (7). After the age of 15, tuberculosis infection was virtually universal. Case rates were very high in late adolescence and early adult life and somewhat lower among older adults. They were similar for males and females except during the peak at 15 to 30 years of age, when the female rates were somewhat higher. Because the likelihood of being infected was similar for both sexes and because virtually everyone had been infected by age 15, the difference in case rates suggests that young adult females are more apt to develop active

[3] Throughout this paper case rates are given as the number of cases occurring during the entire study period per 100 initial population. Dividing the case rates by six will give a close approximation to average annual case rates expressed in per cent.

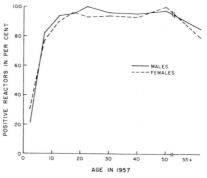

FIG. 2. Percentage of Eskimos with 5 mm. or more of induration to 5 TU of PPD-S, by sex and age in 1957.

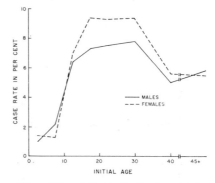

FIG. 3. Tuberculosis case rates in per cent during the study period, 1958 to 1964, among Eskimos assigned placebo by sex and age at start of trial.

disease after infection than young adult males, but that at older ages the risk of active disease after infection is essentially the same for each sex.

The risk of becoming infected with tubercle bacilli decreased considerably during the years after the initiation of the trial, largely as the result of the extensive tuberculosis control program conducted by the Alaska Department of Health and Welfare and the Division of Indian Health of the Public Health Service. The rate of new infections was estimated to be about 1 per cent per year during the first half of the follow-up period and about 0.5

TABLE 1
TUBERCULOSIS CASE RATES DURING STUDY PERIOD AMONG PLACEBO GROUP BY SIZE OF INDURATION TO 5 TU PPD-S AT START OF TRIAL[3]

| Induration (mm.) | Number Tested | Cases | |
		Number	Per Cent
Total	845	38	4.5
0−	275	6	2.2
5−	61	2	3.3
10−	157	9	5.7
15−	215	14	6.5
20+	137	7	5.1

TABLE 2
TUBERCULOSIS CASE RATES DURING STUDY PERIOD AMONG PLACEBO GROUP BY CLASSIFICATION OF INITIAL CHEST ROENTGENOGRAM[3]

| Tuberculosis Classification | Population | Cases | |
		Number	Per Cent
Total	1,699	93	5.5
Negative	1,193	41	3.4
Calcification only	259	13	5.0
Inactive	153	12	7.8
Questionably active	66	14	21.2
Probably active	28	13	46.0

per cent per year during the second half. Although these rates represent a marked improvement for this area of Alaska, they are still at least ten times higher than the estimated rates for the rest of the United States at that time (7).

In spite of high infection rates, the experience of persons tested with tuberculin at the start of the trial and assigned to the placebo group indicates that the risk was greatest for persons who were positive reactors initially. This is shown in table 1. Persons with 5 mm. or more of induration to 5 TU of PPD-S had a case rate over the next six years that was two and one-half times greater than that for negative reactors and accounted for 84 per cent of the tuberculosis that developed among the tested group.

Most of the study population of school age or older who were present in the villages had chest roentgenograms taken near the start of

the trial. These roentgenograms were interpreted by an independent reader who had no information about the subjects except for their name, age, and village. Films considered by physicians of the Alaska Department of Health and Welfare to show obviously active tuberculosis were not always available for review because they had been sent with the patients to the hospital. The initial classification of chest roentgenograms among the placebo group is shown in table 2. Among those whose chest roentgenograms were reviewed, there was a marked correlation of subsequent risk of active tuberculosis with classification of the initial film. Three per cent of those classified as negative developed tuberculosis during the study period. Pulmonary or hilar calcifications were noted in nearly one sixth of the examined population and probably represented healed tuberculous lesions because of the rarity of histoplasmosis in Alaska (8, 9). In contrast to findings in other areas where histoplasmosis is also uncommon (10, 11) the risk of subsequent active tuberculosis was not much higher among persons with calcifications than among persons with negative chest roentgenograms. Active disease occurred among 8 per cent of those initially classified as having inactive tuberculosis and among nearly half of those whose tuberculosis was considered to be probably active. In this respect, the present findings confirm those of others, notably the Danish Tuberculosis Index, that persons with roentgenographic shadows suggestive of tuberculosis have a very high risk of developing active disease (11).

Another related and important risk factor is illustrated in table 3. Practically all persons

TABLE 3
TUBERCULOSIS CASE RATES DURING STUDY PERIOD AMONG PLACEBO GROUP BY INITIAL TUBERCULOSIS STATUS[3]

| Initial Tuberculosis Status | Population | Cases | |
		Number	Per Cent
Total	3,017	141	4.67
Previously known tuberculosis			
Previous treated	611	14	2.3
Never treated	709	75	10.6
No known tuberculosis	1,697	52	3.1

who had been treated for tuberculosis prior to the trial had had adequate chemotherapy and their risk was relatively low. Persons who had been diagnosed as having inactive or suspected tuberculosis, and for whom no treatment was considered necessary at that time, had a very high risk of subsequent reactivation, a finding that has been reported for many other populations. Among this group with untreated tuberculosis, the risk of reactivation increased with extent of disease at the initial examination.

The effect of isoniazid prophylaxis on the tuberculosis experience of the eligible population is illustrated in figure 4. The isoniazid group not only fared better than the placebo group during the year of medication, but it continued to fare better throughout the entire study period of approximately six years. After the first four years, only 8 cases of active tuberculosis occurred among the isoniazid group contrasted with 33 among those who took a placebo.

Isoniazid appeared to have been effective in preventing both reactivations and the development of new disease, as shown in figure 5 in which case rates are indicated for both treatment groups according to tuberculosis status on entry to the trial. For persons who had been previously treated, the difference between the placebo and isoniazid groups could have arisen by chance; the other differences are highly significant both from the statistical and from the public health point of view.

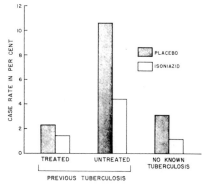

INITIAL TUBERCULOSIS STATUS

FIG. 5. Tuberculosis case rates in per cent during the study period, 1958 to 1964, for placebo and isoniazid groups by tuberculosis status at start of trial.

TABLE 4

TUBERCULOSIS CASE RATES DURING STUDY PERIOD BY MEDICATION ASSIGNED AND INITIAL TUBERCULIN STATUS[3]

Induration to 5 TU PPD-S (mm.)	Placebo			Isoniazid		
	Number Tested	Cases		Number Tested	Cases	
		Number	Per Cent		Number	Per Cent
Total	845	38	4.5	845	4	0.5
0–4	275	6	2.2	299	1	0.3
5+	570	32	5.6	546	3	0.6

The reliability of an estimate of isoniazid's effectiveness in preventing tuberculosis according to initial infection status in this study is sharply limited by the small numbers tested with tuberculin prior to the trial. The case rates by initial tuberculin status shown in table 4 for persons allocated to the placebo and isoniazid groups must be interpreted with caution even though isoniazid appeared to have caused a marked reduction in subsequent tuberculosis for both reactors and nonreactors.

Not all participants took their medication equally well, although there were no significant differences in this respect between the placebo and isoniazid groups. More than a

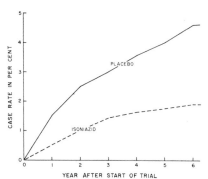

FIG. 4. Cumulative tuberculosis case rates in per cent for placebo and isoniazid groups by year after start of trial.

93

TABLE 5

TUBERCULOSIS CASE RATES DURING STUDY
PERIOD BY MEDICATION ASSIGNED AND
PER CENT OF RECOMMENDED DOSAGE
TAKEN[3]

Per Cent of Recommended Medication Taken	Placebo			Isoniazid		
		Cases			Cases	
	Popula-tion	Num-ber	Per Cent	Popula-tion	Num-ber	Per Cent
Total	3,017	141	4.67	3,047	58	1.90
0—	246	12	4.9	288	8	2.8
20—	345	21	6.1	262	9	3.4
40—	494	24	4.9	514	9	1.8
60—	816	27	3.3	888	15	1.7
80+	1,116	57	5.1	1,095	17	1.6

third of each group did very well indeed, taking 80 per cent or more of the recommended dosage over the year, but others did rather poorly. In part, poor participation resulted from inadequate motivation, but it must be remembered that the design of the trial made it impossible for late starters to complete a full year of medication. The striking result is that at all levels of taking medication the isoniazid group had less tuberculosis. Although the difference in case rates between isoniazid and placebo groups is greatest for those who took medication best, there is a suggestion from the trend among those who took isoniazid that six months of treatment might be enough. Although there were some differences in initial composition between the groups who took medication well and those who took it poorly, these were not marked; adjustments for differences in sex, age, and initial tuberculosis status caused only minor changes in the rates shown in table 5. However, even with the very high case rates among Alaskan Eskimos, there are too few cases in some cells of this table to be certain that a year of treatment is more than is needed. Until these findings can be confirmed, it appears wise to advise that prophylaxis be continued for at least a year. Nevertheless, it does appear that even a little isoniazid is better than none at all.

DISCUSSION

The public health usefulness of a community-wide program of isoniazid prophylaxis can be demonstrated from this study because the entire population of the study area was counted in the original census and because the subsequent tuberculosis experience of virtually all persons in the 30 communities has been ascertained. Only a small handful could not be located at the end of the observation period. By applying the placebo rates to the entire group of participants and adding the 24 cases observed among nonparticipants, it can be shown that a total of 317 new cases would have been expected if no prophylaxis had been given. Conversely, by applying the isoniazid rates to the participants and adding the 24 observed cases among nonparticipants, it can be shown that only 143 cases would have been expected if a complete community program had been attempted without controls. This is a reduction of 174 cases or 55 per cent of the potential new tuberculosis problem after the initiation of the trial.

To prevent these 174 cases required the services of five nurses and two clerks for a period of two and one-half years, or 10 cases prevented for each year of personnel time. Because patients were hospitalized for a period of about ten months on the average, each year of personnel time saved 100 months of hospitalization. This is a tremendous saving. The experience of this trial thus makes it clear that community-wide programs of isoniazid prophylaxis in situations similar to those existing in Alaskan villages are not only feasible and desirable from the humanitarian point of view but excellent financial investments as well.

A persistent concern of some observers has been the possible emergence of isoniazid-resistant strains of tubercle bacilli in the wake of chemoprophylaxis. Although a special study was set up to investigate this phenomenon after the present trial, too few isolations of resistant organisms have been observed to allow any but the broadest conclusions. The first of these is that the infrequency of isoniazid resistance makes it reasonably certain that it is not a major problem. The second is that susceptibility of tubercle bacilli to isoniazid, determined after the patients had been admitted to the study population but before they had received any subsequent chemotherapy (other than the prophylactic regimen), has not been related to prognosis.

The results of tests for drug susceptibility could not have influenced the choice of chemotherapy for these patients, because the only tests done on organisms from these particular patients were those made as part of the special study and the results were not reported to the treatment facilities. In fact, most patients had been discharged from the hospital before the tests were completed. Consequently, all patients in this series received isoniazid and PAS as the basic chemotherapeutic regimen, with short courses of streptomycin reserved for those who had surgery. Patients with resistant organisms and those with susceptible organisms did equally well, both in terms of average length of hospitalization and of lack of relapse over a post-hospital observation period which now ranges from three to six years.

A high rate of acquiring new tuberculous infections is perhaps the best indication that BCG vaccination might play a major role in combating tuberculosis. Consequently, in view of the high infection rates in many areas of Alaska, it is often asked why vaccination has not been given greater emphasis in the tuberculosis control program. As a matter of fact, BCG has not been neglected in Alaska. During the years 1949 to 1952, a major BCG vaccination campaign was conducted by the Alaska Department of Health and Welfare assisted by the U.S. Public Health Service, and BCG was given routinely in some villages for several years thereafter. In 1957, however, when the present trial was begun, it was already clear that most tuberculosis was arising among persons who were not eligible for vaccination and that BCG, even if highly effective, could have no major impact on tuberculosis for many years to come. At the present time, the average annual infection rate has fallen to a fraction of one per cent, and tuberculosis seems even more concentrated among those who were infected years ago. Annual tuberculin testing of school children has become a useful clue to small localized outbreaks of tuberculosis. Spotting incipient outbreaks by tuberculin "conversions" and quenching them with effective chemotherapy and chemoprophylaxis appear to be a most effective means of maintaining maximal pressure against tuberculosis (12).

SUMMARY

In 1957, a controlled trial of isoniazid prophylaxis was initiated in 30 communities in the Bethel area of Alaska, where tuberculosis rates had been among the highest ever reported. More than 85 per cent of the total population of 7,333 persons participated in the trial. Most of the nonparticipants were excluded because they were being treated for tuberculosis or because they came to the study communities late in the medication year; only 3 per cent refused to participate. Half of the participants were randomly allocated to the placebo group and half to the isoniazid group, the latter drug being prescribed in a dosage of 5 mg. per kilogram of body weight daily for one year. The median length of observation is now almost six years.

The risk of active tuberculosis developing during the study period was greatest among young adults, among positive reactors to tuberculin, and among persons with initial evidence of tuberculosis for which treatment did not then seem to be indicated. For all groups this risk was substantially decreased by isoniazid prophylaxis. The reduction in tuberculosis attributable to isoniazid persisted essentially unchanged throughout the entire period of observation, averaging about 60 per cent. Although protection was greatest among persons who took medication regularly for a full year, some protection was noted even among persons who took isoniazid irregularly and for short periods.

Each year of personnel time invested in a program of community-wide prophylaxis has already resulted in the prevention of 10 cases of tuberculosis, accounting for 100 person-months of hospitalization. It is concluded that community-wide prophylaxis is feasible under conditions similar to those in Alaskan villages, and that such programs can be successful both from the humanitarian and economic points of view.

Acknowledgments

Any long-term, population-based study is dependent for its success upon many individuals—subjects, collaborators, and other professional personnel in the same or allied fields. To all of these we are grateful for their freely given cooperation. The group to whom we turned most often for assistance was the staff of the Tuberculosis Case Register of the Alaska Department of Health and Welfare, directed throughout the study period by

Mrs. Clarabelle Johnson. Their conscientious work lightened immeasurably the task of collecting information about the study subjects.

REFERENCES

(1) Aronson, J. D.: The history of disease among the natives of Alaska, Trans. Coll. Physicians, Phila., 1940, *8*, 27.

(2) Weiss, E. S.: Tuberculin sensitivity in Alaska, Public Health Rep., 1953, *68*, 23.

(3) Simmet, R.: Alaska, frontier for health services, Public Health Rep., 1960, *75*, 878.

(4) Comstock, G. W., and Porter, M. E.: Tuberculin sensitivity and tuberculosis among natives of the lower Yukon, Public Health Rep., 1959, *74*, 621.

(5) Porter, M. E., and Comstock, G. W.: Ambulatory chemotherapy in Alaska, Public Health Rep., 1962, *77*, 1021.

(6) Comstock, G. W.: Isoniazid prophylaxis in an undeveloped area, Amer. Rev. Resp. Dis., 1962, *86*, 810.

(7) Comstock, G. W., and Philip, R. N.: Decline of the tuberculosis epidemic in Alaska, Public Health Rep., 1961, *76*, 19.

(8) Comstock, G. W.: Histoplasmin sensitivity in Alaskan natives, Amer. Rev. Tuberc., 1959, *79*, 542.

(9) Edwards, P. Q.: Histoplasmin sensitivity of young men in Alaska, Hawaii, the Phillippines and Puerto Rico, Bull. W.H.O., 1964, *30*, 587.

(10) Pope, A. S., Sartwell, P. E., and Zacks, D.: Development of tuberculosis in infected children, Amer. J. Public Health, 1939, *29*, 1318.

(11) Groth-Petersen, E., Knudsen, J., and Wilbek, E.: Epidemiological basis of tuberculosis eradication in an advanced country, Bull. W.H.O., 1959, *21*, 5.

(12) Fraser, R. I.: Tuberculosis in Alaska in 1965, Alaska Med., 1965, *7*, 12.

An Epidemic in an Eskimo Village Due to Group-B Meningococcus

Part 2. Clinical Features

Thomas H. Corbett, MD, and Jacob A. Brody, MD

S ix cases of group-B meningococcal septicemia occurred in the Eskimo village of Barrow, Alaska, between Oct 25 and Nov 15, 1964. This report discusses the clinical aspects of the outbreak. The epidemiological and laboratory aspects of this outbreak are presented elsewhere in THE JOURNAL (p 383).

Report of Cases

A summary of the significant clinical and laboratory findings in the cases is presented in the Table.

CASE 1.—A 28-year-old Eskimo woman was admitted to the Barrow Hospital on Oct 25, 1964, in a semicomatose and disoriented state. She had been drinking heavily for two days before becoming ill. She noted the onset of nausea and vomiting 24 hours before admission, followed in three hours by chills and fever. Blood-streaked stools were noted 12 hours prior to admission. She became semicomatose and severe pain developed in the abdomen and legs. At admission she was having repeated episodes of explosive diarrhea with mucoid, blood-streaked stools. She periodically became incoherent and maniacal and she tried to bite the nurses several times.

Physical examination revealed the signs of circulatory failure including blood pressure, 60/40 mm Hg; pulse rate, 120 beats per minute; and respirations, 40/min. Bluish-red purpuric spots were seen on the head and neck. The liver was palpable 1 inch below the right costal margin. Meningism was not present.

The white blood cell count (WBC) was 3,100/cu mm, with 54% polymorphonuclear neutrophilic leukocytes (pmn) and 46% lymphocytes. Urinalysis revealed albuminuria (3+). The spinal fluid was clear and under normal pressure. There were 13 pmn per cubic millimeter of spinal fluid.

Considering the symptoms, the history of having eaten fermented whale meat, and the reported cases of botulism from eating the beluga whale,[1] a tentative diagnosis of botulism was made. Because of her desperate condition she was transferred to Anchorage, Alaska, by emergency airlift, but she died en route. Therapy included intravenous administration of potassium penicillin G (10 million units), chloramphenicol (Chloromycetin, 2 gm), and sulfisoxazole (Gantrisin, 2 gm). Pressor agents were also used intravenously.

An autopsy was performed at the Bassett Army Hospital, Fort Wainwright, Alaska. Significant findings were petechiae of the head, neck, and upper extremities; pulmonary and splenic congestion; central degeneration and congestion of the liver; degeneration of the convoluted tubules of the kidneys; congestion of the mucosal and submucosal vessels; and some mucosal hemorrhage in the gastrointestinal tract. Small interstitial hemorrhages were seen to be present in the adrenal glands on microscopical examination, but there was no grossly observable hemorrhage.

CASE 2.—A 46-year-old Eskimo man was admitted to the Barrow Hospital on Nov 1, 1964. He had been drinking heavily for several days before the onset of his illness, and fever and chills developed 36 hours before admission. Abdominal pain, nausea, vomiting and diarrhea commenced six hours later. The stools were black at first and then became mucoid and blood streaked, continuing thus throughout his illness. He noted severe pain in his lower extremities three hours before admission. On admission he complained that his eyes and head hurt.

Physical examination revealed an adult male who appeared critically ill. Signs of circulatory failure included blood pressure, 70/50 mm Hg; pulse rate, 100 beats per minute; and respirations, 40/min. Pinhead-sized petechiae were seen on the forehead and nose. There was blood in the posterior part of the pharynx. The liver was palpable 1 inch below the right costal margin. Bowel sounds were hyperactive. The admission WBC was 2,800/cu mm, with no differential count performed. A stool specimen was watery, yellow, and blood-streaked. Because of his critical condition, further studies were not conducted. Botulism being the tentative diagnosis, the patient received 10 million units of botulism antitoxin and he was taken to the airport for transportation to Fairbanks, Alaska, on a scheduled commercial flight. Intravenous administration of penicillin G (5 million units) and chloramphenicol (1 gm) was started before takeoff. His condition continued to deteriorate, and pressor agents were given during flight. He died 15 minutes after admission to the St. Joseph's Hospital in Fairbanks.

Significant autopsy findings included petechiae of the head, neck, and thorax; pulmonary congestion and edema; congestion of the liver; degeneration of the convoluted tubules of the kidneys; a few petechiae of the gastric and intestinal mucosa with congestion of the intestinal mucosa; and vascular congestion and a small amount of interstitial hemorrhage in the adrenal glands. There was no grossly observable hemorrhage in the adrenals.

CASE 3.—A 25-year-old Eskimo woman with a history of alcohol ingestion was admitted to the Barrow Hospital on

Nov 7, 1964. She complained of weakness, dizziness, vague headache, dry cough, and low back pain of 24 hours' duration. Three hours before admission she suffered chills, fever, shortness of breath, leg pains, sternal chest pain, and difficulty in swallowing. When first seen she was anorexic and semicomatose but had no nausea, vomiting, or diarrhea.

Physical examination revealed blood pressure, 100/60 mm Hg; pulse rate, 120 beats per minute; respirations, 36/min; and temperature, 103 F (39.4 C rectal). There was diffuse tenderness throughout the abdomen. The liver was palpable 1 inch below the right costal margin.

The admission WBC was 26,200/cu mm, with 86% pmn. The results of urinalysis were normal. The spinal-fluid pressure was normal and a blood-cell count showed four pmn per cubic millimeter. A stool guaiac test was negative.

The patient was treated with intravenously administered potassium penicillin G, chloramphenicol, and botulism antitoxin and intramuscularly administered sodium pentobarbital (Nembutal). Circulatory failure developed on the evening of admission and the blood pressure dropped to 88/20 mm Hg. Steroids were given intravenously. No pressor agents were available in Barrow at that time. Supplies of steroids and penicillin for intravenous use were soon exhausted and these drugs were then given orally and intramuscularly, respectively. Botulism antitoxin was discontinued after meningococcus had been isolated from the first patient and established as a probable etiologic agent. Her condition gradually improved. The temperature became normal and the blood pressure stabilized within 24 hours after admission. Her blood pressure again dropped to 78/38 mm Hg 36 hours after admission but rose steadily to normal levels and remained so throughout the remainder of her hospital course. Her sensorium cleared during the second day, but she complained of severe generalized muscle pain for the first four days of hospitalization. She was discharged on the eighth hospital day.

CASE 4.—A 3-year-old Eskimo boy was admitted to the Barrow Hospital on Nov 8, 1964. Twenty-four hours before his admission, fever developed (103 F [39.4 C], rectal) with nausea and vomiting. He was seen at the Barrow Clinic four hours later. Physical examination at that time revealed nothing remarkable. He was sent home with medication to relieve his symptoms. The fever, nausea, and vomiting continued, and he returned complaining of a headache. Physical examination showed nothing of importance. A WBC performed at that time was 45,000/cu mm, with 89% pmn, containing toxic granules. He was admitted for evaluation of this finding. Urinalysis revealed albuminuria (1+) with a few WBCs. The spinal-fluid pressure was normal and a blood-cell count revealed four pmn per cubic millimeter.

He was treated with intramuscular administration of procaine penicillin G, 1.2 million units every 6 hours for 24 hours and then 600,000 units every 12 hours for the remainder of his hospital course. His temperature returned to normal within 24 hours. He was discharged after four days of hospitalization.

Clinical and Laboratory Findings in Six Cases of Meningococcal Disease

Date of Onset of Illness	Case	Age, Yr	Signs and Symptoms	Laboratory Values*†	Cerebrospinal Fluid*	Treatment
10-25-64	1	28	Nausea Vomiting Blood-streaked stools Abdominal and leg pain Chills and fever Purpuric rash Shock	WBC, 3,100/cu mm Pmn, 54% Hgb, 11.5 gm/100 cc Hct, 34% U/a, 3+	Clear Pmn, 13/cu mm Pressure, normal	Penicillin Chloramphenicol Streptomycin Sulfisoxazole Pressor agents

11-1-64	2	46	Chills and fever
			Nausea
			Vomiting
			Blood-streaked stools
			Abdominal and leg pains
			Headache
			Purpuric rash
			Shock
				WBC, 2,800/cu mm
				Hgb, 12 gm/100 cc
				Hct, 38%
					Not tested	Botulism E
						  antitoxin
						Penicillin
						Chloramphenicol
						Levarterenol
						  bitartrate

11-7-64	3	25	Headache Low back pain Chills and fever Anorexia Sternal and leg pains Shock	WBC, 26,200/cu mm Pmn, 86% Hgb, 13.2 gm/100 cc	Clear Pmn, 4/cu mm	Botulism E antitoxin Penicillin Chloramphenicol Sulfisoxazole Steroids Sedatives
11-8-64	4	3	Nausea Vomiting Headache Fever Shock	WBC, 45,000/cu mm Pmn, 89% Hgb, 14.3 gm/100 cc Hct, 42% U/a, 1+	Clear Pmn, 4/cu mm Pressure, normal	Penicillin
11-14-64	5	3	Headache Muscle cramps	WBC, 15,000/cu mm	Not tested	Penicillin
11-15-64	6	37	Malaise Headache Stiff neck Chills and fever Sternal chest pain Meningism Toxic psychosis	WBC, 8,300/cu mm Pmn, 53%	Clear Pmn, 4/cu mm	Penicillin

*Pmn = polymorphonuclear neutrophilic leukocytes.
†U/a = urine reaction for albumin.

CASE 5.—A 3-year-old Eskimo boy was seen in the Barrow Clinic on Nov 15, 1964. He had a temperature of 102.8 F (39.3 C rectal) and had had fever, vague headache, and pain in the upper extremities for 24 hours. The physical examination showed nothing remarkable.

No laboratory examinations were performed, but a blood specimen was obtained for culture, from which group-B meningococcus was isolated.

He was treated with intramuscular administration of procaine penicillin G, 600,000 units each day for seven days on an outpatient basis. He recovered uneventfully.

CASE 6.—A 37-year-old male Caucasian was admitted to the Barrow Hospital on Nov 15, 1964. This man was the driver of the vehicle which transported the first patient to the airport. Several days after this exposure sore throat, fever, and malaise developed, for which he received erythromycin, 250 mg four times a day for five days with improvement of symptoms. Three weeks later, on the morning of admission, he walked five miles in −40 F weather and shortly thereafter complained of general malaise. At 5:30 PM he noted an occipital headache which persisted for several hours. At 7:10 PM his temperature was 99.6 F (37.6 C, oral), and at 8 PM he was babbling incoherently. He complained of chills and fever, a stiff neck, and severe pain throughout the entire anterior chest wall.

Physical examination revealed a normal blood pressure and pulse rate. The respiratory rate was 24/min, and the temperature was 99.6 F (37.6 C, oral). He was semicomatose. The throat was slightly injected. Meningism was present.

The WBC on admission was 8,300/cu mm, with 53% pmn. The urinalysis gave normal findings. A throat smear revealed gram-negative diplococci. The spinal-fluid pressure was normal and a blood-cell count revealed three pmn per cubic millimeter.

He was treated with intravenous administration of potassium penicillin G, 1 million units per hour for 48 hours; this dosage was tapered slowly over the next four days. The temperature became normal several hours after admission and remained so throughout his hospital course. His sensorium also cleared several hours after admission and remained normal. Hysteria was considered a possible diagnosis because of the total lack of objective findings, his mental status on admission, and the marked improvement shortly after admission. (Extreme anxiety was prevalent throughout the village during the outbreak.) He continued to complain of muscle pains in his chest and legs for four days after admission. Group-B meningococcus was isolated from the blood specimen taken at the time of admission.

Comment

Six cases of meningococcal septicemia occurred in Barrow from Oct 25, 1964, to Nov 15, 1964. The organism, a group-B *Neisseria meningitidis* was isolated from the blood in five of the six cases. No cultures were obtained from one of the two patients who died. However, the clinical course, skin hemorrhages, and early death were considered evidence sufficient for diagnosis of meningococcal septicemia.

Symptoms were unusual and confusing to the extent that the admission diagnosis of meningococcal disease was made in only one instance (case 6). Only two of the cases occurred in children. These were so mild they would have been missed had not routine blood culturing for meningococcus been instituted. One was an outpatient, received only minimal doses of penicillin, and recovered uneventfully.

In two of the cases, purpuric rashes developed. Gastrointestinal symptoms were the predominant features in three of the six cases. Nausea, vomiting, diarrhea, and blood-streaked stools were seen with the two fatal cases.

Routine laboratory studies were not helpful diagnostically. The cerebrospinal fluid was normal in all instances when tested, and the WBC was low in two instances (both fatal), normal in one patient, and elevated in three.

Autopsies performed in the two fatal cases yielded no remarkable findings and did not aid in establishing the diagnosis. No adrenal hemorrhage was found on gross examination, and only a small amount of interstitial hemorrhage was noted in the adrenal glands on microscopical examination.

In two of the six cases psychotic episodes occurred in the absence of meningitis. Endotoxemia or anxiety could equally be entertained as possible explanations for this manifestation. Fischer[2] reported two cases in which toxic psychosis was the predominant sign, but in his cases frank meningitis was present.

The picture in the two fatal cases in the Barrow epidemic lends clinical support to the theory of May,[3] Levin and Cluff,[4] and Ferguson and Chapman[5] who ascribe the pathological findings to the effect of endotoxin rather than to destruction of the adrenal gland. In animals,[4] endotoxin caused cortical necrosis of the adrenal gland. In granulocytopenic animals, collapse occurred in the absence of adrenal damage. The fatal cases in our series were markedly granulocytopenic with irreversible circulatory failure, but they showed minimal changes in the adrenal glands.

It has been reported that respiratory infections,

otitis media, extreme fatigue, and excessive use of alcohol may be predisposing factors to meningococcal disease.[6] It was of interest to note that the three adult Eskimo patients in Barrow were heavy drinkers and each had been on a weekend drinking bout before becoming ill. The Caucasian adult had just returned from a fatiguing hike when he became ill.

Rosemary Riebe performed the laboratory studies for this investigation.

Generic and Trade Names of Drugs

Potassium penicillin G—*Dramcillin, Dropcillin, Penalev, K-Cillin, Readicillin, Pentids.*
Chloramphenicol—*Chloromycetin.*
Sulfisoxazole—*Gantrisin.*
Sodium pentobarbital—*Isobarb, Napental, Nembutal Sodium.*
Procaine penicillin G—*Depo-Penicillin, Lentopen, Wycillin.*
Levarterenol bitartrate—*Levophed.*

References

1. Rabeau, I.S.: Botulism in Arctic Alaska: Report of 13 Cases with Five Fatalities, *Alaska Med* 1:6-9 (March) 1959.

2. Fischer, D.S.: Toxic Psychosis Without Fever as Sign of Acute Meningitis, *Arch Intern Med* 111:54-57 (Jan) 1963.

3. May, C.D.: Circulatory Failure (Shock) in Fulminent Meningococcal Infection, *Pediatrics* 25:316-328 (Feb) 1960.

4. Levin, J., and Cluff, L.E.: Endotoxemia and Adrenal Hemorrhage: Mechanism for Waterhouse-Friderichsen Syndrome, *J Exp Med* 121:247-258 (Feb 1) 1965.

5. Ferguson, J.H., and Chapman, O.D.: Fulminating Meningococcic Infections and the So-called Waterhouse-Friderichsen Syndrome, *Amer J Path* 24:763-795 (July) 1948.

6. Laybourn, R.: A Study of Epidemic Meningitis in Missouri: Epidemiologic and Administrative Consideration, *Southern Med J* 24:678-686 (Aug) 1931.

Controlled Trials with Trisulfapyrimidines in the Treatment of Chronic Trachoma

Chandler R. Dawson, Lavelle Hanna, T. Rodman
Wood, Virginia Coleman, Odeon C. Briones, and
Ernest Jawetz

Trachoma is an ancient infectious eye disease which is said to afflict 400 million people in the world and to blind 20 million of them. While most prevalent in Africa and Asia, trachoma is also common among the Indians of the American Southwest and presents a serious health problem there. The etiologic agent, a member of the Psittacosis-Lymphogranuloma-Trachoma group (Chlamydiae), is not a virus and can be inhibited by many antimicrobial drugs in laboratory models [1]. Since the advent of sulfonamides, each antimicrobial drug which became available has found some endorsement for the treatment of clinical trachoma. Until recently, however, there were no careful placebo-controlled trials of drug therapy. Such trials seem essential because the disease manifestations ·of trachoma can be drastically influenced by many environmental features including sanitation, water supply, standards of personal hygiene, and education.

A quarter-century ago Forster and Mc-Gibony [2] administered sulfanilamide 60 mg/kilogram per day for 21 days to American Indian children and estimated on the basis of clinical follow-up examinations that about 75% of "over 20,000 patients" were clinically cured of trachoma. Similar cure rates are quoted in a mas-sive compilation of many subsequent studies on sulfonamide treatment of trachoma [1]. However, when Foster et al. [3] compared oral sulfonamide with placebo in a controlled study in American Indian children, about 60% of each group was significantly improved on clinical grounds 6 months later. Woolridge et al. [4] reported a "cure rate" of 16% in sulfonamide-treated and of 22% in placebo-treated children on Taiwan 6 months after the end of a course of trisulfapyrimidines, 3 g daily for 4 weeks. Thus recent use of sulfonamides has not brought about good clinical response.

Our group introduced another type of treatment evaluation by estimating not only the clinical activity of trachoma but also the prevalence of the infectious agent in the eyes of patients. Direct immunofluorescence microscopy, applied to conjunctival scrapings, appears to be the most sensitive method available for the detection of TRIC (trachoma—inclusion conjunctivitis) inclusions, and often yields positive results when other methods (agent isolation, Giemsa stains of smears) are negative. There are many instances where positive immunofluorescence indicates the presence of the TRIC agent, while all signs of active inflammation are lacking [5, 6].

A mild form of trachoma is endemic among American Indians in the southwestern United States. On many Indian reservations the infection rate is high, yet there is little disabling eye disease, infrequent bacterial conjunctivitis of any severity, and blindness attributable to lifelong trachoma infection is uncommon. Indian children drawn from different reservations attend large boarding schools where medical care is under the supervision of the Division of Indian Health, U.S. Public Health Service. In cooperation with that organization, we began chemotherapy trials in 1965 in such schools in order to evaluate critically the response of mild, often uncomplicated trachoma to various drug regimens. Since a special congressional appropria-

Supported by a grant (NB 00604) from the National Institutes of Health, U. S. Public Health Service, and by a Research Career Development Award (1 K3 NB 31, 781-02) to C. R. D.

We wish to thank the Division of Indian Health of the U. S. Public Health Service; Dr. E. Johnson, Mr. G. Krutz, and Dr. I. Hoshiwara for permission to perform the trials and assistance in their design; and particularly Miss Margaret Hersey, R.N., and Mrs. A. Dilworth, R.N., who supervised administration of all drugs during this study; and Dr. Clyde Olson, Dr. Bruce Ostler, and Mr. Masao Okumoto for their assistance in performing the bacteriologic studies.

Please address requests for reprints to Dr. Jawetz, Department of Microbiology, University of California, San Francisco Medical Center, San Francisco, California 94122.

tion has been provided to finance treatment and eradication programs among Indians, it was important to develop guidelines for the proposed mass treatment. In initial trials we compared the effect of the topical administration of tetracycline (1% drops, 3 times daily for 42 days) or the oral administration of sulfisoxazole (1 g, 4 times daily for 21 days) with their respective placebos [7]. There was no difference in the pattern of clinical response to active drug or placebo, both groups improving markedly during a 6-month period of follow-up. This was attributed to the excellent sanitary environment of the boarding school and the hygienic measures practiced there. However, while the clinical signs diminished, the rate of infection remained unchanged, and the prevalence of positive immunofluorescence was not influenced by drug administration [7, 8].

These initial disappointing results might be attributable to inadequate dose and time of treatment or to the selection of an unusual type of trachoma patients. The mean level of free sulfonamide was only 2.6 mg/100 ml in sulfisoxazole-treated children—a concentration far lower than acceptable for the treatment of other microbial infections. We therefore undertook trials in 2 Indian schools in 1967–1968 with another drug, trisulfapyrimidines U.S.P. The main results are presented here.

Patient Material and Methods

Patients

At the Stewart School near Carson City, Nevada, about 500 students, aged 12–21 years, reside from September to May of each year. Each May the students return to their home

territory for summer vacation, but during the rest of the year they remain at boarding school. A similar time schedule applies to the Sherman Institute at Riverside, California, where there are about 600 students in the same age range. Several Indian tribes, including Navajo, Apache, Paiute, Pima, Papago, and others contribute to the population of the 2 schools.

Schedule of examinations and administration of drugs is given in table 1.

At the beginning of the school year, each student was examined by an ophthalmologist for signs of trachoma. One examiner at each school was responsible for selecting students with clinically active disease who were then assigned at random to treatment or placebo groups. At the Stewart School, a third random group of students without signs of clinical activity in the fall was examined intermittently for 6 months, without treatment, to estimate the development of trachomatous activity in the school population. Follow-up examinations were carried out by the ophthalmologists at intervals of 4, 10, 19, and 20 weeks, as indicated in table 1.

Drug Treatment

At each school, a full-time nurse personally administered all drugs and placebos. All materials were coded, and the identity of drug or placebo remained unknown to subjects, nurse, and physicians throughout the trials until all examination results had been recorded. Trisulfapyrimidines U.S.P. from a commercial source was used, and a lactose-placebo tablet of similar appearance and taste was prepared by the hospital pharmacy, University of California at San Francisco. A daily total of 3.5 g trisulfapyrimi-

Table 1. Schedule of examinations and therapy

	Stewart School	Sherman Institute	Time after completing therapy
	1967	1967	
Preliminary examination	Sept. 18–20	Oct. 2	. . .
Drug administration	Oct. 19–Nov. 8	Oct. 23–Nov. 12	. . .
Follow-up examination	Dec. 4–6	Dec. 11	4 weeks
	1968	1968	
Follow-up examination	Jan. 15	Jan. 22	10 weeks
Follow-up examination	Mar. 18	Mar. 25	19 weeks
Repeat conjunctival smears	. . .	April 2	20 weeks

dines was administered in 3 doses: 1 g at 7–8 A.M., 1 g at 12–1 P.M., and 1.5 g at 5–6 P.M. Corresponding numbers of placebo tablets were administered at the same times. Blood samples were obtained on the fourteenth or fifteenth days of the treatment program from all students 1–2 hr after the second daily dose. Serum was separated, and blood levels of free sulfonamide were estimated by the Bratton-Marshall method, expressing results in terms of a sulfanilamide standard [9].

Assessment of results

Clinical examination. The conjunctiva and cornea were examined with a slit lamp, as described in detail previously [10]. The following signs were recorded and scored for severity at each examination: follicular hypertrophy, papillary hypertrophy, conjunctival scars, trichiasis or entropion, neovascularization of cornea (pannus), corneal scarring, and trachoma stage by the Mac-Callan classification [1]. The examiner was unaware of the previous clinical findings on the subject and of the treatment he received.

The clinical activity of trachoma was judged primarily by the presence of subconjunctival lymphoid follicles on the upper tarsus, particularly in its central portion. An extensive and detailed study of the various changes found in trachoma has convinced us that the classical criterion of follicles on the upper tarsal plate is the best index of clinical activity.

Immunofluorescent staining of conjunctival smears. At each examination, scrapings were obtained from the tarsal (upper) conjunctival epithelium of each eye and smears were examined by at least 2 observers for the presence of TRIC agent by means of specific immunofluorescence. The techniques of preparing fluorescein-labeled antisera in rabbits, and preparing, fixing, storing, and staining the conjunctival smears have been described [6, 11]. A single labeled serum was used for all examinations. Because of the variation in the number of epithelial cells on different slides, no attempt was made to quantify the number of fluorescent inclusions on any 1 examination. Results were recorded as positive or negative immunofluorescence. The vast majority of positive immunofluorescent smears contained 1–5 identifiable inclusions per 100–1,000 cells.

Bacterial cultures. At the Stewart School,

bacterial cultures were taken as described previously [12] from a portion of the students at the September and December examinations, and in March from all the students in the study groups. Cultures were obtained from each eye separately by means of sterile cotton-tipped applicators moistened with trypticase-soy broth. The swab was swept across the lower conjunctival fornix and then streaked onto a segment of a rabbit blood agar plate. The same swab was then touched to the lid margin of the same eye and streaked onto another part of the same plate. Plates were sealed with masking tape, incubated at 37 C for 2–4 days, then transported by car to San Francisco. The plates were then inspected for representative colonies of the more important ocular bacterial pathogens. Only the prevalent bacterial pathogens, if any, were recorded. Because of the crude nature of this bacteriologic sampling, no quantitation of results was attempted.

Results

Assessment of Drug Effect

Stewart School. In September, 1967, 36 students with active trachoma were selected for the chemotherapy trial by examiner A. Eighteen of them received drug, and the alternate 18 placebo, from October 19 to November 8, 1967. An additional 149 students, free from "active trachoma" in September, 1967, but often with scars and other signs of inactive disease, were followed closely throughout the school year without any form of treatment. In this latter group, 13 (8.7%) developed clinically active trachoma (figure 1). This serves as an indication of the conversion rate to clinically active trachoma in this population.

Figure 1 summarizes the clinical and immunofluorescence findings. About 50% of all conjunctival specimens contained TRIC agent by immunofluorescence. The large majority of conjunctival smears contained only 1–5 typical immunofluorescent inclusions per 100–1,000 cells. However, a rare smear contained 10–50 inclusions. There was no correlation whatever between the apparent clinical activity of the patient and the number of inclusions found in repeated specimens. Parenthetically, it should be noted that we have observed a few individuals entirely free of signs of trachomatous activity who had 25 or more inclusions in every smear obtained over a period of 18 months [6]. During the drug trial there was a slight and temporary but not significant decline in the incidence of positive immunofluorescent smears following the course of sulfonamides. None of the incidence figures on any 1 collection date differed significantly from the others. This was also true for the group of students without active trachoma, not included in the trial but observed concurrently. Thus neither treatment nor residence in the environment of the school influenced the prevalence of TRIC agent in the population.

A distinct difference was observed between drug and placebo groups by clinical assessment. Less clinically active trachoma was found among the drug-treated students than among those receiving placebo at each follow-up examination. In spite of the small size of the groups, this difference was statistically significant in January, 1968, 10 weeks after the end of treatment ($\chi^2 = 7.3$; $P = <.01$), but not in December, 1967, 4 weeks after the end of treatment, or in April, 1968, 19 weeks after the end of treatment ($\chi^2 = 2.6$; $P = > .1$).

Sherman Institute. Twenty-nine students with active trachoma were selected by examiner B in September, 1967, for a trial of trisulfapyrimidine treatment. Active drug was given to 15 students and placebo to 14 others from October 19 to November 8, 1967. The clinical appearance of all students improved during their stay in school, but there was no difference between placebo and sulfa groups (figure 2). About 40% of students with active disease had positive immunofluorescence in September, 1967. There was no significant change from this level until April, 1968, and no difference between drug and placebo groups. One week after the first sampling of conjunctival scrapings in April, 1968, the conjunctivae were scraped a second time to obtain smears. There was a striking increase in positive immunofluorescence in this second sampling in both drug and placebo groups, so that 70%–90% of all specimens revealed the presence of TRIC

ORAL TRISULFAPYRIMIDINES THERAPY OF TRACHOMA - STEWART INDIAN SCHOOL
(3.5 GM DAILY ×21)

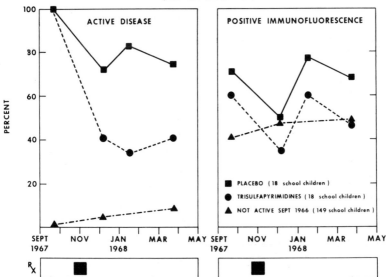

Figure 1. Oral trisulfapyrimidines therapy of trachoma—Stewart Indian School (3.5 g daily ×21).

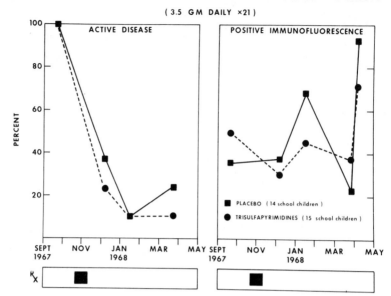

Figure 2. Oral trisulfapyrimidines therapy of trachoma—Sherman Institute (3.5 g daily ×21).

agent. The apparent "provocation" of TRIC agent from latency into activity as a result of trauma is discussed below.

Observer Variation

In previous studies we had observed that the assessment and quantification of trachomatous eye lesions varied markedly from one qualified and experienced ophthalmologist to another. Ideally, the clinical assessment of each patient should be performed independently by at least 2 ophthalmologists on the same day [13, 14]. In anticipation of observer variation, the ophthalmologists involved in the drug trials (examiners A and B) simultaneously examined a group of 27 Indian children and recorded their findings and assessment independently. The comparison in their assessment of "clinically active trachoma" is shown in table 2. Examiner B labeled 22 of the 27 children "active trachoma," whereas examiner A gave this designation to only 15 children. Examiner A found no clinical activity among 8 of the 22 designated "active" by examiner B,

whereas examiner B found no clinical activity in only 1 of the 15 designated "active" by examiner A. This comparison permits the conclusion that examiner A was more stringent in his criteria for "activity" than examiner B and that the latter might tend to include very mild cases in groups selected as "active" for chemotherapy trials. This difference in group selection may have influenced the outcome of the trials. Examiner B at Sherman Institute may have had more very mild cases, which tend to improve spontaneously, particularly under the influence of favorable environment. Examiner A at Stewart School may have restricted his group to relatively severe cases, which are less likely to improve spontaneously and which may benefit from the administration of drugs. We realize that further trials will be necessary to test this hypothesis.

Bacterial Flora

To examine the role of bacterial infections, bacterial cultures were obtained in September,

108

December, and March from a portion of the patients treated for active trachoma with sulfonamide or placebo at the Stewart School. The number of patients with potential pathogens is similar in each group before and after therapy (figure 3). Clinically apparent bacterial conjunctivitis was not found in any of these children. Moreover, ocular bacterial pathogens were equally frequent among patients with clinically active and inactive trachoma in both the treatment and placebo groups at the December and March examinations (figure 3). Only 1 bacterial species, *Moraxella lacunata*, has been associated with a trachoma-like clinical picture. This organism was present in 4 patients in the sulfa-treated group and 3 in the placebo group prior to therapy. It was not found again in the sulfa group, but in the placebo group it was reisolated again from 1 patient in December and March and from

another in March. On only 1 occasion was this associated with clinically active trachoma (table 3), and at that time the patient also yielded inclusion-positive smears from each eye. The persistence of potential bacterial pathogens did not appear to affect the clinical activity of trachoma in either the treatment or control group. Neither could the

Table 2. Observer variation

	Examiner B (Sherman)		
	Active trachoma	Not active trachoma	Total
Examiner A (Stewart):			
Active trachoma	14	1	15
Not active trachoma ..	8	4	12
Total	22	5	27

OCULAR BACTERIAL FLORA AND TRACHOMATOUS ACTIVITY IN PATIENTS TREATED WITH SULFONAMIDE OR PLACEBO

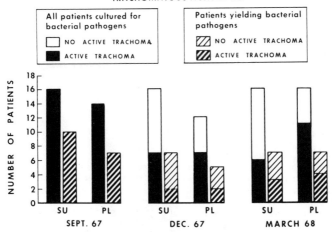

Figure 3. Relative frequency of bacterial pathogens and trachomatous activity in patients treated with oral trisulfapyrimidines (SU) or placebo (PL). At the beginning of the study (September, 1967) all patients had active trachoma and about half had bacterial pathogens on culture. Four weeks (December, 1967) and 19 weeks (March, 1968) after completion of therapy, there was no difference in the prevalence of bacterial pathogens in the sulfonamide and placebo-treated groups. The rates of clinical trachomatous activity in patients yielding bacterial pathogens did not differ significantly from the rates in the whole group at either follow-up visit. Thus bacterial pathogens were unrelated to the persistence of trachomatous activity, and the effect of drug was unrelated to the possible suppression of bacteria.

apparent drug effect observed at Stewart School be attributed to suppression of bacteria.

Sulfonamide Levels

Blood for sulfonamide assay was drawn between 1 and 2 P.M. on the fourteenth and fifteenth days of treatment, respectively, at the 2 schools. One of the students receiving placebo, a girl at the Stewart School, had a measurable sulfonamide level of 5.8 mg/100 ml; she was excluded from the results because it was not clear whether she had received drug rather than placebo, or whether the blood sample had been mislabeled. All of the students receiving sulfonamide had measurable blood levels ranging from 1.7 to 16.2 mg/100 ml. The average level at Sherman Institute was 7.6 mg/100 ml and at Stewart School 7.9 mg/100 ml. Figure 4 shows the distribution of sulfonamide levels in the sera of 36 students. All of them weighed 50 kg or more and received 3.5 g trisulfapyrimidines daily. Only 5 of the 36 students yielded blood levels of less than 5 mg/100 ml, expressed in terms of a sulfanilamide standard. No untoward reactions to sulfonamides were noted.

On each patient, the single blood sulfonamide

Table 3. Ocular bacterial flora in trachoma patients treated with sulfonamides or placebo

Date	Treatment (sulfa)	Placebo
September, 1967	4 Streptococcus	2 Streptococcus
	1 Pneumococcus	
	1 *S. aureus*	2 *S. aureus*
	4 Moraxella (4/4)*	3 Moraxella (3/3)*
	6 No pathogens	7 No pathogens
December, 1967	2 Streptococcus	3 Streptococcus
	3 *S. aureus*	1 Moraxella (0/1)*
	2 Hay bacillus	1 Hay bacillus
	9 No pathogens	7 No pathogens
March, 1968	6 Streptococcus	5 Streptococcus
	1 *S. aureus*	2 Moraxella (1/2)*
	9 No pathogens	10 No pathogens

* Number of patients with clinically active trachoma/total number with Moraxella.

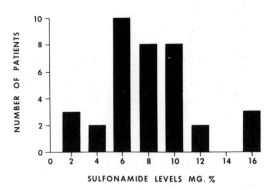

BLOOD SULFONAMIDE LEVELS

IN PERSONS RECEIVING TRISULFAPYRIMIDINES
3.5 GRAMS DAILY

Figure 4. Levels of sulfonamide in the blood of persons receiving trisulfapyrimidines, 3.5 g daily.

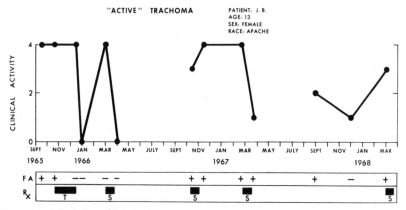

Figure 5. Clinical and microbiological activity of trachoma in an American Indian girl. Clinical activity greater than 2 indicates trachoma of sufficient intensity to be treated. The presence (+) or absence (−) of the agent in conjunctival smears stained by immunofluorescence (FA) was determined at each examination. The patient was treated with tetracycline in oil topically [7] and then with either sulfisoxazole or trisulfapyrimidines [5].

level obtained was compared to clinical outcome at 10 weeks and to frequency of inclusion-positive smears on all 3 specimens taken after therapy had been completed. The sulfonamide level did not appear to be higher in cases without clinical activity at 10 weeks, nor were higher levels associated with fewer inclusion-positive smears. This lack of correlation with clinical outcome and prevalence of inclusion-positive smears is not surprising, since a single blood sulfonamide determination would not necessarily reflect the average level during the 3 week course of therapy. Moreover, since the prevalence of inclusion-positive smears was indistinguishable in the sulfonamide- and placebo-treated patients, it is apparent that this dosage of sulfonamide does not result in marked suppression of the agent.

Effect of Repeated Sulfonamide Treatment on Individual Patients Observed for Several Years

On the basis of a prolonged study of trachoma among American Indian children, we have proposed elsewhere that the severity of eye disease in a given patient was a function of host reaction, varying greatly among different members of the same family, schoolroom, or tribe [5, 6]. Repeated treatment of recurrent trachomatous activity has been advanced as a possible means of eliminating infection from an individual, or from an endemic

area. A number of students examined every year from 1965 to 1968 exhibited positive immunofluorescence regularly and recurrent peaks of clinical activity in spite of 3–5 successive courses of sulfonamide treatment, each consisting of 3–4 g trisulfapyrimidines given daily for 21 days. An example is the 13-year-old Apache girl shown in figure 5. She represents an individual with frequent, intense activity of trachomatous disease in the absence of bacterial superinfection. Sulfonamide treatment ameliorated the clinical appearance each time, but infection (as evidenced by positive immunofluorescence) persisted and led to clinical relapse.

Discussion

In areas of the world where trachoma is widespread and severe, bacterial superinfection is common and often contributes greatly to the progression toward blindness. Many antibacterial drugs suppress bacterial conjunctivitis and thus may be expected to alleviate the signs of active inflammation. The trials conducted by us thus far do not reflect the trachoma problem as it appears in many hyperendemic areas. Our controlled trials of chemotherapy in American Indian children were carried out in the absence of clinically apparent bacterial conjunctivitis. These children have "pure" chlamydial eye infection which infrequently progresses to blindness. Since prevalence of bacterial pathogens did not appear to be related to clinical activity of trachoma after therapy, it is likely that our trials of chemotherapy evaluated only "anti-chlamydial" effects rather than possible treatment of the chlamydiabacteria disease complex.

A central problem in the treatment of chronic trachoma is the well-established host-parasite relationship. The infectious TRIC agent often infects the eye in childhood and may persist there throughout life. TRIC agents, like other chlamydiae, tend to produce infection which may be subclinical for long periods, but relapses into clinical activity eventually. We have demonstrated by immunofluorescence the presence of TRIC infection in apparent "healed" trachoma [5, 6, 11] as well as in repeatedly treated chronic trachoma. Various external influences may precipitate clinical activity in chronic subclinical TRIC infections. The increase in positive smears after trauma as illustrated in figure 2 is one of them. While chronic, established TRIC infection could not be eradicated in our chemotherapy trials, acute TRIC infection can, without doubt, be eradicated by sulfonamide therapy [10].

The results of our controlled trials indicate that trisulfapyrimidines in the dose and time used fail to eradicate chronic TRIC infection, as sulfisoxazole had failed earlier [7, 8]. It is not possible to exclude exogenous reinfection as an explanation for positive immunofluorescence or recurrent clinical activity following extensive drug treatment. However, the likelihood of such an event is small. In September, 1967, about 500 students had been examined, and 36 with "active trachoma" had been found. These were included in the drug trial. In March, 1968, all 500 students were re-examined. Only 23 (4.6%) of those inactive 6 months earlier now showed active trachoma. By contrast, 19 (52.8%) of the original 36 with active disease again had active disease in March, 1968, irrespective of their interval treatment. Since all students intermingled, it would be expected that the active cases developing as a result of reinfection should occur at a similar incidence in all subgroups. The 10-fold higher rate of activity among those with originally active disease suggests that recurrence of persistent infection is a far better explanation than exogenous reinfection. There is a strong suggestion that clinical activity may be suppressed for a period of months after a single 3-week course of trisulfapyrimidines. This effect appears to depend on severity of clinical activity. Mild cases improve in a favorable environment without drug, but severe cases may require additional suppression of TRIC agents by drug for maximal improvement. This improvement may well be only temporary and does not signify permanent "cure." The average sulfonamide levels of 7–8 mg/100 ml in serum may be adequate for antichlamydial effect and are higher than those reported in the past for "successful" trachoma treatment employing sulfonamides [1]. However, we do not know whether prolonged low sulfonamide levels, such as can be achieved by drugs with delayed excretion, may be important [15], whether continuous sulfonamide levels for many weeks are essential, or whether intermittent sulfonamide treatment might be effective, in field trials. In carefully studied individuals (figure 4), repeated courses of sulfonamide in full doses likewise failed to eradicate the TRIC agents from the conjunctiva.

The results presented here emphasize the need for further experimentation to define more effective regimens of chemotherapy. They also stress the need to reassess the value of temporary suppression of clinical activity in trachoma by means of drugs and to give added weight to those environmental factors which favor spontaneous regression and healing.

The differences in clinical findings of 2 observers constitute a problem which could not be satisfactorily resolved in the context of this study. In order to diminish such variation between clinical observers, clear-cut clinical criteria must be agreed upon and different observers must examine all the patients in a study independently on the same day.

Summary

Comparisons of trisulfapyrimidines and a placebo were made in treating mild, uncomplicated chronic trachoma in groups of American Indians in 2 boarding schools. Therapy was evaluated in terms of clinical response and prevalence of fluorescent antibody (FA) staining TRIC agent in conjunctival smears. Blood sulfonamide levels taken once in the 3-week course of therapy were 7–8 mg/100 ml on the average.

Ten weeks after the end of therapy, a significant improvement in clinical trachoma was found by ophthalmologist A in drug-treated cases at the first school (Stewart). In the second school (Sherman Institute), ophthalmologist B found no difference between placebo and drug-treated groups. The prevalence of FA-positive conjunctival smears was not influenced by sulfonamide but was increased significantly following trauma to the conjunctiva. While oral sulfonamide therapy temporarily suppressed clinical activity in 1 school, it did not eradicate the TRIC agent from the conjunctiva. Further experimentation is needed to determine effective therapy for chronic trachoma.

References

1. Bietti, G., and G. Werner. 1967. Trachoma; prevention and treatment. Thomas, Springfield, Ill. 227 p.
2. Forster, W. G., and J. R. McGibony. 1944. Trachoma. Amer. J. Ophthal. 27:1107-1117.
3. Foster, S. O., D. K. Powers, and P. Thygeson. 1966. Trachoma therapy. A controlled study. Amer. J. Ophthal. 61:451-455.
4. Woolridge, R. L., K. H. Cheng, I. H. Chang, C. Y. Yang, T. C. Hsu, and J. T. Grayston. 1967. Failure of trachoma treatment with ophthalmic antibiotics and systemic sulfonamides used alone or in combination with trachoma vaccine. Amer. J. Ophthal. 63:1577-1586.
5. Jawetz, E., L. Hanna, C. R. Dawson, T. R. Wood, and O. Briones. 1967. Subclinical infections with TRIC agents. Amer. J. Ophthal. 63:1413-1424.
6. Hanna, L., C. R. Dawson, O. Briones, P. Thygeson, and E. Jawetz. 1968. Latency in human infections with TRIC agents. J. Immun. 101:43-50.
7. Dawson, C. R., L. Hanna, and E. Jawetz. 1967. Controlled treatment trials of trachoma in American Indian children. Lancet 2:961-964.
8. Dawson, C. R., L. Hanna, T. R. Wood, and E. Jawetz. 1968. Double-blind treatment trials in chronic trachoma of American Indian children. Antimicrobial Agents and Chemotherapy—1967, p. 137-142.
9. Bratton, A. C., and E. K. Marshall. 1939. A new coupling component for sulfanilamide determination. J. Biol. Chem. 128:537-550.
10. Dawson, C., E. Jawetz, L. Hanna, L. Rose, T. R. Wood, and P. Thygeson. 1966. Experimental inclusion conjunctivitis in man. II. Partial resistance to reinfection. Amer. J. Epidem. 84:411-425.
11. Hanna, L., M. Okumoto, P. Thygeson, L. Rose, and C. R. Dawson. 1965. TRIC agents isolated in the United States. X. Immunofluorescence in the diagnosis of TRIC agent infection in man. Proc. Soc. Exp. Biol. Med. 119:722-728.
12. Wood, T. R., and C. R. Dawson. 1967. Bacteriologic studies of a trachomatous population. Amer. J. Ophthal. 63:1298-1301.
13. Assaad, F., and F. Maxwell-Lyons. 1967. Systematic observer variation in trachoma studies. Bull. W.H.O. 36:885-900.
14. Bobb, A. A., Jr. 1966. A critical study of the clinical diagnosis of trachoma. Amer. J. Ophthal. 61:776-782.
15. Bietti, G. B., C. Pannarale, and C. Milano. 1963. Further contributions to the intermittent therapy of trachoma with new long-acting sulfonamides. Amer. J. Ophthal. 63:1569-1573.

113

Diabetes Mellitus in Choctaw Indians

CURTIS C. DREVETS, M.D.

from the Lawton Indian Hospital of the Plains Indians in Western Oklahoma. Diabetics accounted for 4.4 per cent of 9,978 hospital admissions during the period from 1951 through 1955. Schochet did not compare the number of admissions in the different tribal groups.

BACKGROUND

The Choctaw Indians lived in the present states of Alabama and Mississippi until the nineteenth century when most of the tribe moved to the Indian Territory and settled in southeast Oklahoma. Choctaws are smaller and fatter than the average white American and other Indians. They have round faces and brown skin. They do not have the high cheek and red or bronzed skin often found in other American Indians. Intermarriage with non-Indians is common in Oklahoma and admixture for several decades has tended to reduce the percentage of full-blood Choctaws.

The Talihina Indian Hospital, located in southeast Oklahoma, serves as the only Indian Hospital for approximately 10,000 Choctaws in the area. It is a 200 bed general medical, surgical and tuberculosis hospital which was opened in 1937.

METHODS

A retrospective chart review was made of all in-patients and out-patients who registered at the Talihina Indian Hospital between September 1, 1956 and August 31, 1961. The

THE PURPOSE of this paper is to describe the epidemiologic and clinical pattern of diabetes mellitus in the Choctaw Indians of Oklahoma.

The past decade has witnessed a surge of interest in the diverse clinical patterns of diabetes mellitus in different ethnic groups of the world. Before Joslin's[1] survey of diabetes mellitus in Arizona (1940) some observers thought the disease to be uncommon in the American Indian. Joslin found that diabetes is as prevalent among the Arizona Indians as among the non-Indians of that state. He suggested, however, that there might be differences among the tribal groups. This suggestion was confirmed by the observations of Cohen[2] in Arizona.

Data compiled by the Division of Indian Health (U.S. Public Health Service) show that diabetes mellitus accounts for a higher percentage of admissions to hospitals in the Division's Oklahoma City area than in other areas. The only publication on diabetes mellitus from this area is the study of Schochet[3] charts of 7,950 persons having at least one-eighth Choctaw blood were inspected for date of birth, sex, degree of Indian blood, date first and last seen, admissions to the hospital in the past 15 years, and the presence and date of recognition of diabetes mellitus. The charts of all 241 diabetics were further inspected for height and weight at the time of diagnosis, family history of diabetes, complications, associated major illnesses, obstetrical history, laboratory studies, current treatment and degree of control. The criteria for the diagnosis of diabetes mellitus were a fasting venous blood sugar of 130 mg. per cent or a two-hour post-prandial blood sugar of 150 mg. per cent by the Folin-Wu method. Dietary histories were obtained by dietitians from several members of this tribe, both patients and hospital employees. It was not feasible to obtain extensive detailed dietary histories or direct observations of the eating habits from this study.

Prevalence[4] is the proportion of a population who have a disease at a particular instant. Prevalence was determined by selecting from those seen both before and after the arbitrarily selected prevalence point, December 31, 1958, i.e., the persons known to have diabetes on that date. The incidence[4] of a disease is the number of cases which appear during a specified period among a population. By computing the patient years of observation from the initial and most recent visit, the incidence of diabetes mellitus was calculated as the number of diagnoses per 1,000 patient years of observation. Incidence rates reflect the frequency of events

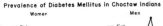
Prevalence of Diabetes Mellitus in Choctaw Indians

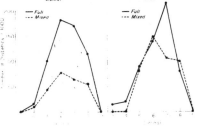

Figure I.

whereas prevalence rates connote existence.

RESULTS: EPIDEMIOLOGY

Three thousand, five hundred and seventy-five persons fulfilled the criteria of the prevalence study; 2,003 (56 per cent) were females, 1,572 were males. There were 1,993 full-blood* and 1,582 mixed-blood Choctaws.

The prevalence rate of diabetes mellitus was 53.2 per 1,000 in full-blood Choctaws and 18.3 per 1,000 in mixed-bloods of all ages. The prevalence rate was slightly higher for males than females. The prevalence rates by decades were computed for both sexes. These are shown in figure I and tables I and II. Diabetes was significantly more prevalent in full-blood Choctaw females than in mixed-bloods in each decade beyond the second. There were no significant differ-

*For purposes of this paper, persons less than full Choctaw but having one-eighth or more Choctaw lineage are spoken of as mixed-bloods. Those with total Choctaw lineage are referred to as full-bloods.

Table I

Prevalence of Diabetes Mellitus in Choctaw Indians

Females

Age (Yr.)	FULL BLOODS			MIXED BLOODS		
	Number	Diabetics	No./1000	Number	Diabetics	No./1000
0-9	195	0	0	213	0	0
10-19	179	0	0	225	0	0
20-29	201	0	0	116	0	0
30-39	179	3	16.8	104	1	9.6
40-49	138	14	100.2	67	3	44.8
50-59	121	22	182.0	51	4	78.5
60-69	88	15	170.8	46	3	65.3
70-79	43	5	116.3	19	1	52.6
80-89	18	0	0	6	0	0
TOTALS	1162	59	50.8	841	12	14.3

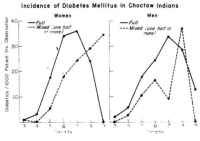

Figure II.

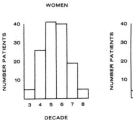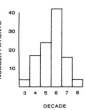

Figure III.

ences between male full-blood and mixed-bloods. There were no diabetics under 20 years of age.

The incidence of diabetes mellitus in Choctaws is shown in figure II and tables III and IV. In each decade having sufficient patient years of observation, the incidence was significantly higher in the full-blood than in the mixed-blood Choctaws. The incidence of diabetes in full-blood Choctaw males and females was similar in each decade except the sixth.

CLINICAL PATTERN

During a study period from September 1, 1956 through March 1, 1962, 241 Choctaw diabetics were observed at Talihina. Women comprised 56 per cent of the diabetics. Three patients had pancreatitis before developing diabetes.

. In women, the age of diagnosis ranged

from 20 to 77 years with an average age of 48.9 years and a median age of 49 years. In men, the age of diagnosis ranged from 23 to 84 years with an average of 50.2 years and a median age of 51 years. Diabetes was found most frequently in the sixth decade in men and in similar numbers in the fifth and sixth decades in women (figure III). The average duration from diagnosis to the most recent visit was 6.0 years. Twenty-one per cent of the patients had been diabetic for ten or more years at their last visit. The family history was recorded on 200 patients. Eighteen per cent of the men and 32.5 per cent of the women had a family history of diabetes.

The age, height and weight at the time of diagnosis were compared with the average weight for various ages and heights obtained from standard tables[5] (table V). Eight per cent of the women and nine per cent of the men were ten per cent less than the average

Table II

Prevalence of Diabetes Mellitus in Choctaw Indians

Males

	FULL BLOODS			MIXED BLOODS		
Age (Yr.)	Number	Diabetics	No./1000	Number	Diabetics	No./1000
0-9	183	0	0	251	0	0
10-19	143	0	0	192	0	0
20-29	72	1	13.9	80	0	0
30-39	104	2	19.2	63	0	0
40-49	90	8	88.9	50	4	80.0
50-59	101	14	138.6	47	7	149.0
60-69	90	19	215.0	38	4	105.2
70-79	38	3	79.0	20	2	100.0
80-89	10	0	0	0	0	0
TOTALS	831	47	56.6	741	17	22.9

116

Table III

Incidence of Diabetes Mellitus in Choctaw Indians

Females

| | FULL BLOODS | | | | MIXED BLOODS* | | |
Age (Yr.)	Pt. Yrs.#	Diabetics	No./1000 Pt. Yrs.#	Pt. Yrs.#	Diabetics	No./1000 Pt. Yrs.#
0-9	1137.5	0	0	938.8	0	0
10-19	1347.5	0	0	925.0	0	0
20-29	2307.5	2	0.9	998.8	1	1.0
30-39	1835.0	6	3.3	813.0	0	0
40-49	1398.8	26	18.6	522.5	3	5.7
50-59	1013.8	35	34.5	480.0	9	18.8
60-69	582.5	21	36.0	286.3	7	24.5
70-79	371.3	9	24.2	101.3	3	29.6
80-89	105.0	0	0	28.8	1	34.7

*—Mixed bloods include only those with one-half or more Indian blood
#—Patient years of observation in decade

weight. Seventy-seven per cent of the women and 63 per cent of the men were ten per cent or more than the average weight. In both sexes obesity was more common in those under 50 years of age. Fifty-three per cent of a group of healthy, non-diabetic Choctaw women and 45 per cent of the men were ten per cent or more overweight by the same standards. Choctaw diabetics were significantly more obese than the non-diabetics ($p < .001$ for women and $< .01$ and $> .001$ for men).*

*Chi square method

THERAPY

At their last visit 80 patients (33 per cent) were being treated by diet alone (table VI). Twenty-nine (12 per cent) were receiving tolbutamide in addition to the diet. One hundred twenty-three (51 per cent) were being treated with diet and insulin. Of those patients receiving insulin 83 (68 per cent) were taking less than 40 units of insulin and only 3 (2.4 per cent) were taking 80 units or more.

DEGREE OF CONTROL OF DIABETES MELLITUS

The degree of control was classified as poor, fair or good in those who had been observed over a period of at least one year. The control was considered good if the majority of the fasting blood sugars were less than 140 mg. per 100 ml. Control was considered fair if the majority of the blood sugars were between 140 and 200 mg. per 100 ml. Thirty-four per cent of 168 dia-

Table IV

Incidence of Diabetes Mellitus in Choctaw Indians

Males

| | FULL BLOODS | | | | MIXED BLOODS* | | |
Age (Yr.)	Pt. Yrs.#	Diabetics	No./1000 Pt. Yrs.#	Pt. Yrs.#	Diabetics	No./1000 Pt. Yrs.#
0-9	995.0	0	0	817.5	0	0
10-19	707.5	0	0	555.0	0	0
20-29	513.8	1	1.9	373.8	0	0
30-39	640.0	4	6.3	372.5	1	2.7
40-49	868.8	16	18.4	372.5	4	10.7
50-59	983.8	24	24.4	358.8	6	16.7
60-69	652.5	22	33.7	221.3	2	9.0
70-79	276.3	8	29.0	53.3	2	37.6
80-89	80.0	1	12.5	7.5	0	0

*—Mixed bloods include only those with one-half or more Indian blood
#—Patient years of observation in decade

betics evaluated by these criteria were in good control and 40 per cent in fair control (table VII). Of those receiving diet alone 63 per cent were in good control and 37 per cent in fair control. Thirty-five per cent of patients on diet plus tolbutamide were in good control and 55 per cent were in fair control. Control was poorer in those on diet and insulin: only 19 per cent were in good control and 39 per cent in fair control. Maximum blood sugars ranged from 118 to 840 mg. per 100 ml. The highest recorded blood sugar in 11 patients was more than 500 mg. per 100 ml.

COMPLICATIONS

There were no known diabetic complications in 199 (83 per cent) of the diabetics. There had been one or more of the following diabetic complications in 42 patients: gangrene, acidosis, retinopathy, nephropathy, neuropathy, and hypoglycemia. Nineteen of 42 poorly controlled patients had 28 complications, 16 of 68 with fair control had 21 complications and only four of 57 diabetics in good control had four complications. The most frequently observed complication was gangrene which occurred in 16 (6.6 per cent). Diabetic acidosis was not observed in the absence of infection. The frequency of various complications is listed in table VIII. There were no significant differences in the frequency of diabetic complications between the full and mixed-bloods.

Table VI
Therapy of Diabetes Mellitus

Therapy	Number	Per Cent
Diet Only	80	33
Diet Plus Tolbutamide	29	12
Diet Plus Insulin	123	51
1-39 units	83	
40-79 units	37	
80 or more units	3	
Unknown	9	4

ASSOCIATED ILLNESSES

The associated illnesses were recorded without time relationship to the patients' diabetes (table IX). Gallbladder disease, diagnosed in 47 (19.5 per cent) diabetics was approximately twise as frequent in the obese as in the non-obese diabetics. The number of severe infections and cardiovascular diseases (all forms) was small. Lens opacities were noted in 43 diabetics (18 per cent). These illnesses occurred in similar percentages in the full and mixed-bloods.

OBSTETRICAL HISTORY

The obstetrical history was adequately recorded on 70 women. A scattergram (figure IV) considering the number of pregnancies, age at diagnosis of diabetes and family history showed no relationship between the age at diagnosis and the number of pregnancies. Patients with more pregnancies did not develop diabetes earlier in life than those who had less pregnancies. Women having a family history of diabetes tended to have fewer pregnancies than those with negative

Table V

Weight at Diagnosis of Diabetes Mellitus Compared to Non-Diabetic Choctaws

	Under Weight < −10%	Over Weight +10 to 29%	Obese > +30%	Normal −9 to +9%	TOTALS
WOMEN					
Diabetics	8%	33%	44%	15%	91
Non-Diabetics	5%	36%	17%	42%	77
MEN					
Diabetics	9%	36%	27%	28%	65
Non-Diabetics	12%	38%	7%	43%	86

Compared with standard table including age and height (see text)
Significance by Chi Square method:
Women — P < .001   Men — P < .01 and > .001

Obstetrical History in Choctaw Diabetics

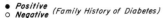

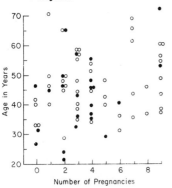

Figure IV.

family histories. A significantly higher percentage of those with a positive family history had four or less pregnancies, while of those with a negative family history almost as many had more than four pregnancies (table X). This seemed to be unrelated to the age at diagnosis. Only three of the 135 women delivered a baby after the onset of their diabetes.

LABORATORY FINDINGS

The average serum cholesterol in 40 diabetic patients was 243 mg. per cent with a range of 89 to 428 mg. per 100 ml. Sixteen (40 per cent) of these were 250 mg. per 100 ml. or more. Persistent proteinuria (1 plus or more) appeared in 36 diabetics (15 per cent). The average interval between the diagnosis of diabetes mellitus and the appearance of proteinuria was 6.1 years. Azo-

Table VII
Degree of Control of Diabetes Mellitus

Therapy	Number Evaluated	% of Evaluated Good*	Fair*	Poor*
Diet Only	51	63	37	0
Diet Plus Tolbutamide	20	35	55	10
Diet Plus Insulin	97	19	39	42
1-39 units	66	23	45	32
40-79 units	29	10	28	62
80 or more units	2	0	0	100

ᵇSee text for definition

Table VIII
Complications of Diabetes Mellitus in Choctaw Indians

	Degree of Control				Per Cent Complications of Total*
	Good	Fair	Poor	Unknown	
Patients with Complications	4	16	19	3	17.4
Gangrene	0	6	9	1	6.6
Acidosis	2	2	6	1	4.6
Retinopathy	0	4	4	0	3.3
Nephropathy	1	4	2	1	3.3
Neuropathy	0	1	2	0	1.2
Hypoglycemia	1	4	5	0	4.1

*Without regard to degree of control

temia (blood urea nitrogen 30 mg. per 100 ml. or more) was observed in 14 (5.8 per cent) after an average interval of 11.4 years from the time of diagnosis of diabetes.

DIETARY HABITS

Inquiry made into the diet of the full-blood Choctaws revealed that their food consists primarily of beans, fat pork, lard and starches. It is common practice for them to fry fat pork and then to fill the frying pan with water and flour. The fat-laden gravy is then either dipped up in several large Choctaw biscuits which are four to five inches in diameter or poured over cooked beans. Whether the Choctaws have two or three meals daily, many eat each meal as if it were their last. Although dietary histories represent hearsay, it is probable that they often consume 4,000 calories or more per day. The diet by average United States standards contains little protein but much carbohydrate and fat. These comments concern the diet of the full-blood Choctaws, however the diet in mixed marriages depends primarily on the ancestry of the spouse.

Table IX

Associated Illnesses in Choctaw Diabetics

Illness	Number Observed	Per Cent*	Degree of Control Good	Fair	Poor
Gallbladder Disease	47	19.5	12	15	15
Cardiovascular Disease	64	26.6	10	24	17
Cancer	7	2.9	2	1	1
Tuberculosis	16	6.6	9	3	2
Genitourinary Infections	14	5.8	2	7	3
Other Major Infections	25	10.3	5	8	8

*Without regard to degree of control

DISCUSSION

Many authors record a variety of figures for the prevalence of diabetes mellitus. Most studies record figures for hospital or clinic admissions or small population samples screened by various means. Wilkerson and Krall,[6] in one of the few noteworthy epidemiological investigations of diabetes, found a prevalence rate of 11/1000 known diabetics and 9/1000 new diabetics. Tullock[7] suggests that the prevalence of diabetes in the tropics varies from 1/1000 in Southern Rhodesians over 14 years of age to 142/1000 in a small series of Mabuiag Islanders of all ages. Sloan[8] found that the prevalence of diabetes varies among ethnic groups from 11/1000 in Caucasians to 78/1000 in unmixed Hawaiian natives in a survey of the Hawaiian labor force. Most surveys report a prevalence of less than 20 diabetics per 1000 of all ages. In 1959 the estimated prevalence of known diabetics in the United States was 9.0/1000 (all ages).[9]

Although a systematic screening procedure was not used, this prevalence and incidence study was based on persons attending a hospital and a clinic which provide almost exclusive care for everyone in the group. An estimated 80 per cent of the Oklahoma Choctaws had registered during the study period. Almost all patients had a blood sugar determination or urinalysis at some time at Talihina. The differences in the observed incidence and prevalence rates between full-blood Choctaws and those having only part Choctaw blood are interesting and significant. Both ethnic groups were observed under the same conditions. Diabetes is considered by some as being transmitted along Mendelian recessive lines.[4, 5] Inbreeding in a minority group would thus increase mating of persons carrying the diabetes trait and intensify the increased prevalence of diabetes. The intermarriage of Choctaws with non-Indians decreased their chances of becoming diabetic.

Scott and Griffith[10] found diabetes to be uncommon in Eskimos. Cohen[2] concluded that prevalence of diabetes varies among the several Arizona tribes. It is difficult to compare tribal variations in the prevalence of diabetes from the available material because each study was conducted in a different manner. Because of the delineation of blood lines, the American Indian offers a unique

Table X

Correlation of Family History of Diabetes Mellitus with Number of Pregnancies

Choctaw Women age 20-48

Family History of D.M.		NUMBER OF PREGNANCIES		TOTAL
		Four or Less	Five or More	
NEGATIVE	Observed	17	13	30
	Expected	20.4	9.6	
POSITIVE	Observed	15	2	17
	Expected	11.6	5.4	

P < .5 and > .02

subject for such studies. There is a particular need for well planned field surveys of various American Indian tribes. Two small field surveys among 100 Choctaw Indians discovered six previously unknown diabetics.[11]

We did not find any type I or juvenile diabetics among the Choctaw Indians despite careful search. Using commonly accepted figures[12] we should have expected approximately 12 juvenile diabetics. The Talihina Indian Hospital has record of only one diabetic under the age of 20 years among more than 300 diabetics of all tribes seen during the period of this study. This was a teenage full-blood Creek boy with typical juvenile diabetes. Cohen[2] did not find any juvenile diabetics among 56 Arizona Indian diabetics. Neither have we observed any Type "J" diabetics of the sort described by Hugh-Jones[13] in Jamaica.

Difficulty in recording diabetic complications probably accounts for the discrepancy in the number of patients having diabetic nephropathy and the number with azotemia and proteinuria. All proteinuria in diabetics is not, of course, caused by diabetic nephropathy. I examined about a third of the diabetics in the study and found their rate of complications was similar to that of the entire group. Physicians working with Oklahoma Indians have had the impression that diabetic complications are less frequent than in non-Indians in this country. Comparison with other published studies is difficult but supports this impression.[13-18]

Do the dietary habits of the Choctaws contribute to the prevalence of diabetes mellitus? I have observed several instances of both marital partners developing diabetes after years of eating at the same table. Since inquiry about the family history for diabetes mellitus usually does not include the spouse, we have no data about the frequency of diabetes mellitus in both marital partners.

SUMMARY

This paper reports the incidence, prevalence and clinical characteristics of diabetes mellitus in Choctaw Indians of Oklahoma. The prevalence of diabetes in full-blood Choctaws of all ages was 53.2/1000 but was 18.3/1000 in Choctaws of less than full-blood. The incidence of diabetes was also greater in full-bloods than in mixed bloods. Juvenile-type diabetes was not observed. The clinical picture of diabetes was similar to non-Indians in the United States. Obesity, gallbladder disease and diabetic gangrene were common. The "average" Choctaw diet appeared to contain less protein but more carbohydrates and fat than the average American diet.

ACKNOWLEDGMENTS

I wish to express appreciation to Hans Wulff, M.D., James A. Hagans, M.D., Ph.D., and Margaret Shackelford of the Departments of Internal Medicine and Public Health and Preventive Medicine and the Biostatistical Unit and Medical Research Computer Center, University of Oklahoma Medical Center, and Herbert A. Hudgins, M.D., M.P.H., and Donald L. Mason of the Oklahoma City Indian Health Area Office for their invaluable assistance in the design of this study, the analysis and statistical work. I also wish to thank Mildred B. Barry, B.S., M.S., Oklahoma City Indian Health Area Office, for the dietary information and Daniel B. Stone, M.B., State University of Iowa Hospitals, for his helpful criticism in the preparation of this paper. □

BIBLIOGRAPHY

1. Joslin, Elliott P.: The Universality of Diabetes, J.A.M.A. 115: 2033, 1940.
2. Cohen, Burton M.: Diabetes Mellitus among Indians of the American Southwest: Its Prevalence and Clinical Characteristics in a Hospitalized Population. Ann. Int. Med. 40: 588, 1954.
3. Schochet, Bernard R.: Five Years Experience with Diabetes Mellitus at the U.S. P.H.S. Indian Hospital, Lawton, Oklahoma, 1951-1955. J. Okla. State Med. Assoc. 51: 459, 1958.
4. McMahon, Brian, Pugh, Thomas F., and Ipsen, Johannes: Epidemiologic Methods, Little, Brown and Co., Boston, 1960.
5. Duncan, Garfield G.: Diseases of Metabolism, 4th Ed., Saunders, Philadelphia, 1959.
6. Wilkerson, Hugh, L. C. and Krall, Leo P.: Diabetes in a New England Town: A Study of 3,516 Persons in Oxford, Mass., J.A.M.A. 135: 209, 1947.
7. Tulloch, J. A.: Diabetes Mellitus in the Tropics. E. & S. Livingstone Ltd., Edinburgh and London, 1962.
8. Sloan, Norman R.: Ethnic Distribution of Diabetes Mellitus in Hawaii. J.A.M.A. 183: 419, 1963.
9. U.S. National Health Survey: Diabetes reported in interviews, United States, July 1957-June 1959; Public Health Service Publication No. 584-B21. Washington, U.S. Government Printing Office, 1960.
10. Scott, E. M. and Griffith, Isabelle V.: Diabetes Mellitus in Eskimos. Metabolism 6: 320, 1957.
11. Fleming, Elizabeth P.: Personal Communication, 1962.
12. Joslin, Elliott P., Root, Howard F., White, Priscilla and Marble, Alexander: The Treatment of Diabetes, 10th Ed., Lea and Febiger, Philadelphia, 1959.
13. Hugh-Jones, P.: Diabetes in Jamaica. Lancet 2: 891, 1955.
14. Parkhurst, Leonard W. and Betsch, Wm. F.: The Incidence and Diagnosis of Diabetes Mellitus in a Diagnostic Clinic, Med. Clinics of N.A. 39: 1571, 1955.
15. MacNeal, Perry S. and Rogers, John: The Complications of Diabetes Mellitus, Med. Clinics of N.A. 39: 1607, 1955.
16. Gifford, Edward S., Jr., The Unsolved Problem of Diabetic Retinopathy, Med. Clinics of N.A. 39: 1671, 1955.
17. Pathania, N. S. and Sachar, R. S.: Cardiovascular Complications of Diabetes Mellitus, Brit. Med. J. 1: 1505, 1961.
18. Cosnett, J. E.: Diabetes among Natal Indians, Brit. Med. J. 1: 187, 1959.

Roentgenographic Evaluation of Temporal Bones from South Dakota Indian Burials

JOHN B. GREGG, JAMES P. STEELE, AND ANN HOLZHUETER

Many diseases of the human body, especially those involving bone directly, so influence the formation, development, or reconstruction of bone that an indelible record of the disease is left in its pattern. Fractures, infections, neoplasms, congenital anomalies, and certain metabolic diseases leave imprints which are usually visible on gross examination or in microscopic sections as long as the bone remains at least partially intact. In the usual archeological specimen the cellular substance is gone and the histological details are largely lost. Despite the loss of histological structure the architecture of the bone, its trabeculations, solid and rarefied parts, and its reconstitution following the ravages of disease, presents patterns in calcium salts which can be easily evaluated by means of x-rays. Roentgenographic examination has the added advantage that the specimen so evaluated is not destroyed or in any way damaged.

In a previous paper (Holzhueter, Gregg and Clifford, '64) the findings relating to middle ear pathology with special reference to fixation of the stapes footplate by otosclerosis as well as other bony abnormalities in ancient Indian skulls from South Dakota were presented and discussed. The examination permitted good analysis of the middle ear and gross skeletal details but dissection and microscopic evaluation was not possible because the skulls were museum specimens and could not be damaged.

Therefore in order to obtain further information concerning possible disease in the temporal bones, each specimen was examined with x-rays. The findings of the radiographic examinations are presented hereinafter.

In the past it has been hypothesized that infections or inflammation (dry catarrh) (Politzer, 1893) (Lindsay, '49) (Shambaugh, '59) were causative, a precipitating or an accentuating factor in the disease otosclerosis with stapes footplate fixation. If inflammatory change in the middle ear and mastoid are influential in the development of otosclerosis it would be of much interest to determine whether the ancient Indians had much in the way of middle ear disease. This should be possible through the use of radiographs of the temporal bones and mastoids.

Some controversy exists as to the exact influence of infections originating in the upper respiratory passages upon the growth and development of the air cells which are usually described as existing in the mastoid and some other portions of the adult temporal bones. It is not the purpose here to discourse upon the subject at length but to bring out the fact that some of these ideas may be open to discussion.

It has been reported (Von Troltsch, 1858), (Von Wreden, 1868), (Zaufel, 1870), (Wendt, 1873), (Gompertz, '06), (Aschoff, 1897), (Gradenigo, 1891), Buck, '64), (McLellan, '64), and others, that the middle ear space of the newborn contains amniotic debris and gelatinous fluid. There is question whether this is an inflammatory or an infectious process. The role of this middle ear infiltrate in the development or severity of middle ear infections in early life has been the subject of considerable debate. Wittmaack ('18) hypothesized that pneumatization of the mastoid bone occurs in three stages: (1) from the fifth foetal month through the first year of life, (2) from two to four years of age, and (3) the remainder of the life of the individual. In the first stage there is an evagination of an epithelium lined recess from the foregut of the embryo into the mesenchyme of the primitive lateral pharyngeal wall which results in the formation of the tympanic cavity, the epitympanic recess and the antrum. During the second stage there is formation of the mastoid area with fusion of the medullary cavities following invasion of the slightly differentiated connective tissue by epithelium, and bone production and replacement. During the third stage which comprises the remainder of the life there is constant bone replacement. Wittmaack believed that the mesenchyme is important in the development of the mastoid bone and the pneumatization thereof. If the mesenchyme is disturbed during this crucial period, pneumatization of the mastoid is altered. He also believed that normoplastic mucosa was important in the pneu-matization of the mastoid area. The ingrowth of this normoplastic mucosa has been supposed to be influenced by the non-bacterial invasion of the middle ear space by amnionic fluid in the pre-natal period. In the event of bacterial penetration into the middle ear space in the neonatal period, the epithelium has been thought to become hypoplastic, resulting in a sclerotic change in the bone of the mastoid. Depending upon the time of the infection and its severity during the mastoid air cell development, the result could be a sclerotic mastoid or a variation of pneumatic and sclerotic bone. Wittmaack hypothesized that the mastoid bone without air cells was pathological and that a sclerotic mastoid was the result of inhibition of development of the air cells. He also felt that pathological mucous membranes which resulted from altered pneumatization were more likely to be affected by chronic and recurrent otitis media, while the normal membrane is resistant.

Cheatle ('06) felt that the acellular mastoid which could be sclerotic or diploic in texture, was the primary bone formation. He also noted that the sclerotic type was more likely to be involved by otitis media. Diamant ('52) reported that variable sized air cells as well as a sclerotic type of bone exist within the substance of a "normal mastoid." He found that the ear with smaller air cell development is more likely to be involved by acute and/or chronic otitis than are ears with larger mastoid air cells. Flisberg ('63) also reported that human ears with poorly developed mastoid air cell systems are more prone to infections. He attributed this to the fact that in a poorly pneumatized mastoid cell system there is less air and a process which obstructs the eustachian tube leads more quickly to evacuation of the air from the middle ear space and mastoid with resultant damage to the drum and middle ear mucosa.

Ruedi ('37) felt that constitutional and idiopathic factors were more important in the development of the mastoid air cells than was amnionic fluid in the middle ears or infections after birth.

In a series of children upon whom mastoid x-rays were taken 6 to 12 months

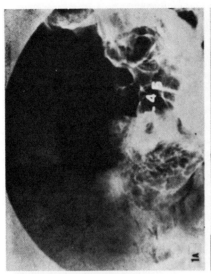

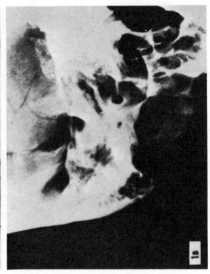

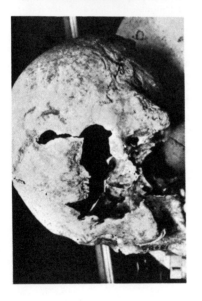

Fig. 1 Specimen no. 13484. Photograph of the left aspect of the skull of an Arikara male 30–35 years of age. Moderate fragmentation of the bones. Stapes was present in this ear.

Fig. 1 A No. 13484. Law View of Mastoid showing good pneumatization, left.

Fig. 1 B No. 13484. Stenvers View, left mastoid. demonstrating good pneumatization.

124

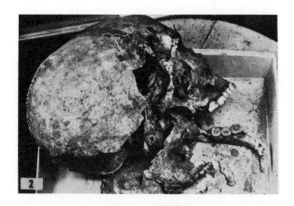

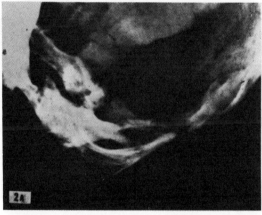

Fig. 2　Specimen 4612. Right aspect of fragmented skull and temporal bone of an 18–22-year-old female, culture undetermined, probably Woodland.

Fig. 2-A　No. 4612. Stenvers View of mastoid showing diploic configuration.

after an episode of purulent otitis media H. W. Schwartz ('51), reported that inflammatory diseases did not have a retarding effect upon subsequent pneumatization of the mastoid. He felt that inherited factors were of primary importance in the type and degree of air cell development.

Compere, ('60) reported that by using a Stenvers view of the temporal bone it is possible to demonstrate the lesions of diffuse otosclerosis "in an appreciable number of cases." These visible changes appear as "(1) Local overgrowths of osseous tissue anywhere in the otic acpsule. (2) Apparent sclerosis of the entire otic capsule, almost obscuring the labyrinthine system in some instances. The opaque area tends to have a nodular outline. (3) Hyperostosis of the entire petrous pyramid."

Despite the controversy which exists, most Otolaryngologists and Radiologists

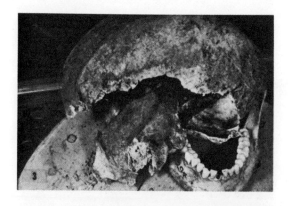

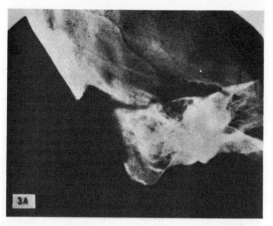

Fig. 3   Specimen 21294. Fragmented skull and temporal bone of Arikara female 21–26-years-old.

Fig. 3-A   No. 21294. Stenvers View showing mixed type mastoid air cell development.

today are of the opinion that pneumatization of the mastoid area is influenced by respiratory infections and that the finding of altered air cell development in radiographs of the mastoids is quite indicative of previous middle ear disease, usually infections from the nasopharynx through the eustachian tubes (Pendergrass, '56), (Meschan, '58), (Meschan, '59), (Caffey, '61), (Shambaugh, '59), (American Otological Society, '35), (Koehler, '28), (Law, '34), (Pancost, '40), (Pendergrass, '56).

METHOD OF STUDY

It has been shown (Farrior, '50), (Etter, '51), and by others, that the anatomy of the normal isolated temporal bones and other bones of the skull can be demonstrated very clearly by radiographic techniques. The methods of examination utilized by these investigators are similar to those which are used in this study.

Following the careful gross examination of each skull, radiographs were made of the mastoids. Two views were taken, a

126

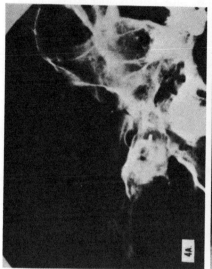
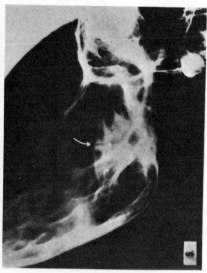

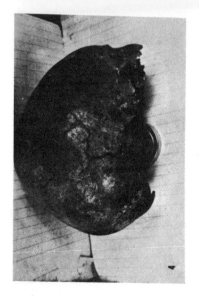

Fig. 4 Specimen 2077. Arikara, 10–15-years, sex undetermined, right lateral aspect of skull.

Fig. 4-A No. 20777. Law View showing a sclerotic mastoid.

Fig. 5 Specimen no. 18151. Woodland. Male, 35–40-years. Stenvers View showing a well pneumatized mastoid air cell system. Note density of bone surrounding superior semi-circular canal (indicated by arrow).

lateral view (Law view) and an oblique posterior-anterior (Stenvers) view. Standard radiological techniques were simulated insofar as positioning the specimens, tube angles, and tube distance from the film. The skulls or temporal bones were fixed into position and held there while the exposures were being made. Although the majority of the skulls were intact and in good condition, a few were badly fragmented, necessitating some ingenuity in positioning the fragments. It was necessary to work out a basic exposure technique and alter it appropriately to compensate for the damaged skulls and those which had thicker bones. The skulls required much less x-ray exposure for good film contrast than that which the mastoid would have required in a living individual. Some of the skulls which had been in the ground for a considerable period of time were partially demineralized and required even less x-ray exposure. For the average intact skull the following exposure gave good results:

	KV	Milli-amperes	Time (sec.)	Tube dist.
Stenvers view	65	60	1/10	40″
Law view	60	60	1/10	40″

TABLE 1

Indian cultures/sex/temporal bones

Culture	Male	Female	Unknown sex	Total skulls	Temporal bones
Arikara	74	52	4	130	251
Sioux Historic	6	6	0	12	24
Middle Plains Woodland	31	17	2	50	88
Miscellaneous	13	10	6	29	54
Totals	124	85	12	221	417

TABLE 2

Roentgenograms showing type of pneumatization in the mastoid area of male temporal bones

		Left				Right				Bilateral			
		P	D	M	S	P	D	M	S	P	D	M	S
Birth to 10 years	Arikara									1			
	Woodland												
	Sioux His.												
	Others												
Eleven to 20 years	Arikara	1				1	1			2			
	Woodland												
	Sioux His.												
	Others	1		1				1					
Twenty-one to 30 years	Arikara	5	2	5	1	3		7	3	14		6	
	Woodland	3	2			2	1	4		4		2	1
	Sioux His.	1	1			2						2	1
	Others			2				1	1	1		2	
Thirty-one to 40 years	Arikara	7		4		1	1	7	2	7		6	
	Woodland			2	1	2		4		2		2	
	Sioux His.									2			
	Others	1								2		1	
Forty-one years plus	Arikara	2		1		1		3		3		3	
	Woodland	2						2		2			
	Sioux His.												
	Others			1				1	1			1	
	Totals	22	3	19	2	12	3	30	7	80		50	4

P: Pneumatic, D: Diploic, M: Mixed, S: Sclerotic.

128

TABLE 3
Roentgenograms showing type of pneumatization in the mastoid area of female temporal bones

		Left				Right				Bilateral			
		P	D	M	S	P	D	M	S	P	D	M	S
Birth to 10 years	Arikara												
	Woodland												
	Sioux His.			none below ten years of age									
	Others												
Eleven to 20 years	Arikara			2		2		1		5		2	1
	Woodland			1		1				2			
	Sioux His.	1		1			1	1					
	Others									2			
Twenty-one to 30 years	Arikara	3		5		5		2	2	13		3	1
	Woodland	2		1		1				3		2	
	Sioux His.			2		1				1			
	Others			2					1	1			1
Thirty-one to 40 years	Arikara	1	1	1		1		1	1	6			
	Woodland	2		2		2		1	1	3		1	
	Sioux His.							1					
	Others					1				1			
Forty-one years plus	Arikara									1			
	Woodland												
	Sioux His.												
	Others												
	Totals	9	1	17		14	1	7	5	76		16	6

P: Pneumatic, D: Diploic, M: Mixed, S: Sclerotic.

TABLE 4
Roentgenograms showing type of pneumatization in the mastoid area of undetermined sex temporal bones

		Left				Right				Bilateral			
		P	D	M	S	P	D	M	S	P	D	M	S
Birth to 10 years	Arikara	1		1				2			1		
	Woodland					1							
	Sioux His.												
	Others												
Eleven to 20 years	Arikara												
	Woodland												
	Sioux His.												
	Others											1	
Twenty-one to 30 years	Arikara	1		3				3		1	1		
	Woodland												
	Sioux His.												
	Others	1		2		1		5	2			1	
Thirty-one to 40 years	Arikara												
	Woodland												
	Sioux His.												
	Others												
Forty-one years plus	Arikara												
	Woodland												
	Sioux His.												
	Others												
	Totals	3		6		2		10	2	2	6	2	

P: Pneumatic, D: Diploic, M: Mixed, S: Sclerotic.

TABLE 5

Temporal bone mastoid air cell development according to age (Arikara/other cultures)

Age		Pneumatic	Diploic	Mixed	Sclerotic
Birth to 10 years	A	3	2	3	
	O	1			
11 to 20 years	A	17	2	7	2
	O	11	3	5	
21 to 30 years	A	73	4	43	8
	O	34	1	40	10
31 to 40 years	A	36	2	25	3
	O	28		18	2
41 years plus	A	11		10	
	O	6		6	1
Totals	A	140	10	88	13
	O	80	4	69	13

A: Arikara. O: Others.

All films were taken with grid casettes and processed in an autoprocessor. Eastman Blue Brand film 10″ × 12″, using one-half a film for each exposure was used throughout.

Each film was interpreted by the authors, first independently and then as a team. The results recorded represent the combined opinions of the Otolaryngologist and the Radiologist.

Utilizing the criteria outlined by Tremble ('29–'34), the mastoid Roentgenograms were classified as: (1) pneumatic, (2) diploic, (3) mixed (pneumatic and diploic), and (4) sclerotic. Results were further categorized according to the various cultures, and by age and sex, for comparison of the radiological patterns in these different groups. Each film was closely scanned for evidence of other pathology in the temporal bones or the bones adjacent to the mastoid visible on the films. The results of the X-ray studies are summarized in tables 1, 2, 3, and 4.

RESULTS AND CONCLUSIONS

(1) It was possible to visualize the internal architecture of the mastoids of Indian skulls taken from the burial mounds of South Dakota with radiographs. Good bony detail was found in skulls which had been in the ground for variable periods of time. As long as at least a portion of the temporal bone and mastoid were available, fragmented skulls were examined about as easily as intact skulls.

(2) The x-ray films could be accurately interpreted and classified as showing the findings of pneumatized, diploic, mixed and sclerotic mastoids. Because the ages, sex and cultures of the individual specimens were a matter of museum record, it was possible to further classify the data.

(3) In total 417 temporal bones were examined. Two hundred fifty one of these, representing 130 separate individuals, were from the Arikara burials, and 166 representing 91 individuals, were from other burials which included Middle Plains Woodland people, Sioux Historic, and miscellaneous cultures. One-hundred-eleven Arikara mastoids (44%) showed evidence of altered cell development (diploic-10, sclerotic-13, mixed-88), while 86 other culture mastoids (51.8%) demonstrated similar changes (diploic-4, sclerotic-13, mixed-69). These findings would suggest that there was no distinct cultural pattern in the pneumatization of the mastoid bones.

(4) Altered mastoid air cell development was found unilaterally and bilaterally; there was no predilection for one side. It was not possible to analyze bilaterality statistically because in 25 instances (Arikara-9, other cultures-16) only one temporal bone was available for study. There was no special sex incidence of altered mastoid cell development.

(5) No findings indicating the residual of cholesteatoma, cancer, antemortum surgery upon the bone, or other bony disease, was seen on any of the x-rays of the temporal bones.

(6) An interesting finding in many temporal bones as seen in the Stenvers projec-

tion was the fact that the bony capsule of the labyrinth of these skulls was considerably more dense than the surrounding bone. In skulls which were partially demineralized the bony capsule was well preserved in outline.

(7) If the hypotheses of Wittmaack, Cheatle, and others, regarding the role of infections in the pneumatization of the mastoid area or their increased incidence in the poorly developed mastoid are applied to the results of this study, the findings would suggest that about 50% of the people represented by the skulls examined must have had a significant amount of middle ear disease during the period of growth of the mastoids.

(8) Infection in the middle ear and mastoid has been blamed as a causative, an accentuating or a precipitating factor in stapes footplate fixation with otosclerosis. If altered temporal bone pneumatization can be blamed upon infection or if a poorly pneumatized mastoid area is influential in the frequency and severity of otitis media, the people studied here must have had considerable middle ear disease and should have shown evidence of stapes footplate fixation, if infections are indeed influential in this disease. In fact, however, they did not (Holzheuter et al., '64).

(9) The specimens represented here are from a rather diversified group of people, both as to the time of their lives in history and as to cultural affiliation. Before attempting to analyze data concerning changes seen in the mastoid air cell development of these skulls by means of more sophisticated statistical methods. A larger sampling, preferably having a greater number of representatives from a single culture should be obtained.

ACKNOWLEDGMENTS

The authors are much indebted to Doctor Walter Hard, Dean, School of Medicine, University of South Dakota for financial assistance, Thomas E. Eyres, M. D., Director of the Student Health Service, University of South Dakota, and his staff for their assistance and the use of their x-ray equipment in the examination of this unusual group of students, and to Doctor Wesley H. Hurt, Mr. Jay Brandon, and Mr. Robert Gant of the William H. Over Museum, University of South Dakota, for their advice and assistance in this project.

LITERATURE CITED

American Otological Society: Symposium on Certain Fundamentals in Regard to Suppuration of the Petrosal pyramid, Ann. Otol., Rhin. and Laryng., 44: 1002, 1935. Normal and Pathological Anatomy of the Petrous Pyramid by S. R. Guild, p. 1011, M. F. Jones, p. 1036, J. G. Wilson, p. 1048, and E. P. Fowler, Jr.; p. 1056.

Aschoff, L. 1897 Die Otitis Media Neonatorum, Ein Beitrag Zur Entwicklungsgeschichte der Paukenhohle, Z. Ohrenheilk, 31: 295.

Buch, N. H., and M. B. Jorgensen 1964 Leukocytic infiltration in middle ear of newborn infants. Arch. Otol., 80: 141.

Caffey, J. 1961 Pediatric X-ray Diagnosis, The Yearbook Publishers Inc., Chicago, p. 120.

Cheatle, A. 1906 Hunterian Lectures, Royal College of Surgeons.

——— 1907 The infantile types of mastoid with ninety-six specimens. Journ. Laryng., London, 22: 256.

——— 1910 The infantile types of the temporal bone and their surgical importance. The Lancet, London, p. 88.

——— 1910 Twenty Specimens of Chronic Middle Ear Suppuration and its Sequelae, Eighteen of the Bones being of the Infantile Types and two Cellular. London Society of Medicine. Proceedings. Otological Section, p. 3.

——— 1911 Three Specimens of Chronic Middle Ear Suppuration in each of which the Opposite Side was Normal, the six Bones being all of the Diploetic Infantile Type. London. Society of Medicine. Proceedings. Otological Section, p. 4.

——— 1913 An Examination of both Temporal Bones from 120 Individuals, made with the view of deciding the Question of Symmetry. London. Society of Medicine. Proceedings. Otological Section, p. 8

——— 1923 The etiology and prevention of chronic middle ear Suppuration. Acta Otolaryngologica, 5: 283.

Compere, W. E. 1960 Radiologic findings in otosclerosis. Arch. Otol., 71: 150.

Diamant, M. 1952 Chronic Otitis, A Critical Analysis, S. Karger, New York, 182.

Etter, L. E. 1950 Radiographic Anatomic Studies of the Skull, Medical Radiography and Photography, Published by the Eastman Kodak Co., Rochester, N. Y., 26: 90.

——— 1952 Radiographic Anatomic Studies of the Skull, Medical Radiography and Photography, Published by the Eastman Kodak Co., Rochester, N. Y., 28: 113.

Farrior, J. B. 1950 Radiographic Anatomy of the Temporal Bone, Medical Radiography and Photography, Published by Eastman Kodak Co., Rochester, N. Y., 26: 69.

Flisberg, K. 1963 Relationship of Middle Ear Disease to Mastoid Hypocellularity. Acta otolaryng., Supp., p. 182.

Gomperz, B. 1906 Pathologie und der Mittelohrenzundungon im Kindesalter, Wien: J. Safar, p. 1–146.

Gradenigo, G., and R. Penzo 1891 Bacteriologische Beobachtungen über den Inhalt der Trommelhöhle in Cadavern von Neugeborenen und Säuglingen. Z. Ohrenheilk, *21:* 298.

Holzhueter, A., J. B. Gregg and S. Clifford 1965 A search for stapes footplate fixation in an Indian population, prehistoric and historic. Amer. J. Phys. Anthrop., *23:* 35–40.

Jackson, C., and C. L. Jackson 1946 Diseases of the Nose, Throat and Ear, W. B. Saunders Co., Phila., p. 204.

Koehler, A. 1928 Roentgenology, William Wood and Co., New York City.

Law, F. M. 1934 Roentgen examination of the mastoid processes, A. J. Roentgenol., *31:* 482.

Lindsay, J. R. 1949 The Influence of Systemic and Local Factors on the Development of Otosclerosis. Trans. Amer. Acad. Ophth. and Otol., Supp. Otosclerosis Study Group, p. 23–28.

McLellan, M. S. et al. 1964 Embryonal connective tissue and exudate, a histological study of ear sections of fetuses and infants. Am. J. Dis. Child., *108:* 164.

Meschan, I. 1958 Roentgen Signs in Clinical Diagnosis, W. B. Saunders, Phila., p. 391–393.

——— 1959 An Atlas of Normal Radiographic Anatomy, W. B. Saunders Co., Phila., Ed. II, p. 308.

Pancost, H. K., E. P. Pendergrass and J. P. Schaffer 1940 The Head and Neck in Roentgen Diagnosis, Charles C Thomas Co., Springfield, Ill.

Pendergrass, E. P., J. P. Schaeffer and P. D. Hodes 1956 The Head and Neck in Roentgen Diagnosis, Vol. I, Charles C Thomas Co., Springfield, Ill., p. 750.

Pendergrass, E. P., J. P. Hodes, R.m Tondreau and P. Marden 1956 The Tympanic Cavity and Ossicles — Roentgen Findings in Health and Disease. Am. J. Roentgenol., *76:* 327.

Politzer, A. 1893 Ueber Primäre Erkrankunz der knöchernen Labyrinth-kapsel, Zeitschrift für ohrenlehe, L.c, *25:* 309.

Rüedi, L. 1937 Die Mittelohrraumentwicklung von 5 Embryonalmonat bis zum 10 Lebensjahr, Acta Otolaryng. (Stockholm) suppl., *22:* 73–131.

Schwertz, H. W. 1951 Influence of heredity on pneumatization of temporal bone. J. Laryng., *65:* 317.

Shambaugh, G. E., Jr. 1959 Surgery of the Ear. W. B. Saunders Co., Philadelphia.

Tremble, G. E. 1929 Bony Labyrinth of the New Born Infant and of the Adult: A Comparative Study. Arch. Otol., *9:* 175.

——— Pneumatization of the Temporal Bone. Arch. Otol., *19:* 172.

Von Tröltsch, A. 1858 Leichbefund in den Gehörorganen Kleiner Kinder. Verh. Physik. Med. Ges Würzburg, *9:* 77.

Von Wreden, R. 1868 Die Otitis Media Neonatorum. Vom Anatomisch-Pathologischen Standpunkte. Berlin, C. Nöhring, p. 12.

Wendt, H. 1873 Über das Verhalten der Paukenhöhle beim Fötus und beim Neugeborenen. Arch. Heilk, *14:* 97.

Wittmaack, K. 1918 Über die normale und die pathologische Pneumatisation des Schläfenbeines. Jena.

——— 1926 Die entzündlichen Erkrankungen des Gehörorgans. Henke-Lubarsch: Handbuch der speziellen pathologischen Anatomie und Histologie. XII: 102. Julius Springer, Berlin.

——— 1927 Zur Histologie der Mittelohrschleimhaut. Monatsschrift für Ohrenheilkunde und Rhino-Laryngologie, *61:* 1357.

——— 1927 Über die Schleimhautkonstitution des Mittelohres in ihren Beziehungen zu den entzündlichen Erkrankungsprozessen. Klinische Wochenschrift, *6:* 1539.

——— 1928–29 Der Einfluss der Anatomie des Mittelohres auf den Verlauf der Mittelohrentzündungen. Acta Oto-Laryngologica. Suppl., *7–11:* 217.

——— 1931 Zur Frage der Bedeutung der Mittelohrentzündungen des frühesten Kindesalters für später. Archiv für ohren- usw. Heilkunde, *129:* 207.

——— 1932 Schleimhautkonstitution und Pneumatisation. Archiv für Ohren-usw. Heilkunde, *132:* 261.

——— 1937 Über die Entstehung der Schleimhautkonstitution des Mittelohres. Acta Laryngologica, *25:* 414.

Zaufel, E. 1870 Sectionen des Gehoroganes van Neugeborenen und Sauglinger. Osterreichtsche Jahr Paediat., *1:* 118.

PARANOID REACTIONS IN CHILDREN

Saul I. Harrison, M.D.,

John H. Hess, Jr., M.D., and Joel P. Zrull, M.D.

In the past eight years we have studied four children in whom the outstanding symptomatology consisted of paranoid delusions superficially resembling the type so frequently seen in adults. A fifth child developed similar delusions during the course of psychoanalysis. The following is a report and discussion of these cases.

Children commonly use projection as a mechanism of adaptation or defense. A multitude of everyday examples could be cited. They would range from the child who indicts his animate or inanimate environment for a shortcoming resulting from his lack of mature skill to the extreme of the imaginary companion phase observed in 13 (Svendsen, 1934) to 20 (Hurlock and Burstein, 1932) per cent of children. Although the "normal" use of projection is observed less frequently in adulthood, one is not surprised to find the week-end golfer blaming his mediocre score on his equipment or the losing bridge player berating his partner. It is our impression that adults may project more frequently in child-like play activities without the question of psychopathology being raised than under any other circumstances. Conversely, the pathologic use of projection resulting in definite paranoid syndromes seems far less frequent in children than in adults. A review of the literature reveals a striking paucity of clinical reports specifically describing paranoid symptomatology in children. In many standard textbooks such reactions are hardly mentioned. The impression gained is that significant paranoid syndromes simply do not occur in children or, if they do, that they are extremely rare and do not constitute the major manifestations of the psychopathology.

Review of the Literature

We shall cite but a few authors as representative of the literature's coverage of paranoid projections in childhood psychopathology. Kanner's (1935) comprehensive treatise on child psychiatry alludes to the subject in the section discussing the clinical picture of schizophrenic children thus: "paranoid delusions, when present, are fleeting, inconsistent, and rarely in the foreground." Bender's (1946) reference to delusions as isolated events in case histories of psychotic children is comparable. Finch's (1960) text mentions that the "child given to excessive use of projection shows chronically irritating behavior.... This tendency in a child may or may not eventually lead to a paranoid personality during adult life." Similarly, Noyes and Kolb (1958) make reference to significant psychogenetic influences in the childhood backgrounds of adults manifesting paranoid symptoms. We could list many other texts in which, when it is not specifically stated, the implication seems clear that paranoid phenomena as the primary symptomatic features are not observed prior to late adolescence, or early adulthood.

The only report of a study specifically devoted to this problem that we were able to find was Despert's (1948) investigation of delusions and hallucinations in children. She found no evidence for true delusions in normal children. Twelve per cent of neurotic children manifested delusions conspicuous for their simplicity, lack of repetition, and their segregation, as it were, from the intact personality. Psychotic children, in her series, beyond the age of ten or eleven had delusions resembling those of adult psychotics except for greater simplicity and a total lack of systematization and organization.

Clinical case reports, specifically designed to focus on the occurrence of paranoid syndromes in children, were equally uncommon. Pearson (1949) described an episode characterized by well organized, systematized, and persistent delusions in an eleven-year-old, latently homosexual albino boy during the course of psychoanalytic therapy. Singer (1960), in describing a borderline patient who had problems with sexual identification and passivity, presents much delusional material which she considered to be "of a paranoid nature." Beres (1956), in another context, describes cases in which the outstanding psychopathology presented was that of delusional states. He points out that this must be viewed in a dynamic and adaptive framework and should not be considered in the same sense that one might conceptualize adult paranoid reactions. Several other case reports are scattered throughout the literature, but these are consistently illustrative of other problems and do not represent attempts to appraise the problem of childhood paranoid reactions.

COMMON FACTORS IN OUR PATIENTS

We shall attempt to summarize briefly the factors common to the five children studied. The similarities among them and the cases reported by Pearson and Singer are striking. All patients were boys, and the age range at referral was from eleven to thirteen years. All had unmistakable evidence of emotional difficulties dating back to early childhood. The most consistent sign was enuresis, which occurred in all our patients except the one whose paranoid manifestations appeared during the course of psychoanalytic therapy. Three were encopretic. All were products of family constellations which, in some way set them apart, not only from peer groups, but, in several instances, from other siblings. This was a consequence of cultural background, socioeconomic status, sibling position, etc. All family constellations revealed either absent, punitive, or culturally unsuitable fathers as patterns for identification. All mothers were in one way or another unusually close to the boys. It seemed that, either overtly or covertly, they prevented their sons from working out the conflicts engendered by the close libidinal mother-son relationship. Hence, all of the patients revealed marked sexual disorientation with striking passive-submissive tendencies, strong latent homosexual trends, and intense castration anxiety. In addition, the family environments were particularly provocative of aggressive impulses, while simultaneously demanding the suppression of overt indications of hostility. All five children had originally attempted to handle both the aggressive and sexual conflicts by typical obsessive-compulsive mechanisms. These proved ineffective. The rigid and crippled personalities, seemingly lacking more suitable ego-adaptive maneuvers, resorted to primitive defenses of projection and denial, resulting in paranoid symptomatology. All the boys, as might be

135

expected, had poor social adjustments, as reflected by school and peer relationships. The nature and content of the delusional symptoms were, in general, similar, having to do with matters of power and control and the infliction of bodily harm, mutilation, or death. Another significant similarity was the apparent rapidity of symptomatic improvement and reportedly adequate adjustment made by these boys following markedly varying types of therapeutic intervention.

CASE REPORTS

Case 1

Joe, a thirteen-year-old American Indian boy, was referred because of persistent running away from his foster home and hostile behavior toward his foster mother and father during the previous year. He reportedly justified his behavior on the basis of reluctantly communicated, unwarranted suspicions. While verbally threatening to kill his foster mother, he would declare that he had a secret and personal connection with the Soviet Union enabling him to enlist the aid of Nikita Khrushchev in controlling his foster parents. He was fascinated with injuries, death, war, and instruments of violence. Strangers were frequently questioned with regard to any killings or injuries in which they might have been involved. The onset of this behavior coincided with the placement of a three-and-one-half-year-old boy in his foster home. Subsequent removal of this foster sibling resulted in only minimal improvement in Joe's difficulties. In spite of his running away and his hostility toward his foster parents, Joe was described as a happy and cheerful young fellow who was never known to cry. He was considered to be somewhat hyperactive. It was stated that he would behave well unless especially excited.

Little is know of Joe's early years, but it was reported that he was a slow speaker and, at age four and one half, used a type of sign language for communication. The medical history reveals a T and A and circumcision at the age of seven years with repair to the circumcision a year later. Joe has never gotten along well with his peers, being the object of a good deal of derision focused on his cultural and racial origin. He ran from fights and refused to participate in athletics. He reportedly played best with younger children. Joe began school at five years of age and progressed adequately with average academic accomplishments, although he was a minor behavioral problem in school.

Minimal information is available regarding Joe's biological parents. Because of neglect, Joe and his twelve siblings were removed from the parents when Joe was less than one year of age. He was placed briefly in two foster homes, and at age thirteen months he was placed in his present foster home, where he has remained. The foster parents are in their seventies and appear well-intentioned, but confused and overwhelmed by Joe's difficulties.

At the time of the initial interview Joe was neatly dressed and cooperative, although somewhat ill at ease. He spoke rapidly, with many interruptions and frequent alterations of ideas. He often would interrupt himself in the middle of a thought with the offhand remark, "Skip it." He was rather grandiose and expansive during the latter part of the interview and frequently implied that he was in some way a powerful person who might influence important events if he so chose. Definite paranoid ideation was evidenced by his impression that perhaps the interviewer was not actually a physician, that the thermostat was a microphone, and that the telephone was directly hooked up to a nearby penitentiary where he might be electrocuted. The remainder of his verbalized thoughts had to do with violent subjects. He appeared to be compelled to examine carefully all objects in the room by touching and smelling, as well as visually. In addition to the disordered thinking, his emotional responses were frequently inappropriate. There was no evidence of organic central nervous system disease.

Psychological testing demonstrated normal intelligence. Extensive use of denial and projection as defensive maneuvers was manifest; the employment of these defenses resulted in paranoid ideation. The testing also revealed an inadequate sexual identification. It was the impression of the psychologist that, while there was no evidence of an overt psychotic process, Joe might be classified as "prepsychotic."

Following this initial psychiatric evaluation, the foster family established contact with a nearby child guidance clinic. However, because of continued difficulties, he was later placed in a state institution which utilizes a therapeutic milieu and individual counseling. He responded favorably to this environment and approximately six months later he was again placed in a foster home. The placement agency continued contact with him. More than two years later he was reported as adjusting, though he continues to be withdrawn and finds difficulty in comfortable peer relationships. Currently, there is no evidence of acting out as previously described. The paranoid delusional material is no longer manifest.

Case 2

Tony, a twelve-year-old boy, was referred because of a three-month history of nightmares, illusions, possible hallucinations, aggressive outbursts, enuresis, and occasional encopresis. He is a first generation American of Italian descent.

Approximately three months prior to referral, following his not qualifying for a music class at school, Tony began to have nightmares consisting of a frightening male figure entering the bedroom and harming him or stealing from him. He stated that at night when he was not asleep he often had the feeling that someone was in, or about to enter, his bedroom. He described seeing shadows of the figure or hearing the floor creak as the figure walked. He would ascribe sinister significance to hearing an automobile pass the house or seeing the lights of an automobile reflected on his bedroom wall. Also, at this time, he became noticeably irritable and aggressive, primarily toward his parents and siblings. His nocturnal enuresis, which had been rare since the age of eight years, again became regular in occurance. Occasionally, he was encopretic. Tony was described as a somewhat isolated, withdrawn boy who had difficulty in peer relationships ostensibly created by their derogatory remarks about his name. He was considered industrious and inordinately interested in earning and saving his money, spending it only on model airplanes.

The background history reveals no abnormalities except for rather early toilet training which was said to have been completed by one year. The medical history was not remarkable. Tony began school at the age of five and had always had some degree of academic difficulty. He had been passed with his group, however. At the time of referral, he was markedly deficient in all subjects. He was scapegoated at school and adjusted best with younger children.

Tony's parents were born in Italy and tended to adhere to rather strict and rigid family customs. There had been considerable marital strife and both parents were capable of extensive outbursts of temper and physical abuse. Tony is the oldest of four children. There was considerable rivalry among the siblings and Tony frequently expressed a feeling that he was least liked. All the children were enuretic and one brother was encopretic.

The initial evaluation revealed Tony to be a small, slight boy who exhibited many feminine mannerisms. At the beginning of the interview he seemed quite shy and bashful, but soon took command of the situation and became quite expansive and omnipotent. He did a good deal of teasing and exhibited considerable aggressiveness, albeit in passive and indirect ways. In his vivid descriptions of the nightmares and the threatening male figures, there seemed to be illusory and hypnogogic elements, but the possibility of hallucinatory phenomena was never ruled out. He remained unshakably certain that he was in physical danger and that unknown persons were after him. In contrast to children suffering from nocturnal anxiety, he felt no safer in the light of day. As far as he was concerned, it was his tormentors who chose the night for their activities. His explanation for this state of affairs was that he was not well liked and that he was perhaps particularly ugly and stupid. On occasion his emotional responses to the material were inappropriate or dulled. He exhibited definite difficulties in terms of his sexual identification. Tony was somewhat feminine both in appearance and behavior, including his speech, gestures, and interests. He appeared to be of average intelligence and there was no evidence of organic central nervous system disease.

The results of psychological testing revealed a normal I.Q. with some interference with intellectual functioning based on emotional conflicts. The primary defensive maneuvers were noted to be denial and projection, resulting in paranoid ideation. There was a good deal of preoccupation with hostility, violence, injury, and death. There was evidence of a marked problem with sexual identification and his orientation was a homosexual one. It was the psychologist's impression that he was not overtly psychotic, but that there was definite evidence of a prepsychotic process.

Tony was seen in outpatient psychotherapy for more than two years following the initial evaluation described above. He was able to discuss and work through his feelings of persecution and the attendant fears and wishes, the problems in his relationship to his parents, especially his father, and some of his sexual conflicts. Throughout the therapeutic contact, his intense feelings of hostility and aggressive impulses were noted and dealt with to a limited extent. During the course of this the enuresis and encopresis halted and his schoolwork improved. Finally, the illusions and delusions regarding the nighttime intruder cleared. It was felt that his sexual identification also improved.

Case 3

Dan, an eleven-year-old white boy, was referred for evaluation because of academic failure, gastrointestinal burning sensations, extensive daydreaming, fears that a person or animal would attack him at night, and a preoccupation with religious matters. Approximately eighteen months prior to referral, Dan began to have difficulty in school, apparently caused by excessive daydreaming, during which time the teacher had difficulty contacting him. At times he would spend hours attempting to write a single sentence. He began to complain of a burning sensation in his stomach and sleep difficulty. He expressed fear that a person, or perhaps a large bear, would come into his bedroom at night and attack him. He stated that he felt someone wished to kill him; perhaps an Egyptian mummy might come to his bedroom at night and take his life. He then insisted that, at one time, he had been an Egyptian king. He described in detail events that he claimed to remember happening in ancient Egypt. Shortly after this, he became extremely interested in religious matters and began to study the Bible extensively. He quoted passages at length. Four months prior to referral, Dan's parents were divorced and Dan remained with his mother. At that time the family began attending a different church and Dan was placed back a grade in school. Concurrently, all of the aforementioned overt symptoms disappeared, though he remained withdrawn and apparently unhappy.

The background material reveals a normal birth and developmental history. Bowel training was accomplished at eighteen months. Nevertheless, Dan remained enuretic to the time of referral. He began school at the age of five, and had done well until the onset of the symptoms. He tended to be an isolated child, having difficulty in forming adequate peer relationships. The medical history is not significant.

Dan's father was a college professor who was described as a rigid, suspicious, and peculiar person given to marked mood swings. At one time he had been given a diagnosis of paranoid schizophrenia. Dan was said to be his favorite child. Dan's mother was noted to be a rigidly controlled individual who was capable of intense hostility and seemed chronically depressed. She responded to stress in a highly intellectual fashion. Dan is the youngest of four children.

The psychiatric interview conducted after the reported disappearance of the presenting symptoms revealed Dan to be a boy of average size who responded to the examiner enthusiastically, by grinning, laughing, and shaking hands for an extended period of time. He smiled constantly throughout the interview, often in a personal secretive way. When he shook hands initially, he stated that he was "shaking hands in the Egyptian way." An initial hesitancy about speaking soon passed as he became quite verbal. He impressed us as being grandiose and omnipotent. In his religious discussion he expressed a good deal of aggressiveness in the form of world destruction fantasies. He intertwined quotations from the Bible with a discussion of planets, rocket ships, and outer space. In commenting on his previous fears and ideas regarding his royal background, he stated that he now knew they were not so and that he must have been just fooling. It was the impression of the examiner that there was a definite sexual malidentification and that his thinking revealed bizarre associations. Affective responses were appropriate, although somewhat extreme and vivid. Dan was considered to be of above average intelligence, and there was no evidence of organic central nervous system disease.

Psychological testing revealed a boy of above average intelligence with marked emotional difficulties. Intense, aggressive, and hostile impulses were noted which were directed primarily toward adult males. Such impulses were handled for the most part by denial and projection, resulting in paranoid ideation. As a corollary of this, there was evidence of considerable fear of retaliation in which some type of homosexual attack might be involved. Dan was thought to be having difficulty in his reality testing and there was evidence of delusional thinking. It was felt that he must be considered actively psychotic, but that he could function to the extent of being followed as an outpatient.

As a result of this evaluation, Dan and his mother were seen at regular, but infrequent, intervals primarily for supportive counseling and maintaining contact. There was continued steady improvement and, after approximately ten months, Dan was not considered psychotic and he was referred to a local child guidance clinic. At the present time it is the impression of this clinic that he is adjusting well.

Jim, a thirteen-year-old white boy, was referred because of poor academic work, exaggerated stories, and aggressive fantasies. The referral was precipitated by his following a male teacher and threatening his life. Jim had been seen by other psychiatrists five years earlier because of aggressive behavior, lying, stealing, and exaggerated story telling. His aggressive behavioral difficulties were first noticed at the age of five, when he entered school. When he was evaluated at eight, he was considered to be a "severely neurotic child, possibly prepsychotic" and institutional placement was recommended. This was not carried out, and at the time of our contact with him, the situation seemed essentially as it had been described five years earlier.

Jim was described as constantly requiring the attention of others and willing to go to any lengths to obtain it. He seemed much concerned with adults and had little interest in relationships with peers. However, he seemed to adjust better with children much younger than himself. He spent long periods of time in isolated activity or simply staring into space. He was readily threatened by competitive activity and was considered a "sissy" by his peers as well as by his mother.

Background material reveals nothing of significance regarding Jim's birth and early development. However, he was enuretic and occasionally encopretic until approximately age six. The mother considered him to have been hyperactive and restless since infancy. There was no significant past medical history. Jim's parents were divorced when he was seven years old. His mother remarried and lived in another section of the country until Jim was twelve. At that time his parents were separated. Jim's mother had been unable to spend much time with him. At the time of the referral she was working as a taxi driver in addition to operating a boarding house. Jim had two older brothers. The first had been seen previously as an outpatient at a child guidance clinic; just prior to Jim's evaluation he had been killed in an automobile accident. Another brother had been a patient at an affiliated clinic and spent two years in a state mental institution.

When Jim was interviewed, he demonstrated a remarkable interest in various objects about the office. His verbalizations about these objects revealed paranoid ideation in that he felt that the pictures on the wall had microphones in them, that lamps secreted recording devices, and that a thermostat contained a button of some kind which could blow up the building. His speech was pressured and his associations were frequently bizarre. At times he seemed to exhibit a flight of ideas. He seemed preoccupied with certain words and numbers and stated that some numbers are significant, mysterious, and have power. He struck the examiner as having marked feelings of omnipotence and grandiosity. It was felt that there was impairment in his sexual identification and that there was definite evidence of homosexual orientation. The content of many of his verbalizations had to do with violence of some sort and he was preoccupied with guns, injury, and killing. He was considered to be of average intelligence, and there was no evidence of organic central nervous system disease.

Psychological testing indicated that Jim was of average intelligence, but functioning at a lower level. Projective testing revealed intense hostile-aggressive impulses with a tenuous control system consisting of inadequate obsessive-compulsive mechanisms, denial and projection, resulting in paranoid delusions. There was evidence of sexual confusion with a homosexual orientation. The impression of the psychologist was that of an overt psychotic process characterized as "paranoid schizophrenia."

Following this evaluation, Jim was placed in a state mental institution where he remained for approximately eight months. He made good progress during that time; he was able to function adequately in school as well as with the available peers. A good deal of his aggressive and hostile ideas and behavior was no longer in evidence. There was also a reduction in his delusional ideation. His emotional responses and reactions became more appropriate and modulated. He appeared to present a more adequate sexual identification. Currently, he is living in the home of a near relative and is said to be adjusting well.

Case 5

Harry, an eleven-year-old boy, was referred by his mother's psychotherapist because he was "not one of the boys," to use the term the mother borrowed from one of his teachers. Harry liked to wear his sister's clothes, did not stand to urinate, and enjoyed making little "bitsy" things. In addition to being effeminate, he had no friends, although he got along famously with all adults except his mother. He was described as being very compliant until a few months prior to referral, when he started indulging in passive resistant behavior, particularly with his favorite teacher. His usually excellent school work had deteriorated in the previous six months. He was afraid of physical injury and did not engage in athletics.

All of the previously mentioned difficulties, with the exception of the poor grades and what we labeled as passive resistance, had always been present, according to his mother. He had been seen by another psychiatrist several years before. Treatment was recommended, but not undertaken.

Harry was the second of four siblings. The siblings were all described as well adjusted, although his mother wondered if Harry's older brother didn't emphasize muscular activities excessively.

His father had been an active, successful professional man, who was described as being too restless to have ever watched a television program. He died of a cerebral hemorrhage in his late thirties, when the patient was eight. His mother was a part-time painter and housewife. She was in psychotherapy for depression at the time of the referral. Her therapist reported that in the course of resolving her depressive feelings, she indulged in a great deal of sexual acting out.

Although the pregnancy was full-term, Harry weighed less than four pounds. This necessitated incubator care, and for that reason Harry was the only one of the children who was not breast-fed. The developmental history was otherwise unremarkable, except for a herniorrhaphy and circumcision at age tnree. There was considerable evidence of Harry having been relatively neglected as an infant as attention was lavished on his older brother.

Psychological testing revealed Harry to be an introspective boy of superior intelligence. His emotional problems interfered with his efficiency. He appeared depressed, passive, sensitive, and terrified of both relations with people and his own fantasies. His associations to masculine sexuality were all negative. Although he appeared more comfortable in a feminine orientation, he seemed to think of himself as neuter. Both sexual and aggressive impulses caused difficulty for him. His superego was considered severe and ego strength was considered good. Harry's paranoid projections appeared during the course of psychoanalytic therapy, which will be summarized below.

The patient initially impressed us as being a good-looking boy who was obviously anxious. His general demeanor could best be described as subdued and sweet. There was no evidence of thought disturbance or other ego deviation. He seemed to recognize his need for help as he expressed the realization that he was "different." He divided children into the "athletic and the chemistry" types, identifying himself with the latter. He was extremely verbal and spent little time in the playroom. When he did, he made designs rather self-consciously. He hoped that treatment would make him popular. Not long after the start of treatment (intervention had been limited up to that point to running comments about his compliance), his difficulties in school were intensified. He, along with all the boys in his class, was suspected of antisocial behavior. This consisted of minor vandalism and thefts. Harry, however, thought he alone was suspect and was convinced that his therapist had somehow influenced the school authorities against him. He was unable to evaluate the reality of this idea, repeating it over the course of several therapeutic hours. He said that he continued to come to his sessions only to check up on his therapist. Subsequently, it was noticed that interspersed between these accusations was evidence of a libidinal and identificatory interest in his therapist. He noted that their shirts were similar and later added that he'd like the title of "Dr." before his name when he grew up. He was not going to marry, ostensibly because the expense involved might preclude the ability to afford pipe tobacco like the therapist smoked. Following statements of this sort, he would intensify his accusations about being betrayed at school. With repeated interpretations of the connection between his interest in and suspicion of his therapist, paranoid material decreased and did not reappear throughout the remainder of his therapy. There has been no recurrence of such ideation in the past eight years.

DISCUSSION

It should be noted that this clinical study was not intended to explore dynamically the question of paranoid reactions in children, to consider the genetics or treatment of such reactions, nor to cover the broad subjects of psychiatric evaluation of children. However, our material suggests to us some preliminary speculations which might serve as a point of departure for further investigation. The first of these concerns the difficulty which all our patients demonstrated with sexual identification. The intense conflict which these boys experience between impulses toward passive submission and a more aggressively dominating masculine role seems to parallel the dynamic formulations

145

offered by Freud (1911) as operable in paranoia. It seemed clear that this intense conflict between the libidinized need to submit or dominate had to be projected and hence was an important factor in the paranoid symptomatology.

However, this does not explain the narrow age range into which our patients fell. Could it be that despite the existence of relatively similar problems for many months and years, it was necessary for these boys to attain a certain age before the paranoid symptoms could flower? If this were so, the physiological resurgence of sexual and aggressive drives ascribed to the prepubertal and pubertal child would appear important. No one is surprised that the child, at this age, utilizes more intense and stringent defensive maneuvers. But this hardly completes the explanation; it emphasizes the need for further investigation.

Another factor regarding the specific age range might be related to the general question of the psychiatric evaluation of children. One wonders how "convincingly" a child younger than ten or twelve years can communicate the kinds of material which our patients were able to offer us. Another consideration is how we view psychopathology at various ages. In other words, should a younger child attempt to communicate the material such as we have outlined, how would we evaluate and handle the child and his productions, and how would the child respond to our maneuvers? Obviously, in our study, we accepted the content as representing a certain psychological mechanism, namely projection, and viewed this as pathological. This premise was then seemingly accepted by the patient, and this tacitly became part of the basis for our contact. Perhaps in a younger child the same content would not be viewed as representing a similar degree of psychopathology and, as a result, we might tend to try to influence the child's thinking by kidding with him about such matters, by firmly pointing to reality, or we might simply ignore such material. Even if we accepted it, as we did with the patients described, it seems possible that a younger child would not agree to his side of the bargain. He might not accept our premise regarding the pathological nature of his communications and simply change the subject, resort to play or some other maneuver. Certainly the younger, nonverbal, psychotic children, some of whom we suspect may be amongst the most florid examples of "paranoid reactions in children," could hardly be viewed within the framework we employed with the five boys reported at this writing.

Our last comment concerns the rapidity of apparent improvement. This is of special interest in view of the aura of pessimism surrounding the diagnosis of a paranoid syndrome in an adult. We believe this phenomenon is related to Beres' (1956) concept of ego deviation in which he points out that rather serious symptomatology may be seen in children and adolescents which, as the unsettled and immature ego's response to internal and external stresses, does not necessarily carry the same implications as similar symptomatic manifestations in adulthood. In this regard, we would like to emphasize that, in describing the occurrence of paranoid reactions in children, we are most assuredly *not* suggesting that this simply be used as a more frequent diagnostic label. We pose these questions not to suggest that we have dealt with them in this clinical study, but to point out that they emerge as possibilities pertinent to our interests in suggesting that paranoid reactions are not so uncommon in children as much of the literature and all of the current texts would seem to indicate.

SUMMARY

Though our clinical study of paranoid delusions in children represents only five cases, the striking similarities between the personality characteristics, the intrapsychic conflicts, the environmental and familial factors, and the age range among these boys seem to be beyond what one would expect by chance. We wonder if these similarities may have significance for further understanding the problem of paranoid reactions not only in children, but in adults. We have also called attention to some considerations in psychiatric evaluation of children. It has been our purpose in this paper to draw attention to the fact that such manifestations do exist, and are not nonexistent or extremely rare as is often suggested. It may be surmised that this awareness would lead to greater interest and increased clinical attention. This in turn might provide the opportunity for further study and enlightenment.

REFERENCES

BENDER, L. (1946), *Techniques in Child Psychiatry*. New York: Grune & Stratton.
BERES, D. (1956), Ego deviation and the concept of schizophrenia. *The Psychoanalytic Study of the Child*, 11:164-235. New York: International Universities Press.
DESPERT, J. L. (1948), Delusional and hallucinatory experiences in children. *Amer. J. Psychiat.*, 104:528-537.
FINCH, S. M. (1960), *Fundamentals of Child Psychiatry*. New York: Norton.

FREUD, S. (1911), Psychoanalytical notes upon an autobiographical account of a case of paranoia (dementia paranoides). *Collected Papers*, 3:387-470. London: Hogarth Press, 1956.

HURLOCK, E. B. & BURSTEIN, W. (1932), The imaginary playmate. *J. Genet. Psychol.*, 41:380-391.

KANNER, L. (1935), *Child Psychiatry*. Springfield, Ill.: Thomas, 1957.

NOYES, A. P. & KOLB, L. C. (1958), *Modern Clinical Psychiatry*. Philadelphia & London: Saunders.

PEARSON, G. H. (1949), *Emotional Disorders of Children*. New York: Norton.

SINGER, M. (1960), Fantasies of a borderline patient. *The Psychoanalytic Study of the Child*, 15:310-356. New York: International Universities Press.

SVENDSEN, M. (1934), Children's imaginary companions. *Arch. Neurol. Psychiat.*, 32:985-999.

Prevalence of Ascariasis and Amebiasis in Cherokee Indian School Children

GEORGE R. HEALY, Ph.D., NEVA N. GLEASON, M.S., ROBERT BOKAT, M.D., HARRY POND, M.D., and MARGARET ROPER, R.N.

PHYSICIANS at the Public Health Service Indian Hospital on the Cherokee North Carolina Indian Reservation diagnosed several cases of severe clinical ascariasis in children in 1964–65 and recorded the death of a child caused by what was believed to be an overwhelming infection with *Ascaris lumbricoides*. A preliminary survey in one part of the reservation in 1963 indicated that 50 percent of the children were infected with *Ascaris* worms.

To determine the prevalence of the roundworm and other intestinal parasites in the Cherokee population, a collaborative study in 1965 between physicians at the hospital and the Parasitology Section of the National Communicable Disease Center, Public Health Service, was initiated. Because of logistical problems in obtaining specimens from persons living in the mountainous area of the reservation, it was decided to examine stool specimens from children attending the elementary school close to the hospital. Moreover, the 655 children in the elementary school would represent a sample of the approximately 5,000 residents of the reservation. More important, such examinations would

indicate the prevalence of intestinal parasites in the group most likely to be affected by any species of clinical importance.

Materials and Methods

One-half pint waxed cardboard cartons labeled with each child's name were distributed to the children at the elementary school along with instructions to bring a stool specimen, preferably a morning one, on the following day. The cartons were collected at the school from each pupil in the morning, and all specimens were processed within 6 hours. The stools were preserved in 10 percent formalin; those which were watery, loose, or soft were also placed in polyvinyl alcohol (PVA) fixative (*1*). When all the stools of a particular day had been preserved, a direct saline and iodine wet mount of the formalinized sediment was examined, as well as a subsequent formalin ether (FE) concentration (*2*). The stools preserved in PVA were stained with Wheatley's trichrome (*3*) and examined for protozoan trophozoites.

To determine the correlation between seropositivity and etiological results, serum specimens were collected from as many children as possible and tested for antibody to *Entamoeba histolytica* and *A. lumbricoides*. Results of the *Ascaris* serology will be reported elsewhere. The amebiasis serology was conducted by using tanned, sensitized sheep red blood cells in the indirect hemagglutination test of Kessel and associates (*4*) as modified by Milgram and associates (*5*). The tests were run in microtitration plates, and titers of 1 : 128 or greater were considered positive. The antigen employed in the test was a sonicated, loyphilized extract of *E. histolytica* strain DKB, grown with *Mycoplasma* organisms. Stock cultures of the amebae had been furnished by Dr. William K. Lewis, University of California, Los Angeles.

Results

Stools were submitted by 631 children (302 boys and 329 girls), representing 96 percent of the 655 students enrolled in the elementary school.

Helminths. The impression of the hospital physicians that *Ascaris* infections were common in the school population was borne out by the observation that 49 percent of the children were infected with the worms. The overall prevalence of *A. lumbricoides* and the other intestinal parasites is shown in table 1. Among the other helminths, only *Trichuris trichiura* was present to a considerable degree (38 percent). All the *Ascaris* and *Trichuris* eggs were detected in the direct wet mount or FE concentrate with the exception of a single infertile *Ascaris* egg found in the PVA stained slide of a stool specimen from an 11-year-old boy. A greater number of hookworm infections would have been detected if a more sensitive technique, such as the culture method of Harada and Mori (*6*), had been employed. Pinworm infections are not generally detected by stool examinations, but the few cases that were detected are included in the results. Although only 14 children had positive *Enterobius vermicularis* infections, 92 percent were infected with one or more parasites; in only one of the infections caused by *E. vermicularis*, did such eggs represent the sole parasitic stages recovered.

Protozoa. Sixty-seven (11 percent) of the children were found to be passing cysts, trophozoites of *E. histolytica*, or both. One-third or

Table 1. **Prevalence of intestinal parasites in stool specimens from 631 Cherokee Indian elementary school children**

Parasite	Specimens positive	
	Number	Percent
Helminths:		
*Ascaris lumbricoides*_____	312	49
*Trichuris trichiura*_____	240	38
Hookworm_____	19	3
Trichostrongylus species_____	1	(¹)
*Enterobius vermicularis*_____	14	2
Protozoa:		
*Entamoeba histolytica*_____	67	11
*Entamoeba hartmanni*_____	220	35
*Entamoeba coli*_____	251	40
*Endolimax nana*_____	289	46
*Iodamoeba bütschlii*_____	34	5
*Giardia lamblia*_____	59	9
*Dientamoeba fragilis*_____	68	11
*Trichomonas hominis*_____	72	11
*Chilomastix mesnili*_____	19	3
Unidentified protozoa_____	7	1
1 or more parasites_____	579	92
No parasites found_____	52	8

¹ 0.2 percent.

more of the children harbored the commensal amebae—*Entamoeba hartmanni*, *Entamoeba coli*, and *Endolimax nana*. Protozoa were detected in seven stool specimens, but specific identification was not possible because of poor fixation or paucity of organisms. No parasitic organisms were detected in 52 (8 percent) of the 631 stools examined.

The prevalence of six parasite species in boys and girls is compared in table 2. Analysis of the data indicated no difference by sex in parasitization by *Ascaris* (154 males, 158 females) or *Trichuris* (112 males, 128 females). The number of hookworm infections was too small for adequate comparison (eight males, 11 females). In the stools of 37 boys and 22 girls, the pathogenic, or potentially pathogenic, protozoan *Giardia lamblia* (*7*) was found. Specimens from 37 boys and 31 girls were positive for *Dientamoeba fragilis*, a parasite with questionable capacity to cause symptoms (*8*). Although the prevalence of *E. histolytica*, *G. lamblia*, and *D. fragilis* appears greater in males than in females, an analysis of parasitization by sex was not possible. Stools from both sexes were examined after FE concentration, but there was a disproportionately larger number of PVA stained slides from boys (62) than from girls (50). The data, therefore, are biased in favor of stool specimens from boys.

The prevalence of the parasites in the children by school grade is presented in tables 3–5. Even though *Ascaris* and *Trichuris* were more prevalent in the lower grades (table 3), at least one-third of the children in the higher grades also harbored roundworms and whipworms. Results in the category "no parasites found" include examinations for helminths and protozoa. The largest number of stools with no parasites found were from children in the fourth, sixth, and seventh grades, a result indicating no specific pattern and certainly no evidence of a diminution of infection in the older children.

Table 2. Prevalence of selected parasites in stool specimens from 631 Cherokee Indian elementary school children, by sex

Parasite	All children		Boys		Girls	
	Number	Percent	Number	Percent	Number	Percent
Ascaris lumbricoides	312	49	154	49	158	51
Trichuris trichiura	240	38	112	47	128	53
Hookworm	19	3	8	42	11	58
Entamoeba histolytica	67	11	39	58	28	42
Giardia lamblia	59	9	37	63	22	37
Dientamoeba fragilis	68	11	37	54	31	46

Table 3. Percentage of 631 Cherokee Indian elementary school children with helminth parasites, by school grade

Parasite	School grade								Overall prevalence
	1	2	3	4	5	6	7	8	
Ascaris lumbricoides	57	56	52	51	60	42	37	33	49
Trichuris trichiura	40	51	36	39	42	29	29	30	38
Hookworm	0	2	5	1	5	5	4	4	3
Trichostrongylus	0	0	0	0	1	0	0	0	[1]
Enterobius vermicularis	1	3	5	3	2	2	0	3	2
No parasites found [2]	4	8	5	14	4	11	15	7	8
Number of students	95	101	64	80	84	62	75	70	

[1] 0.2 percent.
[2] Includes protozoa and helminths.

Table 4. Percentage of 631 Cherokee Indian elementary school children with protozoan parasites, by school grade

Parasite	School grade								Overall prevalence
	1	2	3	4	5	6	7	8	
Entamoeba coli	40	41	39	34	48	47	33	37	40
Endolimax nana	52	37	50	49	51	29	43	56	46
Iodamoeba bütschlii	0	5	3	5	7	3	9	11	5
Giardia lamblia	14	11	9	6	10	13	6	4	9
Dientamoeba fragilis	18	7	8	9	12	11	15	6	11
Chilomastix mesnili	5	3	6	0	2	5	1	1	3
Trichomonas hominis	9	8	6	12	20	16	8	11	11
Unidentified protozoa	0	0	3	0	5	3	3	0	1
Number of students	95	101	64	80	84	62	75	70	

Parasite	School grade								Overall prevalence
	1	2	3	4	5	6	7	8	
Entamoeba histolytica	8	6	9	14	14	8	13	13	11
Entamoeba hartmanni	37	26	33	36	38	37	28	51	35
E. histolytica and *E. hartmanni* combined	39	26	34	40	43	38	35	56	39
Amebic prevalence rate	91	64	77	69	74	69	64	81	74
Number of students	95	101	64	80	84	62	75	70	
Amebiasis hemagglutination test positive (percent)[1]	2	2	2	1	1	2	4	1	2

[1] Indirect HA titers 1:128 or greater.

The seven species of protozoa in table 4 occurred without any appreciable diminution through the eighth grade. *E. coli* and *E. nana* were more prevalent than the other five species.

E. histolytica organisms were found in 67 children (39 boys, 28 girls)—an 11 percent prevalence rate (table 5). Forty-three (64 percent) of the *E. histolytica* infections were diagnosed from cysts found in the FE concentrates; seven (11 percent) were diagnosed from organisms found in both PVA stained slides and FE concentrates; 17 (25 percent) were diagnosed in the PVA stained slide only.

Distribution of the *E. histolytica* throughout the school grades was constant, with more infections in the older children (in the seventh and eighth grades) than in the younger ones (in the first, second, and third grades).

Of particular significance was the observation of an "amebic prevalence rate" (APR) of 74 percent. The APR, first described by Brooke and associates (9), is calculated by considering infections with one or more of the four amebae (*E. histolytica, E. coli, E. hartmanni,* and *E. nana*) as an "amebic" infection. Since the four organisms have comparable but not identical capabilities of surviving in the environment and are transmitted by ingestion of cystic stages, they are indicative of fecal contamination.

Amebiasis serology. Serum specimens were collected from 617 children. Specimens were obtained from all but one of the 67 children whose stools were positive for *E. histolytica.* The following summary of the correlation between etiological and serologic positivity in the 617 children is taken from a table in a previous study by Healy (10).

Test results	Number	Percent
E. histolytica in stools, IHA test positive	2	0.3
E. histolytica in stools, IHA test negative	64	10.4
No *E. histolytica* in stools, IHA test positive	10	1.6
No *E. histolytica* in stools, IHA test negative	541	87.7
Total	617	100.0

Ninety-eight percent of the 617 serums were negative for ameba antibody. Only two (0.3 percent) of the serum specimens were positive with the corresponding *E. histolytica* found in the stool specimens, whereas 10 (1.6 percent) of the serum specimens were positive without demonstration of the amebae in the stool specimens. Organisms recovered in stool specimens from children with positive IHA titers are listed in table 6.

Discussion

Since our survey was concerned with intestinal parasites in elementary school children, no reference can be made to the extent of parasitism in the population of the Cherokee Indian Reservation. Direct examination of a single stool specimen and examination after FE concentration probably resulted in detection of all of the *Ascaris* infections and the majority of the *Trichuris.* The same cannot be said for the intestinal protozoa. Although all specimens were subjected to direct and FE concentrate examinations, only 112 of the 631 stools were preserved in PVA and subsequently examined after trichrome staining. The possibility of more widespread protozoan infections is suggested by table 7, which shows the parasite prevalence in the siblings of three families.

152

Eleven reports of parasitism among North American Indians have been published (11–21). The present study was concerned only with elementary school children from 6 to 16 years of age, whereas most other surveys have included all age groups. *Ascaris* eggs were reported in only three other studies (13, 14, 20); in the study by Fournelle and associates (20), *Ascaris* eggs were found in only one of the 855 stools examined.

A recent survey of intestinal parasitism in the Southeast was conducted by Jeffery and associates (22) in a coastal area of South Carolina in Beaufort County among a rural Negro popula-

Table 6. Parasites recovered from 12 Cherokee Indian elementary school children with positive titers for amebiasis in the indirect hemagglutination test

Child's age, sex, and grade	IHA titer	Parasites found
7, F, 1st	1:256	*Ascaris lumbricoides, Trichuris trichiura, Entamoeba histolytica, Endolimax nana.*
8, M, 1st	1:128	*A. lumbricoides, T. trichiura, Entamoeba hartmanni, E. nana.*
8, M, 2d	1:256	*A. lumbricoides, T. trichiura, E. hartmanni, Trichomonas hominis.*
7, F, 2d	1:128	*A. lumbricoides, T. trichiura, Entamoeba coli, E. nana.*
8, M, 3d	1:128	*A. lumbricoides.*
10, F, 4th	1:256	*A. lumbricoides, E. coli, E. nana, Iodamoeba bütschlii, T. hominis.*
11, M, 5th	1:128	*A. lumbricoides, T. trichiura, E. histolytica, E. coli.*
12, M, 6th	1:128	Unidentified flagellate.
12, F, 7th	1:128	No parasites found.
14, M, 7th	1:128	*A. lumbricoides, T. trichiura, E. hartmanni.*
14, F, 7th	1:128	*T. trichiura, E. coli.*
14, F, 8th	1:128	*E. coli, E. hartmanni, E. nana.*

Table 7. Occurrence of parasites among Cherokee Indian elementary school children from three family groups

Sibling's sex and age	Parasites [1]										
	Al	Tt	Eh	Ehart	Ec	En	Ib	Df	Gl	Th	Cm
Family A:											
Boy, 7	x	x	x	x	x						
Girl, 8	x	x			x		x				x
Girl, 10	x	x		x	x	x	x				
Boy, 11	x	x	x		x	x	x				x
Boy, 13	x	x			x	x	x				
Boy, 14					x	x					
Family B:											
Girl, 6	x	x	x	x		x		x			
Girl, 8	x	x				x		x	x		
Girl, 10	x	x			x			x	x		
Boy, 11	x	x		x	x						
Girl, 12	x	x									
Girl, 15	x	x		x			x				
Family C:											
Boy, 6	x				x						
Girl, 8					x				x		
Girl, 11	x			x	x	x			x	x	
Girl, 13	x					x		x	x	x	
Girl, 14	x				x	x	x		x	x	x

[1] Key: Al—*Ascaris lumbricoides*
Tt—*Trichuris trichiura*
Eh—*Entamoeba histolytica*
Ehart—*Entamoeba hartmanni*
Ec—*Entamoeba coli*
En—*Endolimax nana*
Ib—*Iodamoeba bütschlii*
Df—*Dientamoeba fragilis*
Gl—*Giardia lamblia*
Th—*Trichomonas hominis*
Cm—*Chilomastix mesnili.*

tion. They examined family units and found the following overall prevalence of parasites from 212 stools: *Ascaris* 64 percent, *Trichuris* 37 percent, *E. histolytica* 1.4 percent, *E. coli* 32 percent, *E. nana* 10 percent, *Iodamoeba bütschlii* 0.5 percent, *Trichomonas hominis* 0.5 percent, *Chilomastix mesnili* 1.4 percent, and *G. lamblia* 8 percent. Prevalence for *E. hartmanni* and *D. fragilis* was not given.

In the age groups comparable to those of the Cherokee school children (6–17 years), the survey of Jeffery and associates showed 60 of 74 children (81 percent) positive for *Ascaris* and 38 of 74 (51 percent) positive for *Trichuris*. There was no analysis of parasitization for the protozoa by age groups. Although the sample studied by Jeffery and associates was smaller, both for all persons infected and for children, these persons from South Carolina had a higher prevalence of *Ascaris* (64 percent overall and 81 percent in children) than did the Cherokee children (49 percent).

When our survey is compared with the one of Jeffery and associates, certain differences are noted. Our survey was conducted among American Indian children in western North Carolina in the Great Smoky Mountains while the survey of Jeffery and associates was conducted among American Negro families in the flat coastal plains of South Carolina.

The similar high prevalence of fecally-transmitted intestinal parasites in the two groups, however, emphasizes the important point made by Jeffery and others, that "a high incidence of *Ascaris* in specific groups may not depend so much on the climate or topography, although certain favorable conditions are necessary, as on the particular habits and sanitation of the populations involved."

The survey of the Cherokee Indian children was conducted with three goals in mind. The first was to provide physicians of the Public Health Service Indian Hospital with information on the prevalence of *Ascaris* and other parasites in the school population. As suspected, the prevalence of *Ascaris* infections was high, and the amebic prevalence rate was as high as in some tropical areas.

The second goal was to determine the suitability of serologic tests for ascariasis and amebi-

asis. Evaluation of *Ascaris* serology is in progress. Results of the amebiasis serology enabled us to evaluate the specificity of the indirect hemagglutination (IHA) test for intestinal amebiasis. The results of our evaluation of 617 serum samples taken from infected children indicated no cross reactions with other intestinal parasites. The 617 serums from our survey along with the other serums tested (*10*) also showed that the IHA test was of little value in asymptomatic intestinal amebiasis. Such results are in keeping with the concept that positive serology is evident only where tissue invasion has occurred, as in amebic dysentery or amebic liver abscess. The serologic results corroborated the experiences of physicians from the Public Health Service Indian Hospital, who have recorded only rare instances of clinical amebiasis in the Cherokee Indian population.

The third, and perhaps most useful goal, was to document the prevalence of fecally transmitted parasites. With the exception of hookworm and pinworm, the presence of intestinal parasites indicates the status of a population's sanitation and personal hygiene. Therefore, data on prevalence from our survey would serve as a basis for judging any changes occurring subsequently as a result of improvements in sanitation, intensified health education, or regimens of drug prophylaxis directed against *Ascaris* or other parasites. For example, the effects of certain sanitary improvements that were being provided the Cherokee Indian Reservation under Public Law 86–121 at the time of our survey might be gauged by comparing the prevalence of *Ascaris* or other parasites that we found with the prevalence observed in a similar survey several years from now. (Public Law 86–121 included provisions for the construction of either a well-built, suitably placed outdoor pit privy or the piping in of water for use with an indoor toilet and with facilities for washing and bathing. The Indian householder was required to contribute a certain amount of labor to initiate the construction of either of the two kinds of sanitary facilities.)

Summary

Single stool specimens, collected from each of 631 children at the Cherokee Indian Elementary School, Cherokee, N.C., were examined for intestinal parasites. The organisms identified and their prevalence were as follows: *Ascaris lumbricoides*, 49 percent; *Trichuris trichiura*, 38 percent; hookworm, 3 percent; *Entamoeba histolytica*, 11 percent; *Entamoeba hartmanni*, 35 percent; *Entamoeba coli*, 40 percent; *Endolimax nana*, 46 percent; *Iodamoeba bütschlii*, 5 percent; *Giardia lamblia*, 9 percent; *Dientamoeba fragilis*, 11 percent; *Chilomastix mesnili*, 3 percent, and *Trichomonas hominis*, 11 percent.

Evidence of infection with one or more parasites was found in 92 percent of the children. The amebic prevalence rate, which can be used to measure the extent of ingestion of organisms through fecal contamination, was 74 percent. There was no difference in the prevalence of *A. lumbricoides* or *T. trichiura* between Indian boys and girls. Although there was a slight reduction in the prevalence of some parasites (*A. lumbricoides*, *T. trichiura*, and *G. lamblia*) in children of the higher elementary grades as compared with the lower ones, in many cases an equal or greater number of children in the higher grades were parasitized with *E. histolytica* and *E. hartmanni* as compared with children in the lower grades. In general, the survey revealed a high prevalence of intestinal parasites in children throughout the eight grades of the school.

An indirect hemagglutination (IHA) test for amebiasis was used to detect antibody in the serums of 617 of the children. Results showed no cross reactions with any other intestinal parasites. Only two of the serums (0.3 percent) from children having *E. histolytica* in the stools were positive by IHA; conversely, 10 of the serums (1.6 percent) from children in whom no *E. histolytica* was detected were positive. Results of the indirect hemagglutination test indicated that it was of little value in asymptomatic intestinal amebiasis. They did, however, corroborate the experience of the Public Health Service physicians, who had rarely found cases of clinical amebiasis in the Indian children.

Data obtained in the survey will serve as a basis by which to judge the results of projected activities designed to improve sanitation, intensify health education, and provide drug prophylaxis for ascariasis.

REFERENCES

(1) Brooke, M. M., and Goldman, M.: Polyvinyl alcohol-fixation as a preservative and adhesive for protozoa in dysenteric stools and other liquid media. J Lab Clin Med 34: 1554–1560 (1949).

(2) Ritchie, L.: An ether sedimentation technique for routine stool examinations. Bull U.S. Army Med Depart 8: 326 (1948).

(3) Wheatley, W. B.: A rapid staining procedure for intestinal amebae and flagellates. Amer J Clin Path 21: 990–991 (1951).

(4) Kessel, J. F., Lewis, W. P., Molina Pasquel, C., and Turner, J. A.: Indirect hemagglutination and complement fixation tests in amebiasis. Amer J Trop Med 14: 540–550, July 1965.

(5) Milgram, E., Healy, G. R., and Kagan, I. G.: Studies on the use of the indirect hemagglutination test in the diagnosis of amebiasis. Gastroenterology 50: 645–649, May 1966.

(6) Harada, Y., and Mori, O.: A new method for culturing hookworm. Yonago Acta Med 1: 177–179 (1955).

(7) Brandborg, L., et al.: Histological demonstration of mucosal invasion by *Giardia lamblia* in man. Gastroenterology 52: 143–150 (1967).

(8) Kean, B. H., and Mallock, C. L.: The neglected ameba: *Dientamoeba fragilis*. A report of 100 "pure" infections. Amer J Dig Dis 11: 735–746 (1966).

(9) Brooke, M. M., et al.: Studies of a water-borne outbreak of amebiasis, South Bend, Indiana. III. Investigation of family contacts. Amer J Hyg 62: 214–226 (1955).

(10) Healy, G. R.: The use of and limitations to the indirect hemagglutination test in the diagnosis of intestinal amebiasis. Health Lab Sci 5: 174–179, July 1968.

(11) Owen, W. B., Honess, R. F., and Simon, J. R.: Observations on the protozoan infestations of American Indian children in the United States. J Parasit 19: 178 (1932).

(12) Owen, W. B., Honess, R. F., and Simon, J. R.: Protozoan infestations of American Indian children in Wyoming. J Colorado-Wyoming Acad Sci 1: 78 (1933).

(13) Owen, W. B., Honess, R. F., and Simon, J. R.: Protozoal infestations of American Indian children. JAMA 102: 913–915 (1934).

(14) Spector, B. K., Hardy, A. V., and Mack, M. G.: Studies of the acute diarrheal diseases. II. Parasitological observations. Public Health Rep 54: 1105–1113, June 23, 1939.

(15) Saunders, L. G.: A survey of helminth and protozoan incidence in man and dogs at Fort Chipewyan, Alberta. J Parasit 35: 31–34 (1949).

(16) Kelley, G. W., Jr.: Intestinal parasitism in an irrigated community of western Nebraska. Amer J Trop Med 4: 901–907 (1955).

(17) U.S. Public Health Service: Health services for

American Indians. PHS Publication No. 531. U.S. Government Printing Office, Washington, D.C., 1957.

(*18*) Melvin, D. M., and Brooke, M. M.: Parasitologic surveys on Indian reservations in Montana, South Dakota, New Mexico, Arizona, and Wisconsin. Amer J Trop Med 11: 765–772 (1962).

(*19*) Meerovitch, E., and Eaton, R. D. P.: Outbreak of amebiasis among Indians in northwestern Saskatchewan, Canada. Amer J Trop Med 14: 719–723 (1965).

(*20*) Fournelle, H. J., Rader, V., and Allen, C.: A survey of enteric infections among Alaskan Indians. Public Health Rep 81: 797–803, September 1966.

(*21*) Becke, D.: Enteric parasites of Indians and Anglo-Americans, chiefly on the Winnebago and Omaha Reservations in Nebraska. Nebraska State Med J 53: 293–295, June 1968; 347–349, July 1968; 380–382, August 1968; 421–423, September 1968.

(*22*) Jeffery, G. M., et al.: Study of intestinal helminth infections in a coastal South Carolina area. Public Health Rep 78: 45–55, January 1963.

Tearsheet Requests

Dr. George R. Healy, Parasitology Section, National Communicable Disease Center, Atlanta, Ga. 30333

Incidence of Disease
In the Navajo Indian

A Necropsy Study of Coronary and
Aortic Atherosclerosis, Cholelithiasis,
and Neoplastic Disease

FRANK G. HESSE, MD

It is difficult to obtain an accurate appraisal of the incidence of disease among the 90,000 Navajo Indians, because they live on a 25,000-square-mile reservation equal to the combined areas of the states of Massachusetts, Vermont, Connecticut, and Rhode Island, and they are a rural people who live in family groups at great distances from each other. Native medicine is still widely prevalent, especially among the older generation and in more isolated areas of the reservation. Collection of accurate and complete vital statistics is difficult especially when 41% of the death certificates are not signed by physicians.[1]

Nevertheless, the available vital statistics indicate that the leading causes of death among the Navajo Indians are at variance with that of the rest of the United States population.[2]

There is a higher rate of accidents, pneumonia, tuberculosis, and certain intestinal diseases. Heart disease and malignant neoplasm, however, are conspicuous by their relative infrequency. Vital statistical studies by Smith et al,[1] and clinical studies by Salisbury[3] have reported a relatively low incidence of malignant disease. Bivens et al,[4] however, found that at least the incidence of cancer of the cervix is equivalent to the rest of the US population. A relative frequency of cholecystitis among the Navajo was first reported by Gilbert[5] who also noted the virtual absence of coronary thrombosis.

TABLE 1.—*Leading Causes of Death Among Navajos Percent of Total Deaths* [a]

	% of Total Deaths [*]	
Cause of Death	Navajo 1958-1960	All Races 1959
Accidents	16.1	5.5
Influenza and pneumonia	11.6	3.3
Certain diseases of early infancy	11.9	4.1
Gastritis, duodenitis, enteritis, and colitis	6.4	0.5
Diseases of heart	5.9	38.7
Tuberculosis, all forms	5.0	0.7
Malignant neoplasms	4.8	15.7
Vascular lesions of central nervous system	2.5	11.6
Nonmeningococcal meningitis	2.5	0.1
Congenital malformations	2.5	1.3
Measles	0.8	0.0
All other causes	30.0	19.5

[*] Navajo average, 1958-1960, and US all races, 1959.

TABLE 2.—*Coronary Atherosclerosis, Degree of Severity in 87 Adult Navajo Necropsies*

	No.	Grade				
Age	Cases	1	2	3	4	Average
20-29	14	14	0	0	0	1.0
30-39	10	10	0	0	0	1.0
40-49	15	15	0	0	0	1.0
50-59	16	10	3	2	1	1.63
60-69	15	9	3	2	1	1.67
70-79	12	8	3	0	1	1.5
80 plus	5	5	0	2	0	1.8
Total	87	69	9	6	3	1.34

Streeter et al [6] evaluated 364 Navajo electrocardiograms and the coronary arteries in 45 Navajo autopsies and similarly suggested a low incidence of coronary heart disease.

It should be taken into consideration that malignant neoplasm and coronary thrombosis are usually seen in an older age group. There are over 11,500 Navajos above the age of 45,[2] and it is this group that most frequently will seek the aid of the Navajo medicine man and die at home or arrive in the hospital in a terminal condition often precluding accurate diagnosis of the underlying disease without autopsy study.

In order to obtain more precise data on the incidence of coronary and generalized atherosclerosis, cholecystitis, and malignancy, a study was made of most of the available necropsies performed by qualified pathologists on adult Navajos. Eighty-seven necropsies in patients above the age of 20 were available and reviewed. These included 56 males and 31 females from the records of the Bernalillo County-Indian Hospital, Albuquerque, and the San Juan Hospital, Farmington, NM. While the limitation of statistical data obtained from such a small autopsy series is definitely recognized, it may add to our knowledge of the true incidence of various diseases in the older population.

Results

1. Coronary Atherosclerosis.—In order to evaluate the degree of coronary atherosclerosis, all coronary vessels were graded as to degree of sclerosis as follows: (1) no atherosclerosis to slight lipid streaking; (2) slight atherosclerosis without appreciable encroachment on lumen; (3) moderate atherosclerosis and plaques with less than 75% partial occlusion; (4) marked atherosclerosis with more than 75% occlusion.

Fig 1 shows the average grade of coronary atherosclerosis in each age group. The Navajo has less than half the degree of coronary atherosclerosis found in the similar non-Indian study by White.

2. Aortic Atherosclerosis.—In order to evaluate the degree of atherosclerosis in the

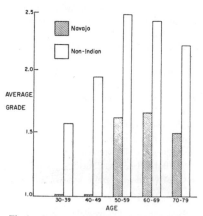

Fig 1.—Average grade of coronary atherosclerosis in each age group, Navajo and non-Indian.[7]

158

TABLE 3.—*Aortic Atherosclerosis, Degree of Severity in 62 Adult Navajo Necropsies*

Age	No. Cases	Grade 0	1	2	3	4
20-29	9	9	0	0	0	0
30-39	6	5	0	1	0	0
40-49	11	7	4	0	0	0
50-59	9	6	3	0	0	0
60-69	11	4	4	2	1	0
70-79	12	4	6	2	0	0
80 plus	4	0	1	3	0	0
Total	62	35	18	8	1	0

peripheral vascular system, the degree of atherosclerosis of the aorta was graded in 62 necropsies in which the aorta was adequately described in the protocol.

The aorta was numerically graded according to the method of Willius et al of the Mayo Clinic.[8] Grade 0, absence of sclerosis; 1, very slight degree of sclerosis; 2, moderate involvement; 3, unmistakable marked sclerosis; 4, extreme sclerosis.

Comparison of the severity of aortic atherosclerosis in the Navajo and the results in the Mayo Clinic series shows that a larger percentage of Navajos had no or slight atherosclerosis. Only 14% of the Navajos had moderate to marked aortic atherosclerosis compared to 37% in the non-Indian Mayo Clinic group.

This study included a 75-year-old diabetic with only slight aortic atherosclerosis, but with complete occlusion of the distal popliteal artery, and a 43-year-old female with slight aortic atherosclerosis who had an old fibrotic iliac artery thrombosis resulting in a previous thigh amputation. There were no other cases indicative of peripheral vascular disease.

3. Cholelithiasis.—The necropsy incidence of cholelithiasis in this series was 24.4% compared to the non-Indian incidence of 9.1% and 11.6% reported by Kozoll[9] and Lieber respectively in a comparable autopsy population over the age of 20.

The incidence for each decade is compared to Kozoll's series. There is a markedly greater incidence of cholelithiasis noted in each age group.

Cancer of the gall bladder here is likewise very common. Three cases were reported, showing an incidence of 3.6% of all autopsies compared to the control autopsy group of 0.32%.

4. Malignant Neoplasm.—In 87 necropsies, 17 patients had a malignant neoplasm. Table 4 shows the general distribution of the neoplasms. In three patients it was an incidental autopsy finding, and 14 died of malignant disease. The necropsy incidence of malignant disease in the Navajo is 19.3% which is comparable to the reported necropsy incidence by Kirschoff and Rigdon[10] of 24.4% for a Caucasian population and 16.8% in a Negro group.

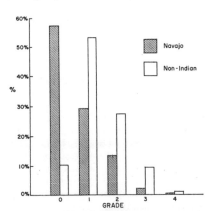

Fig 2.—Severity of aortic atherosclerosis, Navajo and non-Indian.[8]

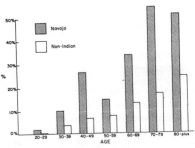

Fig 3.—Percentage of cholelithiasis in each age group, Navajo and non-Indian.[9]

TABLE 4.—*Incidence of Malignant Neoplasm in 87 Adult Navajo Necropsies*

Type of Carcinoma	No.
Pancreas	3
Gallbladder	3
Kidney	2
Stomach	1
Cervix	1
Breast	1
Ovary	1
Bladder	1
Liver	1
Prostate	1
Meningioma	1
Metastatic abdominal adenocarcinoma	1
Total	17

Comment

While the present study consists of only 87 adult necropsies, which are practically all that are presently available due to the infrequency of autopsy permission and the usual unavailability of qualified pathologists on the reservation, it nevertheless shows that a markedly lower incidence of both coronary and aortic atherosclerosis is in full agreement with clinical studies. The Cornell-Many Farms project has found an incidence of coronary heart disease among the Navajo of 8.0 per thousand compared to 32.9 per thousand in the Framingham Study.[11]

It is our clinical impression that arteriosclerotic peripheral vascular disease among the Navajos is extremely rare. All the cases we have seen clinically have been associated with diabetes. Our autopsy findings agree with this impression.

Cholelithiasis, however, is very common among most Indian tribes. Lam [12] reports that it is the most common surgical condition among the Sioux Indians, I [13] have reported a very high incidence among the Pima Indians of Arizona, and Sievers [17] reports a 32% necropsy incidence in a combined group of many southwestern Indian tribes. Discussions with surgeons from other Indian tribes similarly reveals that there appears to be a universally high incidence of cholelithiasis among American Indians. The reason for this is difficult to ascertain as the etiology of cholelithiasis has not been well established.

The diet of the Navajo,[14] Sioux, and Pima Indians [15] are not identical.

Carcinoma of the gallbladder was the most common form of cancer seen among the Pimas.[13] Sievers [16] evaluated all the cancers from southwestern Indian tribes that are cared for at the Phoenix-Indian Hospital and found carcinoma of the gallbladder third in frequency only less than the incidence of carcinoma of the stomach and cervix. This study also indicates that gallbladder carcinoma is among the most common types of cancer among the Navajo. This is unusual considering the relative rarity of this type of cancer in other groups. However, due to the high incidence of cholelithiasis more gallbladder cancer is seen. The Pima and Southwestern tribe studies showed an incidence of gallbladder carcinoma of 2.9% and 2.0% respectively among the cases of cholelithiasis, which is similar to non-Indian studies. The relatively high incidence of malignancy in this small study suggests that this condition may not be as rare in Indians as has been reported and in this study (which is not statistically significant) appears comparable to other ethnic groups. Bivens [4] similarly has found that the incidence of cervical cancer in the Navajo is identical to other groups.

Since there may be bias in the type of case in which autopsy studies are performed, more autopsy examinations are needed to determine the true incidence of cancer and other diseases among the Navajo, as the existing incomplete vital statistics alone may be misleading.

Summary

A study of 87 adult Navajo necropsies showed no coronary atherosclerosis until the fifth decade and much less than a comparable non-Indian group in the older age groups. Aortic atherosclerosis was similarly less frequent and only 14% of Navajos had moderate to marked atherosclerosis compared to 37% in a non-Indian group. Cholelithiasis in the Navajo, however, is found more than twice as frequent in each age group than in comparable non-Indian groups and consequently, carcinoma of the gallbladder is one of the most common cancers in the Navajo. Malignant neoplasms in this necropsy study appeared as frequent as in similar non-Indian studies and may be more frequent than suggested by our present limited vital statistics.

Frank G. Hesse, MD, Medical Arts Square, Suite 15, Albuquerque, NM 87103.

REFERENCES

1. Smith, R. L.; Salzbury, C. G.; and Gilliam, A. G.: Recorded and Expected Mortality Among Navajos With Special Reference to Cancer, J Nat Cancer Inst 17:77-89, 1956.

2. Young, R. W.; Navajo Yearbook: Report No. VIII, 1951-1961, Window Rock, Ariz: The Navajo Agency, 1961.

3. Salzbury, C. G., et al: Cancer Detection Survey of Carcinoma of Lung and Female Pelvis Among Navajos on Navajo Indian Reservation, Surg Gynec Obstet 108:257-266, 1959.

4. Bivens, M. D., et al: Carcinoma of the Cervix in Indians of Southwest, Amer J Obstet Gynec 83:1203-1207, 1962.

5. Gilbert, J.: Absence of Coronary Thrombosis in Navajo Indians, Calif Med 82:114-115, 1955.

6. Streeper, R. B., et al: Electrocardiographic and Autopsy Study of Coronary Heart Disease in Navajo, Dis Chest 38:305-312, 1960.

7. White, N. K.; Edward, J. E.; and Dry, T. J.: Relationship of Degree of Coronary Atherosclerosis With Age in Man, Circulation 1:645-654, 1950.

8. Willius, F. A.; Smith, H. L.; and Sprague, P. H.: Study of Coronary and Aortic Sclerosis: Incidence and Degree in 5,060 Consecutive Postmortem Examinations, Proc Mayo Clin 8:140-144, 1933.

9. Kozoll, D. D.; Dwyer, G.; and Meyer, K. A.: Pathologic Correlation of Gallstones: Review of 1,874 Autopsies of Patients With Gallstones, AMA Arch Surg 79:514-536, 1959.

10. Kirchoff, H., and Rigdon, R. H.: Frequency of Cancer in White and Negro: Study Based Upon Necropsies, Southern Med J 49:834-841, 1956.

11. Deuschle, K., and Adair, J.: Interdisciplinary Approach to Public Health on Navajo Indian Reservation: Medical and Anthropological Aspect, Ann NY Acad Sci 84:887-905, 1960.

12. Lam, R. E.: Gallbladder Disease Among American Indians, J Lancet 74:305-309, 1954.

13. Hesse, F. G.: Incidence of Cholecystitis and Other Diseases Among Pima Indians of Southern Arizona, JAMA 170:1789-1790, 1959.

14. Darby, W. J., et al: Study of Dietary Background and Nutrition of Navajo Indian, J Nutr (suppl 2) 60:1-85, 1956.

15. Hesse, F. G.: Dietary Study of Pima Indian, Amer J Clin Nutr 7:532-537, 1959.

16. Sievers, M. L., and Cohen, S. L.: Lung Cancer Among Indians of Southwestern United States, Ann Intern Med 54:912-915, 1961.

17. Sievers, M. L., and Marquis, J. R.: Southwestern American Indian's Burden: Biliary Disease, JAMA 182:570-572, 1962.

18. Lieber, M. M.: The Incidence of Gallstones and Their Correlation With Other Diseases, Ann Surg 135:394-405, 1952.

Anomaly of the Vertebral Column (Klippel-Feil Syndrome) in American Aborigines

Saul Jarcho, MD

IN 1912 Klippel and Feil[1] described a case of extensive vertebral anomaly characterized by apparent absence of cervical vertebrae. (A slightly earlier and less complete description was reported by Barclay-Smith.[2] The entire spinal column contained only twelve clearly distinguishable vertebrae, but its uppermost part was an osseous mass evidently formed by the fusion of several vertebral elements. A distinct atlas and axis could not be found. The first four pairs of ribs were partly fused at their origin.

As the Klippel-Feil syndrome was elaborated,[3-5] it was recognized to include marked shortening of the neck, the occiput being near the shoulders; fusions of vertebrae en bloc at various levels of the column; presence of hemivertebrae and fragments; anomalies of ribs; and anomalous segmentation of the spinal cord.

In 1938 Jarcho and Levin[6] described the syndrome in two American Negro children, a sister and a brother, whose mother had a defective fifth cervical lamina. This was the third reported family in which the Klippel-Feil anomaly had occurred in more than one person.

Report of a Case

On June 7, 1940, a 38-year-old woman (MSH-40-3476) presented herself at the Outpatient Department of the Mount Sinai Hospital in New York city for the treatment of pain in the wrist. The extreme shortness of her neck (Fig 1) at once attracted attention and she was recognized to have the Klippel-Feil anomaly. The principal findings were short stature (approximately 139 cm [4 ft 7 in]); long oval head held tilted with chin toward the left; mouth nearly horizontal, high, arched palate;

Reprint requests to 35 E 85th St, New York 10025.

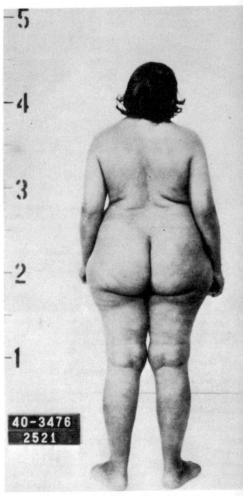

1. Woman of mixed Negro and Cherokee Indian parentage. Note extreme shortness of neck (MSH-40-3476).

neck short; occiput appeared to be resting on shoulders; flexion of neck reduced; prominent right sternomastoid muscle; right clavicle sloping upward and backward more sharply than the left; prominent musculature in left supraspinatus fossa; right shoulder approximately 1.5 cm higher than the left; right nipple approximately 1.5 cm lower than the left. Roentgen examinations, ported on June 21 and Sept 16, 1940, by H. G. Jackson, MD, and A. Melamed, MD, revealed bilateral cervical ribs articulating with the first thoracic ribs; fusion of third, fourth, and fifth cervical bodies and of first and second thoracic bodies; incomplete fusion of posterior arches of sixth and seventh cervical vertebrae; second and third thoracic vertebrae defective; moderate scoliosis of lower cervical and upper thoracic spine, convex to the left; scoliotic deformity in middle lumbar area.

The patient at first appeared to be an American Negro, but her skin was of atypical coppery hue. She was born in Charleston, SC, in 1902 to an American Negro mother and a full-blooded Cherokee Indian father. The latter died in 1937 at the age of 74. The patient

162

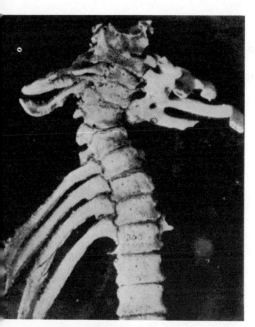

2. Specimen from Paucarcancha, Peru. Note fusion of vertebrae, presence of hemivertebrae, and partial fusion of ribs. (From MacCurdy[7])

Negro-Cherokee sibship described, points to the presence of the Klippel-Feil anomaly in the aboriginal population of the Western Hemisphere over a period of many centuries.

This investigation was supported in part by Public Health Service research grant GM-06392.

Figure 2 is reproduced with permission from the *American Journal of Physical Anthropology* and Wistar Institute, Philadelphia.

References

1. Klippel, M., and Feil, A.: Un cas d'absence des vertèbres cervicales, *Nouv Iconog Salpetriere* **25**:223-250 (May-June) 1912.

2. Barclay-Smith, E.: Multiple Anomaly in Vertebral Column, *J Anat Physiol* **45**:144-171 (Jan) 1911.

3. Lohmüller, W.: Zur Frage angeborener Wirbelsynostosen und primärer angeborener Skoliosen, *Deutsch Z Chir* **242** (No. 11-12):714-722, 1934.

4. Kühne, K.: Die Verebung der Variationen der menschlichen Wirbelsäule, *Z Morph Anthrop* **30** (Heft 1-2):1-221, 1932.

5. Van der Sar, A.: Hereditary Multiple Hemivertebrae, *Docum Med Geog Trop* **4**:23-28 (March) 1952.

6. Jarcho, S., and Levin, P.: Hereditary Malformation of Vertebral Bodies, *Bull Hopkins Hosp* **62**:216-226 (March) 1938.

7. MacCurdy, G.G.: Human Skeletal Remains From Highlands of Peru, *Amer J Phys Anthrop* **6**:217-330 (July-Sept) 1923.

~en of abnormally short stature since childhood but had ~ffered no inconvenience attributable to this. Her father's ~andmother, an American Indian, had a shortened neck; ~is was confirmed by correspondence with the patient's ~other. No other member of the family is known to have ~d a similar anomaly.

In 1923 MacCurdy[7] published his well-known ~udy. In this contribution Plate 44 (Fig 2) is ~ptioned as follows:

~ucarcancha. Adult Male. Very early injury to spinal ~lumn resulting in lateral curvature; fusion of neck ~rtebrae and of ribs; presence of two wedge-shaped ~pernumerary vertebrae; 13 rib scars on the right side; ~e first four ribs on the left side are fused with the ~rtebrae.

In the accompanying text[7(p 261)] Dr. MacCurdy ~marks that the case

~obably has more to do with teratology than with trauma- ~m . . . the vertebrae from the sixth or seventh cervical ~, and including, the twelfth thoracic are still united. ~e first three of the series are fused. . . . At the level of ~e third right rib there is a wedge-shaped undeveloped ~pernumerary vertebra; and at the level of the fifth rib ~ the same side there is a second wedge-shaped un- ~veloped supernumerary vertebra.

It is quite clear that Dr. MacCurdy's specimen ~hibits the principal features of the Klippel-Feil ~omaly, viz, fusion of vertebrae en bloc, with re- ~ction in number; hemivertebrae; and partial fu- ~on of ribs at their origin. (A search for the speci- ~en, conducted with the assistance of friends in ~ew Haven and Lima, has thus far proved fruit- ~ss.) This case, taken together with that of the

Cholecysto-Gastric Fistula Masquerading as Carcinoma of the Stomach

ROBERT E. KRAVETZ, M.D., ALFRED S. GILMORE, M.D., F.A.C.S.

INTESTINAL obstruction due to gallstones is not rare; [1, 7, 9, 15, 16] the etiology, however, is recognized less than one-third of the time.[5] The incidence of gallstone ileus in hospital patients has been estimated at 1 to 2 per cent [7, 9] and it is almost invariably due to biliary-enteric fistula formation. Most frequent sites of fistula formation are the duodenum, colon, jejunum, and stomach. An unusual case of complicated cholecystitis with associated gastric obstruction masquerading as carcinoma of the antrum of the stomach due to gallstones is presented.

Case Report

A 51-year-old Apache woman was admitted to the USPHS Indian Hospital, Phoenix, with progressive nausea, anorexia, weight loss, epigastric pain, and postprandial vomiting. The pain was nonradiating, increased with eating, and was relieved by vomiting. There was no specific food intolerance and only recent mild constipation. She was hospitalized for two weeks at the reservation hospital and was noted to have an enlarged nodular liver and a low grade fever. All laboratory studies of liver function were normal. She had consumed large amounts of alcohol for several years until five years prior to admission.

On physical examination, the vital signs were normal and she was in no acute distress. There was scleral injection, but no icterus. Mild epigastric tenderness was noted without any palpable mass. An irregular, firm, nodular liver edge descended 5 cm. below the right costal margin. There were signs of moderate weight loss.

Urine specific gravity was 1.016, one plus albuminuria, and 8–10 white blood cells per high powered field were found. Hemoglobin was 12.1 Gm./100 ml., and white blood cell count 12,100, with 77 per cent segmented forms, 6 per cent bands, 15 per cent lymphocytes, and 2 per cent eosinophiles. Blood urea nitrogen was 47.5 mg./100 ml. on admission and subsequently 12 mg./100 ml. Fasting blood sugar was 112 mg./100 ml.

The serum cholesterol was 132 mg./100 ml. Serum-glutamic-oxaloacetic-transaminase was 81 units, and serum-glutamic-pyruvic-transaminase was 70 units/100 ml. Prothrombin time was 50 per cent of normal activity. Alkaline phosphatase was 30.9 Shinowara-Jones units/100 ml. (normal 2.8–8.6). A postoperative determination was 8.9 units/100 ml.

The admission diagnostic impression was carcinoma of the stomach with metastases to the liver. An initial upper gastro-intestinal x-ray examination was unsatisfactory because of retained secretions. After 24 hours of gastric suction, repeat examination films revealed a stenosing antral lesion. The stomach was not distensible (Fig. 1). The three-hour study showed some contrast material in the small bowel, but 80 to 90 per cent was retained in the stomach. Radiographic interpretation was carcinoma of the stomach with partial obstruction.

At laparotomy, the omentum, large bowel, and stomach were markedly indurated forming a single mass with an organized exudate over the entire right upper quadrant. After careful dissection, the gallbladder was found adherent to the antrum of the stomach and connected to it by a cholecysto-gastric fistula which admitted one finger. Multiple small gallstones were found both in the gallbladder and impacted in the antrum of the stomach obstructing the pylorus (Fig. 2). Cholecystectomy was performed, and the gastric fistula repaired. A stomach tube was introduced into the duodenum through a narrowed indurated antrum.

164

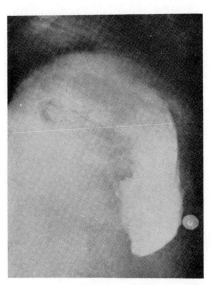

Fig. 1. Gastro-intestinal x-ray examination revealing stenosing antral lesion.

Pathological examination revealed a 6 × 3 cm. thickened gallbladder. The mucosa was ulcerated and edematous with acute and chronic inflammatory changes. Extensive fibropurulent exudate covered the serosal surface. Adjacent peritoneal fibrous and adipose tissue showed extensive chronic inflammatory changes. There was no evidence of carcinoma. A culture taken from the gallbladder at the time of operation was sterile.

The postoperative course was uneventful. On an upper gastro-intestinal x-ray examination performed 26 days after operation there was a constant deformity of the antrum, and the duodenal cap was deformed and spastic. The impression was that of severe antro-duodenitis (Fig. 3). Three months after operation the patient was completely asymptomatic, but has not been able to return for further gastro-intestinal x-ray examination.

Discussion

Perforation of the gallbladder may occur in one of the following ways: 1) into the peritoneal cavity with peritonitis; 2) into adhesions about the gallbladder bed forming a pericholecystic, or subhepatic abscess; or 3) into an adjacent hollow viscus forming a biliary-enteric fistula. These cate-gories are usually referred to as Type I, II, and III of Niemeier.[10, 14] Type III (biliary-enteric fistula) perforation accounts for 19 to 32 per cent of all perforations of the gallbladder with most series supporting the lower figure.[4, 5, 14]

Fistula formation usually follows repeated attacks of acute cholecystitis (obstructive) during which time the serosal surface of the gallbladder becomes inflamed and adheres to the adjacent viscera. With repeated attacks, the ampulla of the gallbladder is obstructed, the arterial supply is reduced, and the venous and lymphatic drainage is compromised; this results in an ischemic wall of the organ and increased intraluminal pressure. The ischemic area becomes necrotic with perforation most commonly occurring at the fundus. The adherent adjacent inflamed intestinal wall is finally penetrated, completing the fistulous tract and resulting in an internal cholecystostomy and decompression.[14]

This condition occurs in older patients, more frequently in women, with a long history of chronic cholecystitis, but not invariably so. Perforation is usually silent, and is frequently followed by decrease in symptoms unless intestinal obstruction intervenes. Biliary-enteric fistulas may be suspected preoperatively, an unexpected finding at cholecystectomy, or associated with intestinal obstruction.

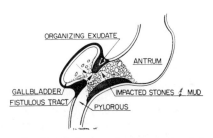

Fig. 2. Artist's conception of operative findings: note biliary gastric fistula and impacted stones in antrum causing obstruction.

The radiographic findings originally outlined by Rigler,[12] if present, should arouse suspicion. They are: 1) visualization of a calculus outside the gallbladder; 2) air or contrast media in the biliary tree; and 3) change of position of a previously observed calculus, especially if the findings are associated with intestinal obstruction. Occasionally a patient may claim that a stone has been vomited or passed per rectum.

Stones are most frequently associated with the fistula and were present in 37 of 40 cases reported by Glenn and Mannix[5] with carcinoma the basis for fistula in the remaining three. Acute noncalculus cholecystitis may rarely cause a fistula.[14] When intestinal obstruction occurs, it usually is in the last 50 cm. of the terminal ileum. In one series of 179 patients with gallstone ileus, 72 per cent of the stones were removed from the ileum, 17 per cent from the jejunum, and 11 per cent from the stomach, duodenum and colon.[1] Four per cent of stones are initially present in the stomach, but may be passed to a more distal point.[2, 3]

One similar report, in which a subacute perforation of the gallbladder with subhepatic abscess simulated a carcinoma of the antrum of the stomach, is noted.[11] In both patients, a preoperative diagnosis of carcinoma of the stomach was suspected, but the findings were subsequently found to be due to complications of a perforated gallbladder. A biliary-enteric fistula was not found in the previously reported patient and this case would be classified as Type II (subacute perforation with abscess formation).

In the present report, no history of previous gastro-intestinal symptoms suggestive of cholecystitis could be elicited, but there was some language barrier. The presenting complaints were highly suggestive of carcinoma of the stomach. This diagnosis was strengthened by palpation of the nodular right upper quadrant mass by at least eight independent observers and thought to rep-

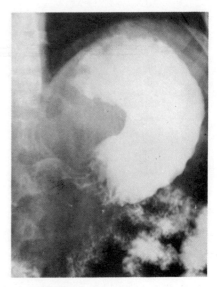

Fig. 3. Postoperative gastro-intestinal x-ray examination showing deformity of antrum of stomach and duodenal bulb.

resent metastatic disease to the liver by all. The elevated alkaline phosphatase and radiographic findings further supported this diagnosis.

The supposed nodular liver was actually organized exudate in the right upper quadrant. Elevation of the alkaline phosphatase in the absence of hyperbilirubinemia may occur in an occasional case of cholecystitis and may be the first clue to a silent common duct stone.[6] Conceivably this patient passed a stone lodged in the common duct prior to surgery. Intrahepatic obstruction was also a consideration, but there was no evidence to support this.

Biliary tract disease is extremely common in Southwestern American Indians with a recent autopsy study reporting an incidence of 52 per cent in adults over 21.[8] Cholecystectomy is the most frequent major surgical procedure performed at this hospital with cholecystitis the commonest cause of acute abdominal disease.[13] De-

166

spite the general awareness by the staff of these facts, biliary tract disease was not considered in this patient because the preoperative findings seemed to be so suggestive of carcinoma of the stomach.

The importance of establishing a tissue diagnosis in every case of suspected carcinoma, no matter how unequivocal the clinical findings may appear, is apparent.

Summary

A patient with chronic cholecystitis, perforation of the gallbladder, and biliary-enteric fistula with a pericholecystic abscess simulating carcinoma of the antrum of the stomach is reported.

The types of perforations of the gallbladder, acute, subacute, and chronic (Types I, II, and III of Niemeier), are listed and the pathogenesis of fistula formation is described.

A history of chronic cholecystitis in an elderly adult with a symptom free period and recurrence of symptoms suggests fistula formation. The radiographic findings of biliary-enteric fistula formation are recounted.

The remarkably high incidence of biliary tract disease (52%) in adult Southwestern American Indians is noted.

Stress is placed upon the importance of establishing a tissue diagnosis in every case of suspected carcinoma, no matter how strong the clinical evidence may appear.

References

1. Brockis, J. G. and M. C. Gilber: Intestinal Obstruction by Gallstones: Review of 179 Cases. Brit. J. Surg.. 44:461, 1957.
2. Chamberlain, B. E.: Incomplete Cholecystogastric Fistula. Amer. J. Surg., 90:153, 1955.
3. DeFoe, E. and S. C. Meigher: Gallstones Impacted in the Stomach and Duodenal Bulb Demonstrated by Roentgenologic Examination. Amer. J. Radiol., 77:40, 1957.
4. Fletcher, A. G., Jr. and I. S. Ravdin: Perforation of Gallbladder. Amer. J. Surg., 81:178, 1951.
5. Glenn, F. and H. Mannix, Jr.: Biliary Enteric Fistula. Surg., Gynec. & Obst., 105:693, 1957.
6. Gutman, A. B.: Serum Alkaline Phosphatase Activity in Disease of the Skeletal and Hepatobiliary Systems. Amer. J. Med., 27:875, 1959.
7. Kirkland, K. C. and E. J. Croce: Gallstone Intestinal Obstruction. J.A.M.A., 176:494, 1961.
8. Kravetz, R. E.: Autopsy Findings in Southwestern American Indians: Review of 211 Cases. Arizona Medicine.
9. McLaughlin, C. W., Jr. and M. Raines: Obstruction of Alimentary Tract from Gallstones. Amer. J. Surg., 81:424, 1951.
10. Miemeier, O. W.: Acute Perforation of the Gallbladder. Amer. J. Surg., 94:772, 1957.
11. Reskoe, J. Y., D. T. Varga and M. M. Stanley: Subacute Perforation of the Gallbladder with Subhepatic Abscess Simulating Carcinoma of the Antrum of the Stomach in a Patient with Pernicious Anemia. J. Kentucky St. Med. A., 59:752, 1961.
12. Rigler, L. G., C. N. Borman and J. F. Noble: Gallstone Obstruction: Pathogenesis and Roentgen Manifestations. J.A.M.A., 117: 1753, 1941.
13. Sievers, M. L. and J. R. Marquis: The Southwestern American Indian's Burden: Biliary Disease. J.A.M.A., 182:570, 1962.
14. Strohl, E. L., W. G. Diffenbaugh, J. H. Baker and M. H. Cheema: Gangrene and Perforation of the Gallbladder. Surg., Gynec. & Obst., 114:1, 1962.
15. Thomas, S. H., J. K. Cherry and B. D. Averbook: Gallstone Ileus. J.A.M.A., 179:625, 1962.
16. Wakfield, E. G., P. M. Vickers and W. Walters: Intestinal Obstruction Caused by Gallstones. Surgery, 5:670, 1939.

An Emotional and Educational Experience for Urban Migrants

BY ROBERT L. LEON, M.D., HARRY W. MARTIN, PH.D.,
AND JOHN H. GLADFELTER, PH.D.

MANY PRINCIPLES and methods developed by psychiatry and other behavioral sciences dealing with human behavior are as applicable in community programs as they are in clinics, and these principles and methods can be used for prevention as well as treatment. This paper illustrates how a team consisting of a psychiatrist, a sociologist, and a clinical psychologist working as consultants to a federal agency was able to develop a program which applied behavioral science theory and methods to the problem of reducing the stress of urban migration.

The Employment Assistance Branch of the Bureau of Indian Affairs has for the last 14 years been helping Indians and Alaskan natives who request this help to relocate to large cities where they may have greater employment opportunities. Some go directly into employment and others first take vocational training before being employed. Funds for transportation to the city and subsistence while the person is in training or seeking employment are provided by the Bureau of Indian Affairs. Many, though by no means all, of the Alaskan Indians and Eskimos who choose to leave are from isolated areas where they have had little or no opportunity to learn the complexities of a modern American city. Although a large number of the migrants are high school graduates, many have less education and very few have attended college. Both single individuals and married couples with children are relocated; almost all are young adults in their late teens and early 20s. Some adjust well, many have adjustment problems which are worked out with the help of the Bureau of Indian Affairs staff in the destination cities, and some develop or bring with them severe problems which necessitate their return to the reservation.

The Seattle Orientation Center[1] was con-

The authors wish to thank Mr. Walter J. Knodel, Chief, Employment Assistance Branch, Bureau of Indian Affairs, for the opportunity to participate in the development of the Seattle Orientation Center, and Mrs. Jimmie Owens, Director of the Center.

[1]The center is physically located in a motel; the clients live in the motel apartments. Staff offices are across a courtyard from the apartments. The motel is adjacent to a shopping center and convenient to bus lines.

ceived by the Bureau of Indian Affairs as a way station for Alaskan natives en route to the large cities in the lower 48 states. Indians, Eskimos, and Aleuts stay two to six weeks, or occasionally longer, until they and the staff feel they can cope fairly comfortably with urban living. The Bureau of Indian Affairs saw the center's purpose as educational and supportive. Many who come are anxious and bewildered and experience what appears to be a feeling of depersonalization when they find themselves alone for the first time on the busy streets of a large city.

Most Eskimos have spent their lives in small villages in western Alaska where they have had close personal relationships with extended families and others in the village. When one Eskimo was asked if he had ever been to a city, he replied, "Yes, I've been to Bethel." Bethel is a town of about 1,500 population. When out hunting and fishing an Eskimo man might be alone or with a few comrades for several days. Airplanes, radios, and boats are familiar to Eskimos; cars, buses, and telephones are strange. For three weeks the staff of the Seattle Orientation Center were unsuccessful in trying to get a shy Eskimo girl to dial a number on a telephone. Finally she summoned enough courage to ask, "How do you dial the dash?"

When an Eskimo or Alaskan Indian is accepted for relocation, he is picked up by a bush pilot in a four-place plane which lands on the river with pontoons in the summer or skis in the winter and flown to the largest nearby town where he takes a commercial plane, usually to Anchorage or Fairbanks. There he boards a jet and in a matter of hours is in a city like Denver, Dallas, San Francisco, Los Angeles, or Chicago. At home he knew and spoke to everyone. Here he knows no one. Few speak or smile. If a person did not speak or smile at home, that meant he was angry.

Migration creates anxiety, demands new skills, and threatens the identity of the migrant. Indeed, the migrant probably undergoes a temporary disruption of the ego and partial loss of identity(1), and to regain his identity he has to experience himself "as something that has continuity"(2).

Weinberg(3), in the conclusion to *Migration and Belonging*, states:

. . . there exists a remarkable similarity between the needs of the new immigrant with those of the newborn human being. The need for belonging, the need to be loved, understood and supported, but not to be dominated, pampered or spoiled, these needs are similar to those enabling the child to develop to a sound, mature person.

A program to aid migrants in making the transition from rural to urban living should meet the emotional needs of the migrant, reduce anxiety, help to restore identity, and provide an opportunity to learn the new skills necessary to urban living.

In the Seattle Orientation Center, Alaskan natives are given the opportunity to learn to find and ride the correct bus. Their first bus ride is with a staff member, perhaps to the zoo or a museum. After this, clients ride buses unaccompanied by staff. They learn to read city maps in the office and in automobiles, where they use the map to direct a staff driver to a predetermined destination. They shop in a supermarket and prepare the sometimes strange foods in the kitchenettes of their motel apartments. Staff members take clients to restaurants to acquaint them with ordering from a menu.

Clients learn to use a telephone, household appliances, and indoor plumbing if they do not already know; and practice banking, budgeting their money, and paying rent. They are introduced to the recreational facilities of a community. They visit industries to learn about various occupations and how to apply for a job by actually making application to several of the major companies in Seattle who are cooperating with the program. All of these learning experiences are straightforward and obviously needed, albeit frequently overlooked, in helping individuals adjust to new situations.

The new learning is important, but it is equally if not more important to deal with clients' anxiety and to help them maintain their identity in the face of potentially depersonalizing experiences. This is accomplished within the context of a modified therapeutic community where clients are encouraged to express feelings in group and individual discussion. Each day begins with a group session led by the director who, while not a mental health professional, has had some training and experience in group dynamics. New arrivals are asked to tell about their home in Alaska, and throughout their stay they are encouraged to relate and contrast new experiences with those at home. The inevitable grief reaction which accompanies leaving home and close relationships is expressed rather than suppressed. Hostility, which is frequently directed toward Bureau of Indian Affairs staff, is accepted by the staff.

Following each new experience is a brief discussion in groups or individually with staff. Again during these discussions the clients are encouraged to talk about the feelings aroused by the experiences. As time approaches for clients to move on to their destination cities their heightened anxiety is acknowledged. An attempt is made to prepare them for what they will experience in the new locale. Those clients who have greater anxiety and have more problems adjusting are given additional time by staff. They may spend the greater part of a day in a staff member's office, where they help with various tasks and receive support from an accepting staff member.

Not all Alaskans come through the Seattle Orientation Center. Those who are better educated and have spent some time in a metropolitan area may go directly from Alaska to their destination city, although some of these individuals have spent time at the center and have found it useful. For the most part, those who come through have had little or no urban living experience. Most have no manifest behavior or personal problems.[2] It was clearly specified that this was not to be a rehabilitation center. Occasionally a client who does have obvious problems but is felt to have a fair chance to adjust to the city is sent to the center.

Discussion

Benefits derived by the clients must await systematic evaluation; the nature of the consultation request did not permit building such evaluation into the program. We have talked with and received reports from many Alaskans who felt their experience at the

center was beneficial, but these are only anecdotal. It would be desirable to compare the urban adjustment of those who come through the center with a control group.

What remains to be discussed are some principles related to working with government agencies in developing community programs. Methods and techniques of mental health consultation are, of course, an important part of such working relationships, but they are not sufficient when a professional is called upon to develop and to a limited extent supervise the functioning of a new program. Here he must knowingly depart from the consultation role and become more directive, recognizing the risks that this departure entails. More and more we will be called upon to work with untrained people who staff community health and welfare programs. We might prefer that these programs be staffed with professionals, but if they are not, are we to turn our backs on them? If we are to be of help, we must be more directive than we have been in consultation with other professionals.

The application of behavioral sciences methodology to designing programs aimed at improving human welfare is in itself somewhat unusual. Not that program planners are unsystematic, but they often do not understand the relationship of personality and social factors. For example, the Bureau of Indian Affairs wisely arranged for us to have a brief but intensive tour of Alaska in order to obtain a firsthand picture of life in that state. It took us several days after our arrival in Alaska to communicate to our hosts that we did not merely want to see villages but that we wanted to interview Eskimos and Indians to learn why they wanted to relocate, what they expected, what were their fears, and how they felt about the Bureau of Indian Affairs. There was no resistance to this, but it is not usual for visitors brought in by public agencies to make such a request; thus, it was not expected that this would be our primary interest.

The anthropological literature is helpful background information, but much of it is not directly useful to Bureau of Indian Affairs program planners because the literature discusses the Alaskan native culture as it existed several decades ago. It is im-

---

[2]Many do have mild or moderate psychiatric problems, but the focus is on functioning in society rather than on psychopathology.

portant to investigate the present problems of Eskimo and Indian cultures, particularly as they relate to the dominant white culture. It is important to know, for example, that the Southeastern Indians would prefer to fish for salmon in the summer but that this cannot be a livelihood for many because salmon are getting to be in short supply. Or it is important to kno · that Eskimos must now have a license to hunt whereas for centuries they have hunted at will and that the duck and geese eggs are no longer to be gathered for food because sportsmen in the states to the south need a good crop for their autumn hunting. In addition, it is interesting that some Eskimo and Indian girls state that they prefer to marry white men because they believe that they will have more beautiful children.

The behavioral scientist's knowledge of human behavior not only allows him to interpret the data he has gathered and predict how clients will react to the program he recommends, but gives him the authority to encourage and help untrained staff with a vital but most often neglected aspect of program—the recognition and expression of feelings. When untrained workers see hostility, anxiety, and grief in clients, they often turn away and communicate that these feelings should be suppressed. The clients' suppressed feelings tend to block necessary learning. Sometimes in order to establish such programs administrators and staff must be told that it is necessary to work with their own feelings about this.

During its operation the center has had numerous visitors. The reactions of the visitors usually fall into one of two groups, one reporting an immediate feeling of warmth and acceptance, the other, although its members may sense the warmth and acceptance, expressing concern over the relaxed and *seemingly* unstructured approach. This latter group would change group discussions to lectures and support to authority. Such a change would immediately shift the prevailing atmosphere, which is an essential part of the design and a great credit to the center's staff, who were able to capture what were to them essentially new concepts of human behavior and put them into action. One Alaskan, after being at the center a while, summed it all up by saying, "I didn't know the BIA cared about me this much."

Summary

This program illustrates the application of behavioral science knowledge to a center for urban migrants. The work of the center is preventive. Education in urban living takes place within a modified therapeutic community so as to promote learning at both the affective and cognitive level in order to prevent possible disorganization and regression which might result from a gross stress reaction precipitated by the migration.

REFERENCES

1. Cumming, J., and Cumming, E.: Ego and Milieu. New York: Atherton Press, 1962.
2. Erikson, E. H.: Childhood and Society. New York: W. W. Norton & Co., 1963.
3. Weinberg, A. A.: Migration and Belonging. The Hague: Nijhoff, 1961.

Effects of High Dietary Calcium and Phosphorus on Calcium, Phosphorus, Nitrogen and Fat Metabolism in Children

Leo Lutwak, m.d., ph.d., Leonard Laster, m.d., Hillel J. Gitelman, m.d., Maurice Fox, m.d. and G. Donald Whedon, m.d., with the technical assistance of Dorothy E. Wolfe, b.a. and Minnie L. Woodson, b.a.

Much controversy exists concerning man's dietary requirements for calcium. Some insist that present recommendations for adequate intakes are much too high[1] and should be lowered; others suggest that these levels are too low and that the average intake should be increased, at least for some persons.[2] Recent studies from this laboratory[3,4] and others[5,6] have shown that considerable variation exists from person to person in the level of dietary calcium needed to maintain balance. Furthermore, of interest is the observation[3] that in some persons an increase in dietary calcium beyond 1,200 to 1,600 mg. per day may actually decrease the absolute retention of calcium.

For optimal nutrition, a daily dietary intake of 1.0 gm. of calcium has been recommended for American children,[7] but the possibility of advising even higher intakes has been raised.[8] No deleterious effects have been observed in man as a result of prolonged intakes of large amounts of dietary calcium[9] but, on the other hand, neither have any benefits been demonstrated.

Recently, as part of a long range study of the effects of high dietary phosphate on dental caries,[10] a group of children became available who presumably had been receiving diets high in calcium and phosphorus for periods of from one to two years. The present report is concerned with the effects of these diets on metabolic balances of minerals and nitrogen in eighteen children from this study.

EXPERIMENTAL METHODS

Subjects and Procedures

In September 1959, a study of the possible role of dibasic calcium phosphate in preventing dental caries was initiated in eight boarding schools associated with Sioux Indian reservations in North and South Dakota, under the sponsorship of the National Institute of Dental Research and the National Institute of Arthritis and Metabolic Diseases of the National Institutes of Health, the Division of Indian Health of the Public Health Service and the Bureau of Indian Affairs of the Department of the Interior with the advice and guidance of the Food and Nutrition Board of the National Research Council. A total of approximately 3,600 children between the ages of six and fourteen years participated in the study. During the nine month school year the children received all their meals at the schools. Each school followed a master menu. The children in some of the schools were control subjects continuing their customary dietary intake; those in the other group ate a similar diet, differing only in the nature of the bread supplied. A special bread was baked with a mix containing added dibasic calcium phosphate which produced a product whose taste and texture were indistinguishable from that of the bread given the control group.

In the spring of 1961 a total of eighteen girls was selected on a random basis from both groups of

TABLE I
Subjects Studied

Subject	Age		Height (cm.)	Weight (kg.)	Body Surface (sq. M.)	Alkaline Phosphatase (King-Armstrong units)	Intestinal Parasites
	yr.	mo.					
Group A							
R. A.	10	11	141.5	31.3	1.12	28	+
A. F.	10	5	134.5	31.0	1.08	31	+
B. G.	10	3	136.0	29.1	1.05	22	−
V. L.	9	10	130.0	27.4	1.01	34	−
C. S.	10	2	142.0	40.2	1.25	50	+
R. S.	8	0*	124.5	23.5	0.90	29	+
A. W.	10	4	137.6	33.1	1.13	33	+
K. W.	10	3	140.2	34.1	1.16	36	+
S. W.	10	3	135.0	31.3	1.08	36	+
Z. W.	9	9	136.6	31.5	1.10	23	+
Average	10	0	135.8	31.3	1.09	32	8 of 10
Group B							
L. B.	9	8	132.4	27.2	1.01	36	+
J. E.	9	10	132.8	31.2	1.07	22	−
R. E.	9	7	133.4	29.6	1.05	42	+
G. F.	11	8	132.5	30.2	1.05	31	−
B. M.	10	7	144.8	44.8	1.33	44	+
R. M.	8	10	132.0	31.6	1.07	28	+
B. W.	9	6	134.7	29.3	1.05	40	+
M. W.	9	9	135.0	30.9	1.08	29	−
Average	9	11	134.7	31.9	1.09	35	5 of 8

NOTE: + = present; − = absent.
* This subject was over eight years of age, but the number of months is not known.

schools using the following criteria: (1) absence of history of illness; (2) continued attendance at the same school for at least one year; (3) normal preliminary physical examination; and (4) parental approval for travel to the National Institutes of Health. [Subsequently, one child (C. S.) was found to have had surgical correction of a congenital heart lesion in infancy, but no evidence of disturbed cardiac function was detectable.]

Ten girls were from schools receiving the supplemented bread (group A), and eight were control subjects (group B). All were evaluated on admission by complete physical examination, blood and urine analyses, electrocardiogram and chest roentgenograms; the results of these examinations were within accepted normal limits except for the presence of occasional asymptomatic intestinal parasitic infestations and blood alkaline phosphatase concen-

trations in excess of reported standards.[11-13] (The mean alkaline phosphatase levels in the two groups were not statistically different.) The physical characteristics and preliminary laboratory studies for each subject are summarized in Table I.

Both groups received diets identical in every respect except for the bread (Chart I). A single menu

CHART I
Diet

Content	Group A	Group B
Calories...............	2,545	2,545
Protein (gm.)............	85.4	85.4
Carbohydrate (gm.).......	283.2	283.2
Fat (gm.)...............	119.0	119.0
Calcium (gm.)...........	2.286	1.295
Phosphorus (gm.).........	2.361	1.593

CHART II
Menu

Daily Menu	Weight (gm.)
Breakfast	
Orange juice	125
Cornflakes®*	15
Butter*	75†
Bread	225
Egg	55
Lunch	
Ground top round beef	60
Rice	14
Peaches	50
Vanilla ice cream	50
Milk	200
Mid-afternoon	
Bread	225
Milk	200
Dinner	
Chicken breast	60
Corn	75
Pineapple	40
Hard candy	15
Milk	200
Bedtime	
Coca-Cola®	200
Bread	225
Jelly	15

* Low sodium.
† For entire day.

was provided, and all meals were totally consumed (Chart II). The subjects were under continuous supervision on the metabolic regimen of the National Institute of Arthritis and Metabolic Diseases Metabolism Unit, as described previously;[14] distilled water was used for drinking and cooking, and a calcium-free dentifrice was provided for oral hygiene. All stools and urine were collected for analysis.

After four days of indoctrination and instruction in metabolic study conduct, a nonabsorbable stool marker was administered; this was repeated four times at six day intervals. A longer period of preliminary adjustment was not used since each child was placed on a regimen of calcium and phosphorus intake similar to that she had been receiving during the preceding year.

Laboratory Methods

All urine was analyzed for creatinine,[15] calcium,[16] phosphorus[17] and nitrogen.[18] All stools were analyzed for calcium, phosphorus, nitrogen and fat.[19] A representative diet for each menu was prepared every four weeks, homogenized and analyzed for fat, calcium, phosphorus and nitrogen. Analyses agreed

with values calculated from tables within 10 per cent. Blood chemistries were measured by the Clinical Chemistry Laboratory of the Clinical Center by standard technics.

RESULTS

The urinary and fecal excretions, the balances of calcium, phosphorus and nitrogen, and the fecal excretions of fat are listed in Table II for the two groups, with the accompanying standard deviations for the values. Individual values are recorded for each subject in Table III. Results were analyzed statistically for significance of difference between the two groups by the analysis of variance developed by Fisher and Yates.[20]

Urinary excretions of calcium were not statistically different in the two groups despite the marked difference in dietary calcium. Fecal excretions of calcium differed significantly in accordance with the dietary intake. Calcium balance was significantly more positive among the subjects in group B (lower calcium and phosphorus intake).

Urinary and fecal excretions of phosphorus differed significantly between the groups, parallel to the dietary intake. As was the case for calcium balance, phosphorus balance was significantly more positive in the group receiving the lower intake (group B).

Urinary and fecal excretions of nitrogen and the resulting nitrogen balances were the same in the two groups, demonstrating independence of nitrogen metabolism from metabolism of calcium and phosphorus.

Fecal fat, on the other hand, was significantly higher in the group receiving larger amounts of dietary calcium and phosphorus as were calcium and phosphorus balances in this study. Figure 1 shows the relationship between calcium balance and fecal excretion of fat plotted for individual six day stool collections. The calculated regression equation obtained for these data is

fecal fat = 4.07 − 3.3 × calcium balance

both fat and calcium expressed as grams per day. The regression coefficient (b) was −3.3 gm. calcium and the calculated correlation coefficient (r) was −0.522. The statistical

TABLE II
Daily Intake, Excretion and Balance in Groups A and B

Dietary Content (gm.)	Urinary Excretion (gm.)	Fecal Excretion (gm.)	Balance (gm.)
	Group A		
Calcium, 2.286	0.180 ± 0.046	2.109 ± 0.095*	−0.003 ± 0.076†
Phosphorus, 2.361	1.277 ± 0.208*	0.944 ± 0.158*	+0.140 ± 0.093†
Nitrogen, 13.66	10.12 ± 0.76	0.76 ± 0.21	+2.73 ± 0.73
Fat, 110.0	...	4.93 ± 0.73†	...
	Group B		
Calcium, 1.295	0.192 ± 0.062	0.830 ± 0.116*	+0.272 ± 0.112†
Phosphorus, 1.593	0.903 ± 0.131*	0.334 ± 0.076*	+0.356 ± 0.111†
Nitrogen, 13.66	10.14 ± 1.16	0.65 ± 0.18	+2.83 ± 1.14
Fat, 119.0	...	2.44 ± 0.61†	...

* Probability difference due to chance < 0.001.
† Probability difference due to chance < 0.01.

TABLE III
Average Daily Excretions and Balances for Twenty-Four Days in Groups A and B

Subject	Calcium (gm.)			Phosphorus (gm.)			Nitrogen (gm.)			Fecal Fat (gm.)
	Urine	Feces	Balance	Urine	Feces	Balance	Urine	Feces	Balance	
				Group A						
R. A.	0.161	2.220	−0.095	1.308	1.020	+0.033	11.03	0.62	+2.02	4.5
A. F.	0.224	2.034	+0.028	1.136	1.010	+0.215	9.53	0.69	+3.44	1.5
B. G.	0.163	2.043	+0.080	1.071	1.014	+0.276	9.90	0.49	+2.75	2.5
V. L.	0.229	2.084	−0.027	1.325	0.915	+0.121	10.23	0.77	+2.68	7.7
C. S.	0.244	2.034	+0.008	1.207	0.910	+0.244	9.93	0.71	+2.95	5.4
R. S.	0.134	2.196	−0.044	1.128	1.170	+0.063	10.14	0.92	+2.60	5.1
A. W.	0.202	1.955	+0.129	1.692	0.655	+0.014	10.94	0.73	+1.97	6.4
K. W.	0.161	2.244	−0.119	1.216	0.993	+0.152	8.56	0.74	+4.36	5.4
S. W.	0.185	2.125	−0.024	1.586	0.701	+0.074	10.97	0.65	+2.04	7.6
Z. W.	0.095	2.157	+0.034	1.097	1.055	+0.209	9.92	1.27	+2.49	3.2
Average	0.180	2.109	−0.003	1.277	0.944	+0.140	10.12	0.76	+2.73	4.9
				Group B						
L. B.	0.269	0.941	+0.085	1.066	0.359	+0.168	11.53	0.35	+1.34	3.6
S. E.	0.189	0.832	+0.274	0.830	0.371	+0.392	9.26	0.81	+3.59	2.9
R. E.	0.131	0.825	+0.339	0.785	0.287	+0.521	8.53	0.74	+4.39	1.6
G. F.	0.088	1.011	+0.196	0.683	0.492	+0.418	8.81	0.68	+4.23	2.1
B. M.	0.244	0.625	+0.426	0.903	0.275	+0.415	10.96	0.42	+2.28	2.1
R. M.	0.166	0.750	+0.379	0.946	0.260	+0.387	10.01	0.89	+2.75	2.5
B. W.	0.256	0.848	+0.191	1.044	0.290	+0.259	10.66	0.68	+2.32	2.1
M. W.	0.196	0.810	+0.289	0.967	0.341	+0.285	11.33	0.63	+1.70	2.6
Average	0.192	0.830	+0.272	0.903	0.334	+0.356	10.14	0.65	+2.83	2.4

probabilities that the observed values for b and r were due to chance were both less than 0.001.

Preadolescent girls eating from 60 to 80 gm. of fat a day excreted 2.0 to 4.0 gm. per day in the feces.[21] Of physiologic interest is the fact that in the present study, all of the periods in which 5 per cent or more of the dietary fat appeared in the stool occurred during simultaneous negative calcium balance. When fat excretion was plotted against fecal excretion of calcium (Fig. 2), the relationship became more apparent, i.e., 5.0 gm. or more of fecal fat (5 per cent or more of dietary intake) were excreted only when fecal calcium was 2.0 gm. or more per day. The converse was not generally true, since there were several instances when high fecal excretion of calcium was associated with low fecal fat. This suggests that high fecal calcium may produce high fecal fat rather than the converse.

The analysis of variance demonstrated significant interindividual variations in the urinary excretions of calcium ($P < 0.001$), phosphorus ($P < 0.001$) and nitrogen ($P < 0.05$) and the fecal excretions of nitrogen ($P < 0.05$) and fat ($P < 0.001$). Nonetheless, comparison of the two groups showed significant differences in fecal excretions of fat, calcium and phosphorus and in calcium and phosphorus balances.

COMMENTS

The relationship between dietary calcium and calcium retention has been reviewed and emphasized,[22] particularly in adults. In children, marked differences in calcium balance have been reported in studies comparing low intakes with adequate or high intakes. Ohlson and Stearns[23] compared the retention of calcium in children at three levels of intake. No significant differences were observed among groups receiving 0.7 to 1.5, 1.5 to 2.0 and 2.0 to 2.4 gm. per day, although all three groups showed greater retention than a group consuming less than 0.7 gm. per day. In the present study, the children receiving 1,300 mg. of calcium per day retained an average of 270 mg., but those receiving 2,300 mg. daily did not retain any. The changes in phosphorus

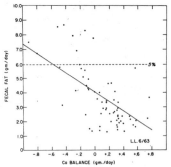

FIG. 1. Relationship between fecal fat and calcium balance: fecal fat = 4.07 − 3.3 (calcium balance).

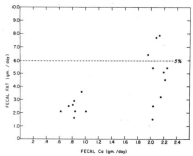

FIG. 2. Relationship between fecal fat and fecal calcium.

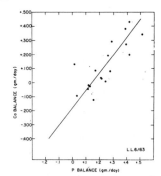

FIG. 3. Relationship between calcium balance and phosphorus balance.

176

balance were parallel to those of calcium balance (Fig. 3) in the ratio of calcium:phosphorus (corrected for nitrogen balance) of 1.27:1 (on a gram basis), the mean value found for normal bone, suggesting that the decreased calcium balance observed was due to a generalized defect in mineral retention rather than to a problem of calcium absorption alone. The dietary calcium:phosphorus ratios of the two groups were not remarkably different, 0.97 at the higher and 0.81 at the lower intake. It has been suggested, however, that in adults[24] better retention of calcium is achieved at lower calcium:phosphorus ratios at dietary calcium intakes above 1,600 mg. per day.

It has been observed in adults with frank steatorrhea[25] that increased dietary calcium may increase fecal excretion of fat. In rats, Kane et al.[26] showed that as the animals approached senescence, dietary fat absorption decreased and fell still further on high calcium diets. Recently,[27] it has been shown that dietary fat absorption may be markedly decreased in young growing rats receiving diets high in calcium. In the present study, elevated fecal excretion of fat approaching chemical steatorrhea (greater than 5 per cent of dietary fat), was found in seven of the ten subjects on the high calcium intakes. The absence of changes in nitrogen balance lends argument against a generalized malabsorption syndrome, however moderate.

Whether the negative calcium balances were the result of a sprue-like syndrome induced by the elevated calcium intake or whether the steatorrhea observed (whatever its etiology) resulted in or from vitamin D deficiency, cannot be differentiated by these observations. The vitamin D contents of the diets used in this study (Table II) were relatively low, of the order of 300 to 400 units per day (primarily from the milk), and may have been liminal for this age. Vitamin D requirements for man have not been accurately defined and may be related to the amount of dietary calcium and phosphorus.[23] This explanation is not likely, however, in view of a possible long-term storage of adequate vitamin D in these children accustomed to outdoor living.

These studies suggest that negative balances

of calcium and the development of steatorrhea may result when high dietary calcium is given. Pancreatic lipase, in vitro, is inhibited by high concentrations of calcium.[28] Thus, the high intestinal concentration of calcium occurring in group A may produce a relative malabsorption of fat. The unabsorbed triglycerides could then be hydrolyzed by intestinal bacteria to form calcium soaps lower in the gut resulting in impaired calcium absorption. In the present studies, the difference in calcium balance between the two groups was about 275 mg. per day. This is equivalent to about 2.5 gm. of fat calculated as butter fat (the major form in these diets), if it were excreted as calcium soaps. The difference in fat excretion actually seen between the two groups was precisely that figure. Further evidence suggesting that the mechanism involved was not initial binding of fat by calcium was the observation that at a calcium intake of 1,300 mg. daily, normal fecal excretions of fat were observed.

The mean urinary excretion of calcium of the group receiving the higher calcium intake was actually lower than that of the control group, contrary to what might have been expected. The minimal correlation between dietary and urinary calcium has been well demonstrated in the past,[29] but in view of the occasional question raised concerning the possible effects of elevated dietary intakes of calcium on urinary levels of calcium, this observation is again emphasized. Of further interest and without explanation is the relatively high level of urinary excretion of calcium observed in these children (average for all eighteen, 185 mg. per day) as well as the wide interindividual variability.

SUMMARY

Calcium, phosphorus, nitrogen and fat balances were measured in eighteen American Indian children, ten of whom were on a dietary intake of 2,300 mg. calcium and 2,400 mg. phosphorus and eight on dietary intakes of 1,300 mg. calcium and 1,600 mg. phosphorus. Both groups had been on diets similar to the experimental regimens for at least one year prior to the balance studies. Urinary calcium

177

levels varied from person to person and were unrelated to dietary calcium. Both calcium and phosphorus storage were markedly diminished on the higher mineral intakes. Chemical steatorrhea (greater than 5 per cent of dietary fat) was seen in seven of ten subjects on higher intakes of calcium and phosphorus but in none of the other group. Nitrogen balances were unrelated to the excretions of fat, calcium or phosphorus. An hypothesis was suggested for the relationship between dietary calcium, phosphorus and fat and the altered absorption of calcium, phosphorus and fat observed in certain subjects on high dietary calcium intake.

ACKNOWLEDGMENT

We wish to express our appreciation to Miss Helen Biesecker and the Nursing Staff of Unit 9-W of the Clinical Center, Miss Jeanne Reid and the staff of the Metabolic Kitchen for the National Institute of Arthritis and Metabolic Diseases and Mrs. Jessie Dowling and the Social Service Staff serving this Institute.

REFERENCES

1. HEGSTED, D. M. Calcium requirements. Nutrition Rev., 15: 257, 1957.
2. WHEDON, G. D. and LUTWAK, L. Contribution to symposium on human calcium requirements. J.A.M.A., 185: 591, 1963.
3. LUTWAK, L. and WHEDON, G. D. Mineral metabolic balance and Ca⁴⁶ kinetic studies in osteoporosis: effects of dietary calcium, vitamin D and estrogens. Fed. Proc., 22: 553, 1963.
4. LUTWAK, L. Osteoporosis, a disorder of nutrition. New York J. Med., 63: 590, 1963.
5. NORDIN, B. E. C. Calcium balance and calcium requirement in spinal osteoporosis. Am. J. Clin. Nutrition, 10: 384, 1962.
6. HARRISON, M., FRASER, R. and MULLEN, B. Calcium metabolism in osteoporosis: acute and long-term responses to increased calcium intake Lancet, 1: 1015, 1961.
7. Food and Nutrition Board. Recommended Dietary Allowances, publication No. 589. Washington, 1958. National Academy of Science-National Research Council.
8. HARRISON, H. E. Contribution to symposium of human calcium requirements. J.A.M.A., 185: 589, 1963.
9. WHEDON, G. D. Effects of high calcium intake on bones, blood and soft tissue: relationship of calcium intake to balance in osteoporosis. Fed. Proc., 18: 1112, 1959.
10. MICKELSEN, O., SHIP, I., LIKINS, R., ZIPKIN, I., LUTWAK, L. and SHUCK, C. To be published.

11. VERMEHREN, E. Variationen in phosphatasegehalt des plasmas im anschluss an die verschiedenen lebensalter. Acta med. scandinav., 100: 244, 1939.
12. CLARK, L. C., JR. and BECK, E. Plasma "alkaline" phosphatase activity. I. Normative data for growing children. J. Pediat., 36: 335, 1950.
13. HARRISON, A. P., RODERUCK, C., LESHER, M., KOUCHER, M., MOYER, E. Z., LAMECK, W. and BEACH, E. F. Nutritional status of children. VII. Blood serum phosphatase. J. Am. Dietet. A., 24: 503, 1948.
14. CEGLAREK, M. M., BRYANT, B. E. and WHEDON, G. D. A Manual for Metabolic Balance Studies. Washington, D. C., 1958. U. S. Department of Health, Education and Welfare.
15. HAWK, P. B., OSER, B. L. and SUMMERSON, W. H. Practical Physiological Chemistry, 13th ed., p. 899. New York, 1954. Blakiston Co.
16. LUTWAK, L. and SMITH, P. Flame photometric determination of calcium in biological materials. To be published.
17. HAWK, P. B., OSER, B. L. and SUMMERSON, W. H. Practical Physiological Chemistry, 13th ed., p. 951. New York, 1954. Blakiston Co.
18. BALL, J. S. and VAN METER, R. Determination of nitrogen in shale oil and petroleum. Anal. Chem., 23: 1002, 1951.
19. VAN DE KAMER, J. H. Total fatty acids in stool. In: Standard Methods in Clinical Chemistry, vol. 2. New York, 1958. Academic Press, Inc.
20. FISHER, R. A. and YATES, F. Statistical Tables for Agricultural, Biological and Medical Research. Edinburgh, 1953. Oliver & Boyd, Ltd.
21. STIER, L. B., TAYLOR, D. D., PACE, J. K. and EISEN, J. N. Metabolic patterns in preadolescent children. IV. Fat intake and excretion. J. Nutrition, 73: 347, 1961.
22. LUTWAK, L. and WHEDON, G. D. Osteoporosis. Dis. Month, April 1963.
23. OHLSON, M. A. and STEARNS, G. Calcium intake of children and adults. Fed. Proc., 18: 1076, 1959.
24. LUTWAK, L. and WHEDON, G. D. Relationship between calcium and phosphorus balances in man. Clin. Res., 11: 223, 1963.
25. BASSETT, S. H., KEUTMANN, E. H., HYDE, H. V. Z., VAN ALSTINE, H. E. and RUSS, E. Metabolism in idiopathic steatorrhea. I. The influence of dietary and other factors on lipid and mineral balance. J. Clin. Invest., 18: 101, 1939.
26. KANE, G. G., LOVELACE, F. E. and McCAY, C. M. Dietary fat and calcium wastage in old age. J. Gerontol., 4: 185, 1949.
27. WERNER, M. and LUTWAK, L. Dietary influences on fat absorption. Fed. Proc., 22: 553, 1963.
28. DRENICK, E. J. The influence of ingestion of calcium and other soap-forming substances on fecal rat. Gastroenterology, 41: 242, 1961.
29. KNAPP, E. L. Factors influencing the urinary excretion of calcium. J. Clin. Invest., 26: 182, 1947.

Peritonsillar Abscess and Cellulitis

Observations from Cases on Navaho Reservation

GERALD LEE MANDELL, M.D.

LEONARD R. PROSNITZ, M.D.

WHILE WORKING at the U.S. Public Health Service Hospital at Tuba City in Northern Arizona, the authors noted that peritonsillar abscess and cellulitis was seen relatively frequently in Navaho and Hopi Indian patients. Possible explanations for this and a discussion of modes of treatment follow.

Clinical picture

Acute tonsillitis rarely leads to peritonsillar abscess or cellulitis (quinsy sore throat).[1,2] Chamovitz et al.[3] found that none of 522 patients with streptococcal sore throat treated with antibiotics developed peritonsillar abscess or cellulitis, while 7 of 391 untreated patients developed this complication.[3]

The initiating pharyngitis or tonsillitis may be mild or severe. Dysphagia becomes a major problem, and the patient complains of pain in the throat and neck and earache on the affected side. There is marked trismus, and saliva may run from the corner of the mouth. Tender cervical nodes are often palpable. The pharynx is difficult to visualize because of the trismus. The breath may be foul. The pharynx and tonsils are erythematous and hyperemic, with or without exudate. The greatest swelling is anterior and superior to the tonsil. Palpation is difficult because of the trismus and tenderness.

Often one cannot differentiate between abscess and cellulitis. Fluctuance is difficult to determine in the boggy, edematous, and tender peritonsillar mass, and an incision may miss a small nidus of pus deep in an area of cellulitis. Thus, we shall refer to peritonsillar abscess and cellulitis.

Comparative incidence

There are 30,000 admissions to The New York Hospital annually. From July, 1960, through June, 1965, 30 cases of peritonsillar abscess or cellulitis were seen. The Tuba City Indian Hospital has 2,300 admissions yearly, but there were 69 cases of peritonsillar abscess or cellulitis during the same period. There are several factors that may explain this difference.

Beta hemolytic streptococcal sore throats are more common in the Navaho than in the United States population as a whole. The United States rate is 170 per 100,000, and the Navaho rate is 1,185 per 100,000 per year.[4]

Nearly all adult Navahos have intact tonsils. In a study of 407 military personnel with acute streptococcal sore throats, only 1 of 111 previously tonsillectomized men, as contrasted with 20 of 296 men with intact tonsils, developed peritonsillar abscess or cellulitis.[3]

The development of peritonsillar abscess

or cellulitis is less likely after antibiotic treatment of acute pharyngitis than after no treatment.[3] Many Navahos and Hopis distrust "Anglo medicine" and often live great distances from medical facilities. Thus, treatment of pharyngitis is either nonexistent or comes late in the course of the disease.

There were no recurrences in The New York Hospital series, but in Tuba City there were 11 patients who had two episodes, 6 with three episodes, and 1 man who had five episodes of peritonsillar abscess or cellulitis. This probably reflects the unwillingness of the Indian patient to return for tonsillectomy after the acute illness is over.

Bacteriology

Cultures of tonsillar swabs of patients with peritonsillar abscess or cellulitis done at Tuba City showed that of 23 cases, 13 were positive for group A beta hemolytic streptococci. The culture results at The New York Hospital in 27 patients showed that 14 grew group A beta hemolytic streptococci. Where both throat swab and actual pus from an abscess were cultured, the results were nearly identical. The percentage of recovery of group A beta streptococcus patients remained about 50 per cent.

Treatment

Surgical drainage is the time-honored method of treatment for peritonsillar abscess. Most of the standard textbooks state that this is the present treatment of choice.[5-12] All sources agree that antibiotics, especially penicillin, should be used. Incision and drainage is not without risk. Hemorrhage,[13] aspiration, and the complications of anesthesia are the greatest dangers. It is very difficult to evaluate fluctuance in an area of boggy hypervascular tissue, and therefore early surgical incision would probably mean that cellulitis without pus would inadvertently be surgically treated.

Eighteen of the 30 patients from The New York Hospital were treated with surgical incision, but the records of only 7 patients stated that pus was present. Four of the 69 patients from Tuba City were so treated,

and 3 had pus. All were treated with antibiotics. There was no significant difference in length of hospital stay or in days of intravenous fluid therapy between surgically and nonsurgically treated patients. The majority of patients received penicillin alone in doses varying from 250 mg. of phenoxymethyl penicillin orally four times per day to 10 million units of aqueous penicillin intravenously daily. The addition of other antibiotics in a few cases (tetracycline, novobiocin, and erythromycin) did not seem to be of added benefit.

There were no complications in either group, and even the 13 cases of the total of 99 that drained spontaneously went on to uneventful recovery. From April, 1963, through June, 1965, all 20 of the cases seen at Tuba City by the authors were treated with penicillin alone and all did well.

The large number of recurrences in the Tuba City group for this five-year period and the absence of any recurrences after tonsillectomy in the New York group is a strong argument for peritonsillar abscess and cellulitis being a definite indication for tonsillectomy.[12]

Conclusion

The authors feel that incision and drainage are indicated in peritonsillar abscess and cellulitis only where there is gross and obvious fluctuance. In a situation where there is any doubt as to the presence of pus, conservative (penicillin) therapy has proved successful. In a situation where a competent throat surgeon is not available, our experience has been that penicillin treatment alone is satisfactory even in the fluctuant abscess.

Summary

Sixty-nine episodes of peritonsillar abscess and cellulitis from Tuba City, Arizona, and 30 from The New York Hospital from the years 1960 through 1965 were studied. Peritonsillar abscesses and cellulitis are seen frequently in the Indian population where beta hemolytic streptococcal infections are common, medical care is delayed or absent, and most of the population has not had tonsillectomy. Fifty per cent of cases grew group A beta hemolytic streptococci on throat or abscess pus culture. Treatment with penicillin alone produced satisfactory results. Incision and drainage appears to be only rarely necessary. Peritonsillar abscess tends to recur, and tonsillectomy should be performed after the acute episode.

ACKNOWLEDGMENT. The authors wish to express their gratitude to Edward W. Hook, M.D., for his comments and suggestions.

References

1. Rantz, L. A.: The natural history of hemolytic streptococcus sore throat, California Med. **65:** 265 (1946).

2. Brink, W. R., Rammelkamp, C. H., Jr., Denny, F. W., and Wannamaker, L. W.: Effect in penicillin and aureomycin on the natural course of streptococcal tonsillitis and pharyngitis, Am. J. Med. **10:** 300 (1951).

3. Chamovitz, R., Rammelkamp, C. H., Jr., Wannamaker, L. W., and Denny, F. W., Jr.: The effect of tonsil-lectomy on the incidence of streptococcal respiratory disease and its complications, Pediatrics **26:** 355 (1960).

4. Indian Health Highlights, U.S. Department of Health, Education, and Welfare, Washington, D.C., Government Printing Office, 1964.

5. Austin, F.: Peritonsillar abscess, in Davis, L., Ed.: Christopher's Text of Surgery, 7th ed., Philadelphia, W. B. Saunders Company, 1960, p. 324.

6. Parrott, R., and Nelson, W.: in Nelson, W., Ed.: Textbook of Pediatrics, 8th ed., ibid. 1964, p. 81.

7. Bennett, I., in Harrison, T., Ed.: Principles of Internal Medicine, 3rd ed., New York, McGraw-Hill Book Company, Inc., 1962, p. 963.

8. Ballenger, H. C., and Ballenger, J. J.: Diseases of the Nose, Throat and Ear, 10th ed., Philadelphia, Lea & Febiger, 1957, p. 268.

9. Baies, L.: Fundamentals of Otolaryngology, Philadelphia, W. B. Saunders Company, 1959, p. 357.

10. Rantz, L.: in Beeson, P., and McDermott, W., Eds.: Cecil Loeb Textbook of Medicine, 11th ed., ibid. 1963, p. 173.

11. Dolowitz, D. A.: Basic Otolaryngology, New York, McGraw-Hill Book Company, Inc., 1954, p. 198.

12. Jaakkola, S., and Johnsson, G.: The treatment of peritonsillar abscess by incision and tonsillectomy" a froid" at the Oto-Laryngological Hospital, University of Helsinki, Acta oto-laryng. supp. **188:** 266 (1964).

13. Gage, E. L., Nelson, R. W., and Gatherum, R. S.: Beware the branchial bistoury. Aneurysm!, Med. Times **92:** 209 (Mar.) 1964.

A Survey of Chronic Disease and Diet in Seminole Indians in Oklahoma

Ruben H. Mayberry, m.d., m.p.h. and Robert D. Lindeman, m.d.

The navaho and Pima Indians have been reported to have a high incidence of diabetes and gallbladder disease and a low incidence of coronary artery disease, hypertension and malignancy.[1-9] Serum cholesterol values were lower in Navaho Indians than in white subjects but were not significantly lower in a group of Pima Indians.[2,10] Pima Indians were reported to ingest a diet slightly lower in fat content but otherwise similar to that consumed by the average white person; Navaho Indians were reported to ingest a "typically American diet."[2,10] Little else has been reported about the dietary habits and incidence of chronic disease of other Indian populations in this country.

Two concentrations of Seminole Indians remain in this country. About 900 Seminole Indians remain isolated on three reservations in Florida. Another 2,400 Seminole Indians are integrated with the white population of Seminole County, Oklahoma. Data on incidence and factors influencing the incidence of chronic, primarily cardiovascular, diseases were gathered on a sample of Seminole Indians and on a control sample of white subjects from Seminole County and compared with data provided on a similar sample of Seminole Indians surveyed in Florida.

METHODS

Of the 302 Seminole Indians surveyed from Seminole County, Oklahoma, about 150 were seen on visits to the Seminole County Health Department or one of its branch offices. Indians specifically attending the diabetes clinic were not included in an attempt to avoid bias of the sample. Another 100 subjects were seen on visits to the outpatient facilities of the Indian Hospital at Shawnee, Oklahoma. The remaining fifty were seen by the Public Health nurses in the schools and communities. All 422 white control subjects were seen in the Seminole

County Health Department or one of its branch offices. Many of the white subjects visited the health department specifically to obtain the following tests after hearing of their availability. All subjects were fourteen years of age or older.

Age, height and weight were recorded first for each subject. Single blood pressure determinations were obtained by a public health nurse, and a blood specimen was drawn for determination of hemoglobin (Leitz photometric method), serum cholesterol[11] and postprandial blood sugar levels (modified Folin-Wu) and for performance of the serologic test for syphilis. Information concerning the presence of known diabetes also was obtained. All subjects with an elevated or borderline elevated postprandial blood sugar level were asked to return for a glucose tolerance test.

Data on 221 Seminole Indians living on reservations in Florida (Big Cypress, Dania and Brighton) were provided for comparison with our data.[12] Bartlett's test for homogeneity of variances was computed for each of the variables for the three groups. Correcting for differences in the ages of each group by analysis of covariants, the significance of differences in height, weight, systolic and diastolic blood pressures, hemoglobin and cholesterol levels were tested for the three groups.

Interviews about diet were completed on fifty-four Seminole Indian and sixty white subjects from Seminole County. A qualitative and quantitative analysis was made of food ingested during the day prior to the interview, estimating total caloric, protein, carbohydrate and fat intake.[13,14]

Death certificates on all Indian and white subjects over age twenty-five who died in Seminole County between 1950 and 1959 were examined. The numbers of deaths due to coronary artery disease (category 420), stroke (categories 330 to 334), hypertension with and without heart disease (categories 440 to 447), all cardiovascular disease (categories 330 to 334 and 400 to 468), diabetes (category 260), primary lung cancer (category 162) and all other causes were tabulated.[15] Due to the problems encountered because of mixed blood in separating Indians from white subjects in census reports and on death certificates, death rates could not be considered reliable. Therefore, the per cent of all death certificates filed for Indians and for white persons according to disease category is reported.

RESULTS

Considerable difference was found in the mean age of the Seminole Indians as compared to that of the control group of white subjects. The mean age for the Seminole Indians studied in Oklahoma was thirty-three and a half years, for the Seminole Indian in Florida 36.2 years and for the control group 44.2 years. In all three groups, there were more female than male subjects. Of the 302 Oklahoma Indians studied, 203 (67.2 per cent) claimed to be full-blooded Seminole Indians. The remainder claimed to be half Seminole Indian or more.

The mean height, weight, systolic and diastolic blood pressures, and hemoglobin and cholesterol levels in the age groups fourteen to twenty-nine, thirty to forty-nine, fifty to sixty-four and sixty-five and over are shown by sex and race in Figure 1. Data on the Seminole Indians in Florida are included except for cholesterol levels when differences in methods of determination prevented direct comparison.

The mean heights of male and female Oklahoma and Florida Seminole Indians were significantly less than that of their white counterparts (p < 0.01). The mean weights, when corrected for height, of both Indian groups also were significantly greater (p < 0.01) than those of the white subjects. Table I shows the incidence of overweight in the two groups of male and female Indians and male and female white subjects. The mean systolic and diastolic blood pressures were similar in the three groups (p > 0.05) except for a slightly lower diastolic pressure of borderline significance (p < 0.05, > 0.01) in the female Florida Indians. Actually thirty-three (10.9 per cent) of the 302 Seminole Indians in Oklahoma and twenty-one (9.5 per cent) of 221 Indians in Florida had blood pressures above 160 mm. systolic or 100 mm. diastolic. This compared with an incidence of hypertension of 12.3 per cent in the white subjects. Difference in age distribution in the groups studied could easily account for the difference in incidence of hypertension observed.

The mean hemoglobin levels in both Indian male populations were significantly higher (p < 0.01) than in the male white subjects. Since hemoglobin values for Seminole Indians in Florida were determined in a different

183

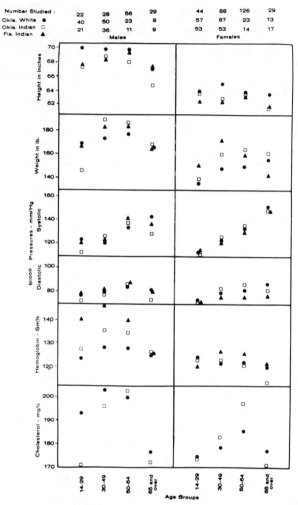

Fig. 1. Comparison of height, weight, systolic and diastolic blood pressures, and hemo-globin and cholesterol levels in Florida and Oklahoma Seminole Indian and Oklahoma white subjects in Seminole County. Data are shown for men and women by age groups.

184

TABLE I

Incidence of Overweight in Male and Female Seminole
Indian and White Subjects*

Subjects	No. Studied	Per Cent of Subjects Overweight	
		25% or More	40% or More
Men			
Oklahoma Indian......	121	23.1	8.3
Florida Indian.........	77	19.5	7.8
Oklahoma white	135	10.4	1.5
Women			
Oklahoma Indian......	181	34.3	19.3
Florida Indian.........	137	39.4	25.5
Oklahoma white.......	287	16.4	9.8

* Based on height and age.

laboratory, the significance of higher levels in this group may be questioned. In the women, however, the hemoglobin levels were similar in the three groups.

There were no significant differences (p > 0.05) in serum cholesterol levels between male and female Oklahoma Seminole Indian and white subjects. The incidence of hypercholesterolemia (above 260 mg. per 100 ml.) was 9.1 and 5.4 per cent in the male and female Oklahoma Indians and 15.6 and 9.1 per cent in the male and female white subjects. Most of this difference in incidence is attributed to the older mean age of the white subjects studied. Although a different method of determining cholesterol levels was used in the Florida study, determination in a small number of samples was carried out by both the Oklahoma and Florida laboratories. The values ran about 10 per cent higher in the Florida laboratory. If this difference could be considered constant in all studies the cholesterol levels in the Seminole Indians in Florida would be similar to those obtained from the two groups in Oklahoma.

The subjects first were asked if they were known to have diabetes and the time interval since their last meal. A blood sugar level was determined in all persons. A blood

sugar value of over 210 mg. per 100 ml. up to two hours postprandially or over 160 mg. per 100 ml. after two hours was considered elevated. Blood sugar values of between 180 and 210 mg. per 100 ml. up to two hours postprandially and between 130 and 160 mg. per 100 ml. after two hours were considered to be borderline elevations.

Glucose tolerance tests were carried out on thirty of 113 persons with borderline elevations in postprandial blood sugar levels. Nine of these showed curves consistent with a diagnosis of diabetes (blood sugar levels two hours postprandially greater than 130 mg. per 100 ml.), two showed borderline curves, and nineteen showed no evidence of diabetes. The results of the interviews and postprandial blood sugar determinations are shown in Figure 2. There were fourteen known diabetic Oklahoma Indians and nine known diabetic white subjects in the study. There were also thirteen Indians and ten white persons with definitely elevated blood sugar levels. In the Florida study there were ten known diabetic subjects. There were, in addition, fifteen subjects with a blood sugar value of 130 mg. per 100 ml. or higher two hours postprandially. Of these, glucose tolerance test results confirmed the presence of diabetes in three and excluded the diagnosis in five. The other seven persons were not retested.

Twenty-two Seminole Indians in Oklahoma had positive serologic test results for syphilis as did seven Indians in Florida. Only four of the white control subjects had positive reactions. No confirmatory Wassermann tests were drawn.

Table II shows the mean dietary intake for male and female Indian and white subjects for the day prior to the interview. The Indians had a slightly higher mean total caloric intake than the white subjects. This may be related to the younger mean age of the Indians studied. The per cent of the diet made up of carbohydrate, protein and fat was similar in the Indian and white subjects although the Indians may have ingested a slightly higher ratio of polyunsaturated to saturated fats. The Indians consumed more fat pork and lard. The

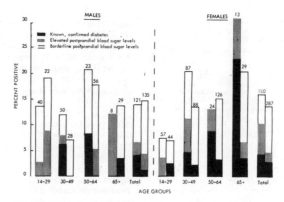

FIG. 2. Incidence of previously known diabetes and elevated and borderline elevated postprandial blood sugar levels in Seminole Indian and white subjects in Seminole County, Oklahoma. Data are shown for men and women by age groups. The bar on the left is for the Seminole Indians and the bar on the right for the white subjects. The value at the top of each bar represents the number of persons studied in that group.

white subjects commonly used milk as a beverage, whereas the Indians rarely did. Use of other meats such as lean pork, beef, chicken and fish was about equal in the two groups. Use of eggs, potatoes, vegetables, legumes, breads and desserts also was similar in the two groups.

Death certificates were filed for 266 Indians who died in Seminole County between 1950 and 1959. The mean age at death of this group was 48.9 years as compared to a mean age at death of 64.8 years for all white persons who died in the state. Much of the shortened life expectancy in the Seminole Indian in Oklahoma was due to the large number of death certificates (19.2 per cent) filed for persons

TABLE II

Comparison of the Daily Food Intake of Indian and White Men and Women

Data	Indian Men		White Men		Indian Women		White Women	
No. of studies.............	20		17		34		43	
Mean age (yr.)............	41		57		39		57	
Diet								
Total calories...........	2,484		1,861		1,864		1,690	
Carbohydrate (gm.)*.....	256	(41)	197	(42)	205	(44)	180	(43)
Protein (gm.)*...........	86	(14)	71	(15)	59	(12)	58	(14)
Fat (gm.)*..............	124	(45)	88	(42)	90	(44)	82	(44)
Fatty acids								
Total saturated (gm.)*..	44	(16)	34	(17)	32	(16)	34	(18)
Unsaturated (gm.)*....	58	(20.5)	39	(18.5)	45	(21)	37	(19.5)
Oleic (gm.)*..........	48	(17)	34	(16)	38	(18)	32	(17)
Linoleic (gm.)*.......	10	(3.5)	5	(2.5)	7	(3)	5	(2.5)
P:S ratio†	0.23:1		0.15:1		0.28:1		0.14:1	

* Numbers in parentheses = per cent; numbers outside parentheses = mean.
† Polyunsaturated:saturated fat ratio.

TABLE III
Deaths Among Indian and White Subjects Aged Twenty-Five and Over in Seminole County, Oklahoma*

Data	Indian Men		White Men		Indian Women		White Women	
Population†	1,159		11,246		1,184		11,725	
Mean age at death (yr.)	63.1		67.6		64.1		70.4	
Total deaths	116	(100.0)	1,361	(100.0)	90	(100.0)	799	(100.0)
Disease category								
Coronary artery disease	18	(15.5)	422	(31.0)	10	(11.1)	165	(20.7)
Stroke	16	(13.8)	175	(12.9)	7	(7.8)	124	(15.5)
Hypertension	11	(9.5)	69	(5.0)	2	(2.2)	76	(9.5)
Total cardiovascular disease	52	(44.8)	730	(53.6)	28	(31.1)	392	(49.1)
Diabetes	5	(4.3)	22	(1.6)	3	(3.3)	22	(2.8)
Lung cancer	1	(0.9)	39	(2.9)	0	(0)	12	(1.5)

NOTE: Figures outside parentheses = number; figures inside parentheses = per cent.
* Based on death certificates filed between 1950 and 1959.
† Based on the 1960 census reports.

who died during the first five years of life. In order to minimize the effect of this excessive early mortality on the chronic disease statistics, only those death certificates filed on persons age twenty-five years and older were examined. Even so, there still was a younger mean age at death in the Indian (Table III). Table III lists the per cent of all deaths by sex attributed to arteriosclerotic heart or coronary artery disease, stroke, hypertension, all cardiovascular disease, diabetes and lung cancer in the Oklahoma Indian and white subjects over the age of twenty-five occurring in Seminole County between 1950 and 1959.

COMMENTS

Differences in the incidence of certain chronic diseases between Indian and white populations have been described previously.[1-9] The influence of environment is often difficult to separate from racial or hereditary factors. In this study, the relatively isolated, inbred Seminole Indians in Florida and the integrated Seminole Indians in Seminole County, Oklahoma were compared with their white counterpart in Seminole County. Hopefully, some cultural, educational and economic differences might exist in these racially related. Seminole Indians showing the effects on the two populations. Differences in methods used in performing the hemoglobin and cholesterol determinations in the two laboratories makes interpretation of these data difficult; however,

other comparisons particularly of body build and blood pressure should be valid.

The mean ages of the two Indian groups were significantly less than those of the white group in Oklahoma, making necessary correction for age differences between the three groups. Subjects in the older age groups would be expected to have a higher incidence of hypertension and diabetes and probably obesity and elevated cholesterol levels.

The high incidence of obesity seen in our Indian populations was similar to that reported in other Indian populations. The striking lack of hypertension seen in the Navaho Indians was not seen in either group of Seminole Indians.[8] The hemoglobin levels in the male Seminole Indians were significantly higher than those in the male white subjects. This difference was not apparent in the female subjects. The serum cholesterol levels in both male and female Seminole Indians in Oklahoma were similar to those seen in their white counterparts. This is in contrast to the lower levels reportedly seen in the Navaho Indians.[2] The incidence of diabetes appears to be higher in both Seminole Indian groups than in the white group and is consistent with reports of others that there is a higher incidence of diabetes in Indian populations.[1,5,7]

Four factors then have been evaluated which presumably influence the incidence of coronary artery disease: Obesity and diabetes were more common in the Seminole Indians although blood cholesterol levels and blood pressure determinations were similar in Indian and white subjects. The diet of the Seminole Indians in Oklahoma was similar to that of their white counterparts. The incidence of coronary artery disease in the Seminole Indians in Oklahoma still was less than that observed in the white subjects even after differences in life expectancy were taken into consideration. Deaths from stroke and hypertension, on the other hand, were higher in the male Seminole Indian than in the male white subject. However, the size of the sample may be too small from which to draw conclusions. The incidence of deaths attributed to coronary artery disease, stroke, hypertension and other cardiovascular diseases is much higher and in striking contrast with the low death rates for the same diseases seen in the Navaho and Pima Indians. Whether racial or hereditary characteristics or environ-

ment are responsible for these differences remains to be determined.

The wide variations in death rates existing between the Indians of other counties or tribes in Oklahoma for coronary artery disease and other cardiovascular disease are shown in Table IV, tabulating death certificates filed in these counties for male Indians twenty-five years of age and older. The highest death rates for coronary artery disease were seen in Miami, Kay and Osage counties. These counties all have Indian populations which have integrated extensively with the white populations and have accepted many of their educational standards and cultural influences. Although the Cherokee Indians (Adair, Cherokee and Muskogee counties) have the lowest death rates from coronary artery disease, they have the highest death rates from stroke and hypertension.

The Seminole Indians were found to have a

TABLE IV

Percentage of Male Indian Deaths* From Various Categories of Cardiovascular Disease in Some Counties in Oklahoma with Large Indian Populations

County	Male Indian Population†	Principal Tribes	Male Death Certificate Filed (no.)	Per cent of Total Deaths Attributed to			
				Coronary Artery Disease	Stroke	Hypertension	All Cardiovascular Disease
Adair.........	1,555	Cherokee	186	15.6	8.6	7.5	41.4
Blaine.........	451	Cheyenne, Arapaho	43	23.3	9.3	0.0	37.2
Caddo.........	1,520	Caddo, Wichita, Comanche, Kiowa, Apache	105	15.2	9.5	3.8	44.8
Cherokee.......	1,529	Cherokee	132	12.1	10.6	9.1	45.5
Comanche......	1,272	Comanche, Kiowa, Apache	57	17.5	14.0	1.8	45.6
Delaware.......	1,067	Cherokee, Delaware, Senecas	83	23.0	14.5	7.2	50.6
Hughes.........	668	Creeks	47	25.5	4.3	6.4	38.3
Kay...........	830	Ponca, Oto-Missouri, Kaw, Tonkawa	52	32.7	1.9	1.9	40.4
McCurtain......	1,015	Choctaw	76	13.1	11.8	1.3	36.8
Muskogee.......	890	Cherokee	62	12.9	16.1	8.1	45.2
Osage.........	835	Osage	114	26.3	5.3	1.8	39.5
Ottawa........	558	Quapaws, many northeastern small U. S. tribes	36	33.3	11.1	5.6	61.1
Pottawatomie...	839	Shawnee, Pottawatomie, Kickapoo	67	22.4	3.0	3.0	43.3

* Based on death certificates filed between 1950 and 1959.
† Based on 1960 census.

lower death rate from primary lung cancer than their white counterparts in Oklahoma. This same low incidence of lung cancer was also seen in other Indian populations in Oklahoma. Of 1,060 death certificates filed for male Indians in the thirteen counties listed in Table IV, only ten cases of lung cancer (0.9 per cent) were reported. This is consistent with the findings reported in other Indian tribes in this country.[5,9]

Several problems present themselves in evaluating death certificate data. The possibility exists that in some Indians the popular diagnoses of coronary artery disease or stroke were recorded as the cause of death when death was actually due to something else. Clinically, one is impressed, however, that the occurrence of cardiovascular diseases is much more frequent in the Seminole Indians than in the Navaho and Pima Indians.

Another problem in evaluating these death certificate data is determining who represents an Indian. This is left up to the attending physician, as there is no standard definition as to how much Indian blood must be present. A person who has part Indian and part white blood can be listed as either on the death certificate.

SUMMARY

Body build, blood pressure determinations, hemoglobin and cholesterol levels, the incidence of diabetes, dietary habits and causes of death are compared in Seminole Indians and white subjects in Seminole County, Oklahoma. Similar data were made available for comparison on Florida Seminole Indians.

Indians were shorter and heavier than white subjects. Mean blood pressure determinations, serum cholesterol levels and dietary habits were similar in Indian and white subjects. More diabetes was found in the Indian populations. Coronary artery disease as a cause of death was less frequent in the Indian than in the white subject in Oklahoma but much more frequent than that reported for Navaho and Pima Indians. Hypertension, stroke and diabetes ranked relatively high and lung cancer low as causes of death in the Oklahoma Indian.

ACKNOWLEDGMENT

We wish to thank Dr. Gerald Powley of the Florida State Department of Health for supplying the information on the Seminole Indians in Florida. We also wish to thank Miss George Goss Smith, Nutrition Consultant, Oklahoma State Department of Health, Misses Janis A. Sopher, Nell Williams and Emma Dulay for conducting and compiling the dietary interviews and Dr. James A. Hagans, Biostatistical Unit and Medical Research Computer Center, Department of Preventive Medicine and Public Health, Oklahoma University Medical Center for statistical assistance.

REFERENCES

1. PARKS, J. H. and WASKOW, E. Diabetes among the Pima Indians of Arizona. *Arizona Med.*, 18: 99, 1961.
2. PAGE, I. H., LEWIS, L. A. and GILBERT, J. Plasma lipids and proteins and their relationship to coronary disease among Navajo Indians. *Circulation*, 13: 675, 1956.
3. SMITH, R. L. Cardiovascular-renal and diabetes deaths among the Navajo. *Pub. Health Rep.*, 72: 33, 1957.
4. GILBERT, J. Absence of coronary thrombosis in Navajo Indians. *California Med.*, 82: 114, 1955.
5. HESSE, F. G. The incidence of cholecystitis and other diseases among the Pima Indians of southern Arizona. *J. A. M. A.*, 170: 1789, 1959.
6. STREEPER, R. B., MASSEY, R. U., LIU, G., DILLINGHAM, C. H. and CUSHING, A. An electrocardiographic and autopsy study of coronary artery disease in the Navajo. *Dis. Chest*, 38: 305, 1960.
7. COHEN, B. M. Diabetes mellitus among Indians of the American Southwest. Its prevalence and clinical characteristics in a hospitalized population. *Ann. Int. Med.*, 40: 588, 1954.
8. COHEN, B. M. Arterial hypertension among Indians of the southwestern United States. *Am. J. M. Sc.*, 225: 505, 1953.
9. SIEVERS, M. L. and MARQUIS, J. R. Duodenal ulcer among southwestern American Indians. *Gastroenterology*, 42: 566, 1962.
10. HESSE, F. G. A dietary study of the Pima Indian. *Am. J. Clin. Nutrition*, 7: 532, 1959.
11. PEARSON, S., STERN, S. and McGAVACK, T. H. Determination of total cholesterol in serum. *Anal. Chem.*, 25: 813, 1953.
12. POWLEY, G. Unpublished data, 1962. Florida State Department of Health.
13. Nutritive value of foods. In: Institute of Home Economics Agricultural Research Service, Home and Garden Bulletin No. 72. Washington, D. C., 1960. U.S. Department of Agriculture.
14. BOWES, A. DEP. and CHURCH, C. F. Food Values of Portions Commonly Used, 7th ed. Philadelphia, 1951. College Offset Press.
15. Manual on the International Statistical Classification of Diseases, Injuries and Causes of Death. vol. 1. Geneva, 1957. W. H. O.

189

Surveillance of Respiratory Virus Infections Among Alaskan Eskimo Children

James E. Maynard, MD, Elmer T. Feltz, MS, Herta Wulff, PhD,

Robert Fortuine, MD, Jack D. Poland, MD, and Tom D. Y. Chin, MD

Morbidity and mortality due to respiratory disease are significant health problems for Alaska Aleuts, Indians, and Eskimos. Of the leading nonviolent causes of death for these people in 1950, influenza-pneumonia ranked second, exceeded only by tuberculosis.[1] In 1960, tuberculosis had been relegated to sixth place in the list of leading nonviolent causes of death, and influenza-pneumonia achieved first place. In a recent study of Alaskan Eskimo infant morbidity and mortality, infant deaths were reported to exceed 120/1,000 live births.[2] Of all neonatal deaths 15% were due to respiratory infections as contrasted with 75% for the postneonatal period. In this same study, acute respiratory disease constituted the major source of morbidity during the first year of life. One author, in a study of lower respiratory tract illness among Alaskan Eskimo children, reported that 35% of the children surveyed had at least one episode of pneumonia or bronchitis during the first year of life.[3]

The role played by respiratory viruses in the production of acute respiratory disease in Alaskan natives has not heretofore been adequately assessed. This has been in large part due to the lack of virus laboratory facilities in Alaska and to logistic problems attendant on effective specimen collection and transport in remote areas. The only virus diagnostic laboratory in the State of Alaska was established in 1955 at the Arctic Health Research Laboratory in Anchorage. Since 1963, the laboratory has engaged, with increasing intensity, in studies of acute respiratory disease in Alaskan native populations. The following study represents the first surveillance program undertaken in a remote population of Alaskan Eskimo children in an attempt to determine the relative importance of viruses in the production of acute respiratory disease.

Materials and Methods

The Study Population.—Subjects for study consisted of Eskimo children, 6 years of age and under, resident in the village of Bethel, Alaska, who presented to the outpatient clinic of the Public Health Service Alaska Native Hospital, Bethel, with symptoms of acute respiratory disease of less than five days' duration. Surveillance began on Jan 16 and ended on May 15, 1966. In December 1965, prior to the initiation of the surveillance program, serum specimens were collected from 122 Eskimo children, 6 years of age and under, to establish the prevalence (by age group) of antibody titers to respiratory syncytial virus and parainfluenza virus types 1, 2, and 3. Although some of the children, from whom serum specimens were collected in December and in whom acute respiratory disease developed during the ensuing surveillance period, were included in the diagnostic study, the serologic survey population was not followed on a routine basis, and no attempt was made to precisely define the denominator population from which the outpatient clinic subjects derived. The total population of Bethel native children in the 6 years and under age group was estimated at 300 in December 1965.

Table 1.—Prevalence of Antibodies to Respiratory Syncytial and Parainfluenza Viruses in Alaskan Eskimo Children*

Age of Children, yr	Respiratory Syncytial Virus			Neutralizing Antibody Titer ≥ 1:8 for Parainfluenza Virus Type								
				1			2			3		
	Number of Children	Number Positive	% Positive	Number of Children	Number Positive	% Positive	Number of Children	Number Positive	% Positive	Number of Children	Number Positive	% Positive
<1	6	0	0	7	0	0	7	1	14	7	3	42
1	17	6	35	19	10	53	19	9	47	19	9	47
2	27	12	44	28	18	64	28	19	68	27	24	89
3	19	8	42	21	20	95	21	14	66	20	16	80
4	25	14	56	27	18	67	27	16	59	27	27	100
5-6	19	9	47	20	16	80	20	11	55	20	20	100
Total	113	49	43	122	82	67	122	70	57	120	99	82

*Bethel, December 1965.

At time of clinic visit, an illness questionnaire was filled out by the admitting physician, a combined throat and nasal swab was collected for viral isolation studies, and a blood specimen was drawn during the acute phase of the illness. A convalescent period blood specimen was obtained from 15 to 45 days later. An attempt was made to include in the study every child seen in the clinic who fulfilled study criteria. It was evident, however, that clinic physicians did miss collecting specimens on a number of children who otherwise would have been included.

Laboratory Methods.—Specimens for virus isolation were collected in a transport medium consisting of tryptose phosphate broth with 0.5% gelatin and 1.0% chicken serum added. Antibiotic additives per milliliter of medium consisted of penicillin G, 250 units, streptomycin sulfate, 250µg, neomycin sulfate, 250µg, and bacitracin, 2.5 units. Specimens were aliquoted at the point of collection and then placed at −70 C. Throat swabs and serum were shipped to the virus laboratory in Anchorage once a week on dry ice, with aliquots of materials transhipped to the Kansas City (Kan) Field Station of the Communicable Disease Center for parallel viral studies. All throat specimens underwent one cycle of freeze-thaw prior to attempts at virus isolation. Specimens were passed in primary rhesus monkey kidney, HEp-2, and the Wistar 38 line of human fetal diploid cells at both Anchorage and Kansas City, and were subject to two to five blind passes before being discarded as negative. Hemadsorbing agents were identified by neutralization with monospecific commercial antisera with end points determined by hemadsorption inhibition. Influenza isolates were also typed by hemagglutination inhibition with A_2/Taiwan/1/64 and B/Singapore/3/64 antisera obtained from the Respirovirus Unit of the Communicable Disease Center, Atlanta. Respiratory syncytial virus, adenovirus, and herpes simplex virus isolates were identified by neutralization with commercial antisera.

Titers of neutralizing antibodies to respiratory syncytial virus (Long strain), and parainfluenza virus types 1 (HA 2 strain), 2 (CA strain), and 3 (HA 1 strain) were determined from the December survey. Sera obtained during the acute and convalescent phases from the January to May surveillance study were tested for neutralizing antibodies to respiratory syncytial virus and parainfluenza virus types 1, 2, and 3. In addition, these sera were tested for hemagglutination-inhibiting antibodies to A_2/Taiwan/1/64 and B/Alaska/1/66 influenza viruses.

Results

Table 1 shows the prevalence of neutralizing antibody titers at screening level or above to respiratory syncytial and parainfluenza viruses for the children sampled in the December serologic survey. The distribution of sera positive for respiratory syncytial virus antibody appeared rather constant with age except for infants, where no antibodies were detected in the six children sampled. The overall prevalence of sera positive for respiratory syncytial antibody was 43%. For parainfluenza viruses, relative frequency of antibody-positive sera was lowest for parainfluenza type 2, with only 57% of all sera designated as positive. This contrasted with 67% and 82%, respectively, for parainfluenza virus types 1 and 3.

During the January to May surveillance study,

Diagnostic categories and distribution of cases by week of onset of illness. RS = respiratory syncytial.

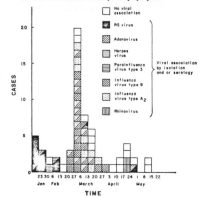

Table 2.—Clinical Findings for 12 Cases of
Illness Associated With Respiratory Syncytial Virus*

Findings	No. of Children Manifesting
Cough	12
Temp ≧ 100F (37.8C)	10
Rhinitis	10
Rales and/or rhonchi	7
Pharyngitis	4
Tracheobronchitis	4
Laryngitis	1

*Bethel surveillance study of 1966.

clinical information and laboratory specimens were collected from 63 children. One child was seen on two separate occasions with two distinct episodes of acute respiratory disease. For study purposes, this child was counted twice to produce a total of 64 separate illnesses. A total of 38 viruses were recovered from 36 children ill with acute respiratory disease. This included two illnesses from each of which simultaneous recoveries of two agents were made. The isolation rate for the 64 illnesses was 56%. Viral isolates included influenza virus types A2 and B, respiratory syncytial virus, parainfluenza virus type 3, adenovirus types 2 and 5, rhinovirus, and herpes simplex virus. In addition, serologic evidence of infection based on fourfold or greater rises in titer of paired sera against the agents tested brought the total of laboratory-confirmed virus-associated illnesses to 48 or 75% of total illnesses. The Figure shows the diagnostic categories and distribution in time by week of onset of cases admitted to the study. Three distinct increases in incidence of acute respiratory disease occurred. These included an outbreak associated with recoveries of respiratory syncytial virus in January, a mixed influenza A2 and B epidemic in February and March, and a clustering of illnesses in April from which rhinoviruses, respiratory syncytial virus, and adenovirus type 5 were recovered.

Twelve cases of illness associated with respiratory syncytial virus were confirmed during the study period. In six cases respiratory syncytial virus was recovered from the throat swab, and serum specimens obtained during the acute and convalescent phases of illness showed fourfold or greater rises in neutralizing antibody titer to both the isolated virus and Long strain of respiratory syncytial virus. Six additional cases showed fourfold or greater rises in neutralizing antibody titer to Long strain

Table 3.—Prevalence of Neutralizing Antibody to
Respiratory Syncytial Virus by Age*

Age, yr	Number of Children	Antibody Titer ≧ 1:8	
		Number Positive	% Positive
<1	11	6	54
1	4	4	100
2	13	13	100
3	7	6	86
4	9	9	100
5	5	5	100
6	5	5	100
Total	54	48	89

*In sera obtained during acute phase of illnesses of Bethel children in 1966.

in sera from the acute and convalescent phases. Thus, virus was isolated from 50% of laboratory-confirmed infections. Ten of the 12 infections occurred in illnesses with onsets prior to Feb 20.

Table 2 gives the predominant clinical findings for the 12 children infected with respiratory syncytial virus. Cough, fever, and rhinitis predominated in the clinical picture with more than half of the children also manifesting signs of lower respiratory tract involvement. Five of the children were less than 1 year of age. Three of these were clinically diagnosed as having bronchiolitis and two as having mild viral upper respiratory tract infection. Respiratory syncytial virus was recovered from throat swabs in these latter two cases. In one 6-month-old child with bronchiolitis, adenovirus type 5 and respiratory syncytial virus were simultaneously isolated from the throat specimen, and paired sera produced diagnostic rises in neutralizing antibody titer to both agents. Parainfluenza virus type 3 was isolated from a 1-month-old child with bronchiolitis who demonstrated simultaneous neutralizing antibody titer rises to both respiratory syncytial virus and parainfluenza type 3. The remaining illnesses associated with respiratory syncytial virus were evenly distributed across the age range of 2 to 5 years. These included three cases diagnosed as upper respiratory tract infections, three cases of pneumonia, and one case of acute bronchitis. Adenovirus type 2 was recovered from the throat swab and simultaneous diagnostic rises in neutralizing antibody titer to the isolated virus and respiratory syncytial virus were found in one child with bronchopneumonia.

That an outbreak of respiratory syncytial virus infection had occurred during the study period is also demonstrated in Table 3, which shows prevalence of neutralizing antibody titer to respiratory syncytial virus equal to or greater than 1:8 in sera (from acute phase of illness) of 54 of the 64 children seen during the January to May surveillance period. In contrast to a prevalence of 43% derived from the December survey, 89% of children in the surveillance group demonstrated respiratory syncytial antibody in sera obtained during the acute phases of illness. It is evident that the surveillance study began at or just after the peak of the respiratory syncytial virus outbreak. This may be inferred from the fact that of the 51 illnesses seen with dates of onset after Feb 20, diagnostic rises in neutralizing antibody titer to respiratory syncytial virus in paired sera were demonstrated in only two cases. This contrasted with diagnostic titer rises in paired sera from 11 of the 13 cases with dates of onset prior to Feb 20. In addition, seven children from whom sera were obtained in the December survey were subsequently admitted to the surveillance study after Feb 20. All seven of these children showed high stationary neutralization titers to respiratory syncytial virus in their paired sera. Repeat respiratory syncytial virus neutralization tests were performed in the December survey and on sera from these seven cases during the acute phase following Feb 20, and diagnostic titer rises to respiratory syncytial virus were found in all seven.

Of the 39 cases of illness with dates of onset between the weeks ending Feb 27 and March 27, thirty-three were associated with influenza virus infections. Influenza B viruses were recovered and concurrent fourfold rises in influenza B HAI antibody titer were found in 19 instances. Influenza A2 virus was recovered from three cases. Serologic evidence alone of influenza virus infection was obtained in the remaining 11 cases. The mixed nature of the influenza epidemic and probability of occurrence of dual influenza virus infections was demonstrated by the fact that 13 children showed simultaneous fourfold or better rises in HI antibody titer to both A₂Taiwan/1/64 and B/Alaska/1/66 antigens. These results are shown in Table 4. In all but one of the cases blood was drawn in the convalescent phase, between 20 and 28 days after samples were obtained during the acute phase. Influenza B virus was isolated from throat swabs in 11 of the 13 cases. In no instances were simultaneous influenza A2 and B isolations made.

The three children from whom influenza A2 virus was isolated showed diagnostic rises in serum antibody titer to the Taiwan antigen alone. Evidence of simultaneous infection with other viruses in addition to influenza virus was obtained in two instances. These included one 2-year-old child with febrile upper respiratory tract infection, from whom herpes simplex and influenza B viruses were simultaneously isolated, and a 2-year-old child with pneumonia, in whom there were simultaneous diagnostic rises in antibody titer to influenza B virus and respiratory syncytial virus.

Typical clinical findings for the 31 children infected with influenza virus types A2 or B or both only consisted of fever, cough, and coryza. Evidence of lower respiratory tract involvement indicated by signs of tracheobronchitis or chest rales was found in 16 (52%) of these. Table 5 relates clinical severity of the 31 influenza cases to type of influenza infection. Only two of the 10 cases shown by isolation or serology or both to be associated with influenza B virus infection alone gave evidence of lower respiratory tract involvement. This contrasted sharply with the clinical picture seen in the A2 infections alone and the simultaneous A2 and B infections, where a much higher frequency of lower respiratory tract involvement obtained.

Of particular interest was one infant who apparently had a true influenzal pneumonia. This 6-month-old boy was admitted to the hospital three days after onset of an illness consisting of fever, cough, and tachypnea. Influenza B virus was isolated from the throat swab, and paired sera showed diagnostic rises in HI antibody titer to both influenza A2 and B antigens. The admission chest film showed infiltrates along the right cardiac border and white blood cell and differential counts performed at the same time revealed a total cell count

Table 4.—Virus Isolations and Results of HI Tests in Paired Sera From 13 Cases of Influenza*

Case No.	Influenza Virus Isolated	HI Titer Reciprocals†			
		A₂/Tai/1/64		B/Ak/1/66	
		Acute	Convalescent	Acute	Convalescent
1	B	20	320	< 10	40
2	B	< 10	80	< 10	40
3	...	< 10	160	< 10	160
4	B	< 10	80	< 10	80
5	B	< 10	20	< 10	160
6	B	10	160	< 10	160
7	B	< 10	40	< 10	40
8	B	20	320	< 10	80
9	...	< 10	40	< 10	20
10	B	< 10	80	< 10	160
11	B	< 10	80	< 10	40
12	B	< 10	80	< 10	160
13	B	< 10	80	< 10	40

*Bethel surveillance study of 1966.
†Lowest serum dilution tested 1:10.

of only 12,500/cu mm, with 29% neutrophils, 5% band cells, and 66% lymphocytes.

The two illnesses with onsets in May, which were associated with isolations of rhinovirus, occurred in girls, one 7 months and the other 2 years of age. Both cases were diagnosed as mild upper respiratory tract infections with body temperatures of 100.2 F (37.9 C) and 100.4 F (38 C), respectively, cough, and rhinitis as the only clinical manifestations. The isolated virus strains were not inhibited by 25 available rhinovirus antisera.

Comment

The extreme sensitivity of respiratory syncytial virus to freezing has been emphasized by Beem, et al.[4] These workers found that slow freezing of virus at −30 C resulted in complete loss of infectivity, and that rapid freezing at −70 C resulted in a large decrease in infectivity. More recently, Jordan[5] reported that Long strain of respiratory syncytial virus maintained in a medium consisting of 5% chicken serum, 25% tryptose phosphate broth, and 70% Eagles minimum essential medium survived quick freezing at −70 C for as long as six

Table 5.—Clinical Severity of 31 Cases of Influenza by Type of Influenza Infection*

Virus Infection Category	Cases With LRI†/Total Cases	%
Influenza B only	2/10	20
Influenza A2 only	6/8	75
Both influenza A2 and B	9/13	69
Total	17/31	55

*Bethel surveillance study of 1966.
†LRI = lower respiratory tract involvement.

months without significant loss of infectivity. Wulff et al[6] showed that Long strain, when preserved in high cystine altered Eagles medium with 50% glycerin, was stabilized at both −20 C or −70 C with no appreciable loss of titer for a period of nine months. However, this medium is not suitable for initial virus isolation because of toxicity of glycerin to tissue culture at the concentrations used and the resulting necessity for dilution of specimens prior to inoculation. In our laboratories, Long strain has survived for as long as three months without significant loss of infectivity when stored after quick freezing at -70 C in medium with 0.5% gelatin and 1% chicken serum added as stabilizers. The present study has demonstrated that nonlaboratory adapted "wild" strains of respiratory syncytial virus in this same medium will survive a single quick freeze at -70 C for periods as long as ten days, and that frequency of respiratory syncytial viral isolation under these circumstances may reach 50% of serologically confirmed respiratory syncytial infections.

The serologic evidence of simultaneous influenza A2 and B virus infections during the mixed influenza epidemic in Bethel is worthy of note. Lack of ability to demonstrate both viruses in throat specimens from children with diagnostic rises in both A2 and B virus serum antibody titers could be related to a viral interference phenomenon or to closely spaced, rather than simultaneous, infections. With regard to the latter possibility, none of the 13 children with dual serologic infections had history of a second respiratory illness closely following the reference illness. Another possible reason for failure to isolate both viruses may relate to laboratory technique. During the study period, influenza B viruses were isolated with ease and produced marked cytopathic effect in primary monkey kidney tissue culture by the sixth day of first passage incubation. Total destruction of cell monolayers usually occurred within ten days. In contrast, influenza A2 viruses were difficult to isolate, produced no cytopathic effect in cell monolayers, and hemadsorbed late, usually at ten days or beyond. Influenza A2 virus might have been revealed by longer tissue-culture incubation, with suppression of influenza B cytopathic effect by use of monovalent B antiserum. Further attempts at isolation of A2 virus from 13 throat specimens positive for B virus are currently in progress.

Our finding that clinical illness associated with influenza B virus infection in young children is generally less severe than that associated with influenza A2 infection provides confirmation of a generally accepted clinical impression which has not heretofore been adequately documented. The extremely high rate of lower respiratory tract involvement seen with influenza A2 infections in Bethel children would also support consideration of the prophylactic use of influenza vaccines in pediatric practice in this area, where socioeconomic and nutritional deprivation is associated with a generally sustained high risk of morbidity and mortality from infectious disease.

Rhinovirus antisera were provided by Jacob C. Holper, PhD, of the Infectious Disease Research Division, Abbott Laboratories, Chicago, through the Vaccine Development Program, National Institute of Allergy and Infectious Diseases.

References

1. Parran, T.: *Alaska's Health: A Survey Report*, section 6, University of Pittsburgh (Pa), 1954, p 110.

2. Maynard, J.E., and Hammes, L.M.: *A Study of Morbidity and Mortality Among Eskimo Infants of Western Alaska: Administrative Report*, Anchorage, Alaska: Arctic Health Research Center, May 1964.

3. Brody, J.A.: Lower Respiratory Illness Among Alaskan Eskimo Children, *Arch Environ Health* 11:620-623 (Nov) 1965.

4. Beem, M., et al: Association of the Chimpanzee Coryza Agent With Acute Respiratory Disease in Children, *New Eng J Med* 263:523-530 (Sept) 1960.

5. Jordan, W.S.: Growth Characteristics of Respiratory Syncytial Virus, *J Immunol* 88:581-590 (May) 1962.

6. Wulff, H.; Kidd, P.; and Wenner, H.A.: Respiratory Syncytial Virus: Properties of Strains Propagated in Monkey Kidney Cell Cultures, *Proc Soc Exp Biol Med* 115:458-462 (Feb) 1964.

194

INTRADERMAL TEST IN THE DETECTION OF TRICHINOSIS

Further Observations on Two Outbreaks Due to Bear Meat in Alaska

James E. Maynard, M.D., and Irving G. Kagan, Ph.D.

DURING the fall and winter of 1960-61, among Eskimo families at Bethel and Goodnews Bay, Alaska, there was an outbreak of trichinosis, totaling 24 cases, due to the ingestion of the meat of both black and brown bear. All cases were confirmed serologically and epidemiologically, and included 18 clinical and 6 subclinical infections. A report of these 2 outbreaks, with an evaluation of serodiagnosis and a review of the Arctic ecology of *Trichinella spiralis*, has been published elsewhere.[1] In the original epidemiologic investigation, an intracutaneous test using a standard commercial preparation§ was performed in 23 documented cases one to five months after ingestion of bear meat. Tests were performed on the volar surfaces of the forearms, with an injection of 0.10 ml. of 1:10,000 concentration of the antigen in one arm and the same quantity of diluent saline control in the contralateral arm. The responses were read at fifteen minutes using the standard antigen-control wheal-diameter comparison to determine the character of the reaction. Positive results were obtained in only 14 of the 23 documented cases. In addition, a skin-test survey of 26 persons from the involved villages with negative serologic reactions, no clinical illness but a history of possible ingestion of implicated meat yielded positive reactions in 10 cases.

The high rate of false-negative reactions in confirmed clinical infections, coupled with the high rate of positive reactions in persons with no clinical illness, considerably complicated the interpretation of the skin-test readings for diagnostic purposes.

A review of the literature on trichinella skin-testing indicated that lack of suitable case and control-group studies, as well as of consistent standardization of skin-test antigens and standard interpretation of the skin-test reaction itself, has precluded adequate evaluation of the role of the intradermal test both in epidemiologic survey and as a diagnostic adjunct.

The presence of a relatively large number of cases in which the clinical and epidemiologic diagnosis was clear cut and the existence of a comparable control group in the area led to the initiation of a controlled study of two trichina skin-test antigens prepared at the Communicable Disease Center, in series with the commercial antigen administered and interpreted according to rigorously defined criteria. This paper presents the results of this study.

MATERIALS AND METHODS

Two skin-test antigens prepared at the Communicable Disease Center were used for the study. The first, an acid-soluble protein-fraction antigen, was prepared according to the method of Melcher.[2] Two grams of lyophilized trichina larvas was extracted with petroleum ether in a Soxhlet apparatus for seven days. The dry delipidized larvas were triturated with 50 ml. of borate buffer (pH 8.3) overnight at 4°C. with shaking, and centrifuged at 10,000 × g for thirty minutes. The clear supernatant was precipitated in the cold at pH 4.8 with 0.2-normal hydrochloric acid, and the precipitate discarded. The acid-soluble fraction was used as the antigen.

The second, a metabolic-products antigen (LXS), was prepared from viable larvas. The larvas recovered after three hours of digestion were washed thoroughly in three saline rinses, the middle rinse also containing 1:10,000 thimerosal (merthiolate). Dilutional counts were made, and 500,000 larvas were placed in an Erlenmeyer flask with 5 ml. of ox ultrafiltrate, 10 ml. of Simms-X6 balanced saline

§In the form of trichinella extract, Lederle Laboratories, Pearl River, New York.

195

solution, 15,000 units of penicillin G and 15 mg. of streptomycin sulfate. The larvas were incubated at 37°C. for three days with shakings twice a day to ensure more even distribution of the metabolic products. After the third day the supernatant fluid was collected by centrifugation for use as antigen.

Nitrogen content of both antigens was determined by a modified Nessler method after Lang.[3] By adjustment of nitrogen content 2 concentrations of each of the antigens were prepared. The 2 Melcher antigens contained 20 microgm. and 10 microgm. of nitrogen per milliliter each. The 2 LXS antigens contained 30 microgm. and 15 microgm. of nitrogen per milliliter each. These 4 solutions, in addition to diluent controls and commercial antigen and control, were used for the skin tests.

The test group consisted of 22 confirmed infections from Bethel and Goodnews Bay. Sixteen of these subjects had clinical manifestations of disease as well as positive serologic reactions on serial bentonite flocculation tests. Six persons partook of infected meat, had serologic evidence of infestation and were classified as having subclinical infections.

The contact group consisted of 26 persons from Goodnews Bay who had a history of ingestion contact with contaminated meat but no clinical illness, and in whom serologic evidence of infection could not be demonstrated by bentonite flocculation test. The control group of 60 was chosen from Eskimos inhabiting the village of Mekoryuk, located on Nunivak, an island in the Bering Sea in proximity to the case and contact villages. No trichinosis was known to have occurred in this village. Figure 1 shows the geographic relations of these villages.

For injection of the Melcher and LXS antigens and controls, a dose of 0.05 ml. was administered with 0.25-ml. syringes with 27-gauge 0.95-cm. platinum needles. The standard dose of 0.1 ml. of commercial antigen and control was given in 1-ml. tuberculin syringes with the use of similar platinum needles. Injections, placed evenly across the back in the area of the scapulas, were administered by Public Health nurses experienced in the administration of tuberculin tests. We read reactions at the end of fifteen minutes by outlining the wheals with ballpoint pen and transferring these tracings to paper

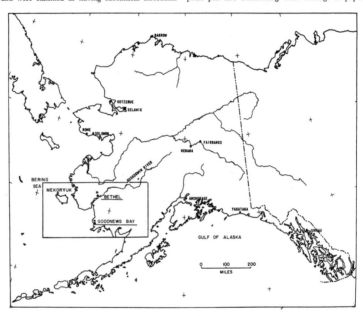

FIGURE 1. *Map of Alaska.*

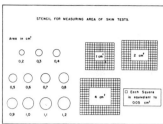

FIGURE 2. *Stencil for Measuring the Area of Skin Tests.*

slightly moistened with alcohol. Determinations of wheal area were made independently by 2 persons, who had no knowledge of the sequence of antigen and control injections, according to a standardized method described by Kagan and Pellegrino[4] and used extensively in the evaluation of the intradermal test for bilharziasis. Figure 2 shows the stencil used in the measurement of wheal area.

Analysis of the case, contact and control data revealed that the wheal-area comparison giving the highest rate of reactivity in the case group and the lowest rate in the control group for all antigens employed was a test wheal at least twice the area of the control wheal. Accordingly, this ratio was considered indicative of a positive reaction, and all results were based on this criterion.

RESULTS

Table 1 gives the skin-test results for the case, contact and control groups. In the Bethel case group the mean wheal area obtained with the antigens employed was 1.83 square cm. for Melcher 20, 1.78 square cm. for Melcher 10, 2.79 square cm. for LXS 30, 1.63 square cm. for LXS 15 and 1.28 square cm. for the commercial antigen. The mean areas for the 3 control solutions were 0.57 square cm. for Melcher control, 0.65 square cm. for LXS control and 0.85 square cm. for the commercial control. The relatively high mean wheal area for the LXS 30 antigen was influenced greatly by 1 subject, whose test reaction measured 12.35 square cm. The fact that the mean test wheal area of the commercial antigen was less than twice the mean area of the corresponding control wheals is a reflection of the low frequency of positive reactions for this antigen in the case group. With the Melcher 20 antigen

3 of the 4 negative tests were negative with all the antigens employed. One negative Melcher 20 test was positive with the other antigens. The case group showed that the Melcher 20 and Melcher 10 antigens were somewhat more sensitive than the corresponding LXS antigens and much more sensitive than the commercial antigen.

In the Goodnews Bay contact group 7 of the 8 tests positive with the Melcher 20 antigen were also positive with the Melcher 10 antigen. Only 4 of these subjects were positive with the LXS antigens. The intermediate reactivity of this group was consistent with the long-term intermittent ingestion contact with bear meat in the village. Again, commercial-antigen reactivity was considerably below that of the other antigens.

Because of the lack of demonstrated superior sensitivity of the LXS antigens to the Melcher antigens in the case group, and because of their difficulty in preparation in contrast to Melcher antigen, it was decided to dispense with further evaluation of this material and to use only Melcher and commercial antigen in the control group. At Mekoryuk 12 tests were positive with the Melcher 20, and only 3 with the Melcher 10 antigen. All 3 positive with the Melcher 10 antigen were also positive with the Melcher 20 antigen, and only 1 was positive with the commercial antigen.

For all positive Melcher skin tests in the 3 groups, test wheal areas measured at least 0.8 square cm. Of the 29 subjects with positive Melcher 10 skin tests 26 (90 per cent) had areas 1.0 square cm. or greater.

The rates of reactivity in the case, contact and control groups indicated superiority of the Melcher antigens over commercial antigen. Sensitivity of the Melcher 10 antigen was equivalent to that of the Melcher 20 in both case and contact groups. However, the rate of reactivity of the Melcher 20 antigen in the control group was high enough to indicate unacceptable nonspecificity for this material. The low rate of reactivity of the Melcher 10 antigen in the control group suggested acceptable specificity.

In the interpretation of the skin tests it was important to determine the range of reactivity of the control wheals. Table 2 gives the distribution of control wheal areas in the series as well as the distribution of positive Melcher 10 test wheal areas. The median area for control wheals was in the range of 0.70 to 0.89 square cm. whereas the median area for positive test wheals was in the range of

TABLE 1. *Trichina Skin-Test Results.*

SUBJECT STATUS	MELCHER 20 REACTIVITY		LXS 30 REACTIVITY		MELCHER 10 REACTIVITY		LXS 15 REACTIVITY		COMMERCIAL-ANTIGEN REACTIVITY	
	x/n	%	x/n	%	x/n	%	x/n	%	x/n	%
Confirmed cases	18/22	82	16/22	73	17/22	77	12/22	55	6/22	27
Goodnews contacts	8/26	31	6/26	23	9/26	35	3/26	12	2/26	8
Mekoryuk controls	12/60	20	—	—	3/60	5	—	—	4/60	7

WHEAL AREA	CONTROL WHEALS		POSITIVE TEST WHEALS	
	NO.	PERCENTAGE	NO.	PERCENTAGE
sq. cm.				
0.00-0.29	0	0	0	0
0.30-0.49	15	14	0	0
0.50-0.69	28	26	0	0
0.70-0.89	24	22	3	10
0.90-1.09	29	27	1	4
1.10-1.29	12	11	7	24
1.30 & over	0	0	18	62
Totals	108	100	29	100

1.30 square cm. or greater. There was a considerable overlap, however, in the distribution of control wheal and positive test wheal areas. A total of 11 positive tests (38 per cent) and 65 control tests (60 per cent) fell between wheal areas of 0.7 to 1.29 square cm.

DISCUSSION

In the choice of a skin-test control group for trichinosis it is not sufficient simply to accept as controls persons who have no clinical history of illness compatible with the disease. The existence of subclinical infection has been well documented in the past and was shown to exist in the Bethel and Goodnews Bay outbreaks.[1] Furthermore, seronegativity is not in itself an adequate criterion for a control-group construction. For both the Suessenguth–Kline slide flocculation test and the bentonite flocculation test, serum specimens from infected human patients may revert to negative as early as twelve months after infection. Gould[5] has also noted that complement-fixing antibodies disappear in many cases as early as one year after infection. The same considerations apply to the precipitin test. Control groups should be assembled from persons living under ecologic conditions that favor little or no ingestion contact with faunal sources known to commonly harbor trichina larvas. Furthermore, infection with helminthic agents known to cross-react antigenically with *Trichinella spiralis*, such as *Ascaris lumbricoides* and *Trichuris trichiura*, must be absent or at a minimum in the control population. Racial and ethnic characteristics of the test and control populations should also be similar since differences, particularly in the skin, may introduce unevaluated variables.

In this study the case and control groups were similar in racial and ethnic characteristics and lived under equivalent ecologic conditions. Both groups belong to the Kuskokwim Eskimo linguistic grouping, whose members inhabit the delta and tundra country of western Alaska from the Yukon River south to Bristol Bay. The entire economy is still basically one of hunting and fishing. These Eskimos do not eat pork, but the mainland peoples, from whom the case group was drawn, do have

ingestion contact with the nonporcine boreal faunal reservoirs of trichina present in Alaska such as black and brown bear. These reservoirs do not exist on Nunivak Island, and the relatively nonmobile group at Mekoryuk depend largely upon a local reindeer industry for meat. The islanders do utilize walrus and seal for food. Rausch and his associates[6] found no evidence of trichinous infestation in autopsy examination of 51 walrus from St. Lawrence Island and the Alaska coast, and trichinella larvas were found in only 2 of 310 seals obtained from the same area.

Hitchcock,[7] in a parasitologic study of Eskimos in this area of Alaska, was repeatedly unable to recover the eggs of *A. lumbricoides* or *T. trichiura* in human stool samples. Fournelle et al.,[8] in a subsequent study in the area, found a low incidence of trichuris and ascarid infection in dogs but no evidence of ascaris infection in human beings. Of over 1000 human stool examinations, they reported infection with trichuris in only 1. From the foregoing, it may be concluded that contact with the larvas of *T. spiralis* was minimal in the control group, and that nonspecificity, introduced through the presence of other known helminthic cross-reactors, was unlikely.

The intradermal test as a diagnostic tool in the detection of trichinosis has been a subject of interest since Bachman,[9] in 1928, demonstrated reactivity in infected guinea pigs after injection of dried pulverized larvas extracted with Coca's solution. Subsequently, both immediate and delayed skin reactivity was demonstrated in patients with clinical histories of the disease. Considered most specific has been the immediate reaction, which usually occurs within fifteen minutes of infection and is said to represent an example of atopic hypersensitivity not unlike that seen in hay fever or asthma. Introduction of a small amount of exciting agent produces a characteristic wheal, often with pseudopods, surrounded by a zone of erythema reaching maximum proportions in ten to twenty minutes. Gould[5] has cited the earliest appearance of a positive immediate reaction in man as sixteen days after infection but has generally believed that most skin tests do not become positive until the end of the third week. Kagan[10] has reported sensitivity that lasted as long as twenty years after infection.

The interpretation of the skin reaction itself has varied considerably over the years. McCoy et al.,[11] injecting 0.1 ml. of a 1:10,000 dilution of antigen, used both wheal diameter and erythema diameter as criteria. They considered a positive reaction one in which the wheal diameter was at least 7 mm. and the diameter of the zone of erythema at least 20 mm. Schapiro, Crosby and Sickler,[12] using an antigen of 1:10,000 dilution, regarded test wheals of 5-mm. diameter or greater as positive. Although they used a control injection in their studies it is not clear how it was interpreted in relation to the test injection. Harrell and Horne,[13] injecting 0.02 to 0.03 ml. of a 1:10,000 dilution of antigen, called a reaction positive if the diameter of the test wheal and erythema exceeded that of the control by 5 mm. or more. Frisch, Whims and Oppenheim,[14] using 0.05 ml. of antigen diluted 1:10,000, regarded any test wheal that exceeded 8 mm. in diameter as positive. More recently, the production of erythema has been considered too unreliable to be included in the diameter reading, and the formation of a test wheal whose diameter exceeds that of the control wheal by 3 mm. or more using 0.05 to 0.1 ml. of a 1:10,000 dilution of antigen has been considered to represent an adequate interpretive criterion.

Actually, there is reason to doubt the reproducibility of readings based upon wheal diameter in trichinosis. As with skin tests for bilharziasis, wheal outlines, using trichina antigen, tend to be irregular, and, not uncommonly, the wheals demonstrate pseudopodia. Furthermore, it is possible to vary a diameter reading according to whether widest cross-sectional diameter or simple transverse diameter is measured. In our series of wheal outlines it was possible to vary the diameter readings of a single wheal by as much as 5 mm. according to which diameter was used. The literature on trichina skin testing is usually not explicit in the definition of diameters. Because of these facts we consider measurement of wheal area to represent a better standardized and more reproducible method of defining the skin reactivity of the antigen.

The back was chosen as the site of injection for these studies because of indications that it may be more sensitive in the production of reactions than the skin of the arm. In the evaluation of an intradermal test for bilharziasis in Brazil Pellegrino et al.[15] showed a significant difference in response when children were tested on the arm or the back, with the back always being more sensitive. Kagan and his associates,[16] using bilharzia antigen in adult males and females, demonstrated the same increased sensitivity on the back. The likelihood that this phenomenon of increased sensitivity is not limited to 1 helminthic antigen made the choice of a back site for trichina skin testing seem indicated.

The high rate of reactivity of the Melcher 20 antigen in the control group indicated a lack of specificity that may preclude its use as a diagnostic tool. The acceptable specificity of the Melcher 10 antigen invited the speculation that degree of specificity could have been related to the nitrogen content of the material.

The use of control injections in skin testing detracts from the ease with which these tests can be administered. If control reactivity in this series had been slight and the frequency distribution of control wheal areas more confined and definitely de-

marcated from that of the test wheal areas, the data would have favored the concept of dispensing with the control injection. The significant overlap in these distributions, however, indicated that it would have been impossible to dispense with the control injection and still maintain the degree of sensitivity attained through test-control wheal-area comparison.

The 16 negative tests with the commercial antigen in confirmed cases was evidence of a lack of sensitivity of this antigen great enough to preclude its usefulness as either a diagnostic or survey tool in this series. All tests in cases and contacts were performed at least five months after ingestion of bear meat, and these 16 tests should represent true false-negative tests since there is little evidence that a postulated positive skin reactivity early in illness could revert to negative by the time of testing. Certainly, a negative skin test with commercial antigen would not have ruled out a diagnosis of trichinosis.

SUMMARY

In 2 outbreaks of trichinosis in western Alaska due to ingestion of infected bear meat, 2 trichina skin-test antigens prepared at the Communicable Disease Center were evaluated with a commercially available skin-test antigen. When injections were placed across the back of subjects and measurements of wheal area made in infected patients, contacts and control groups a test wheal at least twice the area of the control wheal was found to be the most reliable means of identifying positive reactors. Frequency distributions of control and positive test wheal areas showed significant overlap and indicated that adequate sensitivity could be obtained only when skin-test interpretation was related to a comparison of test-control wheal area. A 10-microgm. nitrogen concentration of an acid-soluble protein fraction of trichina larvas (Melcher's antigen) showed good sensitivity and specificity in the series and was considered useful as a diagnostic and survey tool in trichinosis investigations. The lack of sensitivity of the commercially available antigen precluded its diagnostic usefulness in this evaluation.

REFERENCES

1. Maynard, J. E., and Pauls, F. P. Trichinosis in Alaska: review and report of two outbreaks due to bear meat with observations on serodiagnosis and skin testing. *Am. J. Hyg.* **76**:252-261, 1962.
2. Melcher, L. R. Antigenic analysis of Trichinella spiralis. *J. Infect. Dis.* **73**:31-39, 1943.
3. Lang, C. A. Simple micro determination of Kjeldahl nitrogen in biological materials. *Analytical Chem.* **30**:1692-1694, 1958.
4. Kagan, I. G., and Pellegrino, J. Critical review of immunologic methods for diagnosis of bilharzias. *Bull. World Health Organ.* **25**:611-674, 1961.
5. Gould, S. E. *Trichinosis.* 356 pp. Springfield, Illinois: Thomas, 1945. Pp. 55-62 and 133-164.
6. Rausch, R., Babero, B. B., Rausch, R. V., and Schiller, E. L. Studies on helminth fauna of Alaska. XXVII. Occurrence of larvae of Trichinella spiralis in Alaskan mammals. *J. Parasitol.* **42**:259-271, 1956.
7. Hitchcock, D. J. Parasitological study on Eskimos in Bethel area of Alaska. *J. Parasitol.* **36**:232-234, 1950.

8. Fournelle, H. J., Wallace, I. L., and Rader, V. Bacteriological and parasitological survey of enteric infections in Alaskan Eskimo area. *Am. J. Pub. Health* **48**:1489-1497, 1958.

9. Bachman, G. W. Intradermal reaction in experimental trichinosis. *J. Prev. Med.* **2**:513-523, 1928.

10. Kagan, I. G. Trichinosis: review of biologic, serologic, and immunologic aspects. *J. Infect. Dis.* **107**:65-93, 1960.

11. McCoy, O. R., Miller, J. J., Jr., and Friedlander, R. D. Use of intradermal test in diagnosis of trichiniasis. *J. Immunol.* **24**:1-23, 1933.

12. Schapiro, M. M., Crosby, B. L., and Sickler, M. M. Correlation of clinical diagnosis and postmortem findings in trichinosis. *J. Lab. & Clin. Med.* **23**:681-687, 1938.

13. Harrell, G. T., and Horne, S. F. Trichinella skin tests in tuberculosis sanitariums, hospitals for mental diseases, and general hospitals: comparison of results in tuberculous and non-tuberculous patients. *Am. J. Trop. Med.* **25**:51-58, 1945.

14. Frisch, A. W., Whims, C. B., and Oppenheim, J. M. Intradermal reactions in trichinosis. *Am. J. Clin. Path.* **17**:16-23, 1947.

15. Pellegrino, J., Rezénde, C. L. de, Memoria, J. M. P., Mourao, O. G., and Brener, Z. Diagnóstico de laboratório da esquistossomose mansoni na criança. *J. Pediat.* **24**:211-230, 1959.

16. Kagan, I. G., Pellegrino, J., and Memoria, J. M. P. Studies on standardization of intradermal test for diagnosis of bilharziasis. *Am. J. Trop. Med. & Hyg.* **10**:200-207, 1961.

Autopsied Cases by Age, Sex, and "Race"

C. A. McMahan, Ph.D.

The investigator usually begins preliminary epidemiologic studies with gross descriptive variables. Initially, he may make use of demographic and quasi-demographic variables, such as age, sex, race, residence, occupational status, educational status, economic status, combinations of variables called socioeconomic status, religious affiliation, and marital status. To obtain research leads, he would like to demonstrate an association between a specified disease and one or more of these variables. To illustrate from the present International Atherosclerosis Project (IAP), the investigator would like to demonstrate the association between arterial involvement with atherosclerotic lesions and a specified variable by identifying differential involvement among subgroups of that variable.

This particular report is concerned with only three of the descriptive variables listed above, namely, age, sex, and "race" (or ethnic group), where these variables characterize the autopsied cases from which arterial specimens were collected. Clearly then, this paper concerns demography, not findings related to arterial involvement.

BASIS OF DESCRIPTIVE EPIDEMIOLOGY

Associations involving descriptive variables are of fundamental importance to the epidemiologist in developing hypotheses. Probably the most important descriptive variable concerns passage of time as related to an individual, usually measured in years since date of birth. Moreover, the combination of this variable of age with the two variables sex and race might be considered a basic triad for descriptive epidemiology.

METHOD OF COMPARISON

One objective of this international study is to identify variation in average arterial involvement according to geographic residence. In the study of atherosclerosis, opinions regarding differential arterial involvement by age, sex, and race are held by many experienced pathologists; in fact, a major portion of the methodology of this study was designed to take into account these views by making comparisons among similar age-sex-race groups when possible. In other words, the attempt was made to study average arterial involvement while holding age, sex, and race more or less "constant"; unfortunately, race and geographic residence were confounded in many situations, making it necessary to attempt to hold only sex and age constant.

PURPOSE

Among the purposes of this paper are the following: (1) to post again a danger sign with regard to generalizing from a group of autopsied cases to a living population; (2) to provide a frame of reference in terms of what is hypothesized about autopsied cases in the United States; (3) to examine the age distribution of the autopsied cases utilized in the IAP; (4) to examine the sex ratio of the autopsied cases used in the IAP; (5) to indicate why certain analytic procedures were followed in the IAP; and (6) to provide a more meaningful framework for interpreting the results relevant to arterial involvement.

Superficial reading of this paper may suggest negative overtones relating to the International Atherosclerosis Project; no such implication is intended. Data obtained at autopsy concerning the severity and the qualitative characteristics of a chronic disease, such as atherosclerosis with its "iceberg" phenomenon, deserve intensive study and warrant major efforts.

BACKGROUND

ORIGINAL PLANNING

In 1958, at the request of the sponsors of this project, suggested topics to be included in a protocol for the then embryonic international study of atherosclerosis were outlined. For each topic, detailed procedures were suggested. Schedules (data collection forms) were drafted to be pretested. The investigators then took the necessary steps to expand and add details to the protocol and to test the data collection procedures. These procedures were considered prepilot studies, they were "homework" to provide working data and documents for discussion at future planning conferences.

One of the major problems facing such a proposed study was the complex relationship between a sample composed only of autopsied cases and a population of living persons; admittedly this was a problem, but no substitute procedure for collecting the required data appeared feasible. Had resources been available, an attempt would have been made to circumscribe the problem. In fact, the plan was to make a hospital census at each large collection hospital on at least two specified dates during the study; to collect demographic data on all deaths and all autopsied cases for short periods of time during the study (up to a year); to utilize data from hospital records; to use local population census data and vital statistics data when available; and to visit each collection facility and systematically observe the local population, the hospital patient "population," as well as the "populations" of dead persons and autopsied cases at each location.

Limitations of population census data and vital statistics data are well known for many of the areas from which it was planned to collect specimens for the Project. These limitations were carefully considered before drafting the initial plans for the study, the outline of the protocol, and the tentative data collection forms. "Memoranda for the record" indicate that (in 1958) professional demographers and other personnel were consulted at the United States Bureau of the Census, the United States National Office of Vital Statistics, the Pan American World Health Organization, the United Nations, and at other institutions, on the matter of circumventing problems involving inferences based on autopsied cases. In fact, Professor Felix Moore of the University of Michigan in Ann Arbor visited the Louisiana State University Medical Center in New Orleans as a consultant on these problems.

STUDIES OF PERSONS DYING AND AUTOPSIED CASES AT EACH LABORATORY OF PATHOLOGY. Original plans called for collection of data on each death, as well as on each autopsied case, at each collection center. A pilot study for calendar year 1959 was designed and conducted. Explicitly, in New Orleans, Louisiana, a majority of the specimens collected for the Project was expected to originate in Charity Hospital of Louisiana at New Orleans; some cases would obviously be "coroner's cases." During the last 3 months of 1958, Elizabeth J. Moore and others pretested a survey to collect data on all deaths as well as autopsied cases at Charity Hospital (Fig. 1). The study was conducted during the period January 1 to December 31, 1959.[289]

PREPLANNING CONFERENCE, GUATEMALA CITY, GUATEMALA, DECEMBER 1959. At this conference, dangers were described of attempting to make inferences about disease conditions in a living population based only upon data obtained from autopsied cases. The proposal (suggested in the foregoing remarks) was made for collecting data on the indigenous population for each area.

PLANNING CONFERENCE, JANUARY 1960. Prior to this conference, the protocol and collection procedures had already been structured and, hence, were supplemented, strengthened, clarified, critically appraised, and revised by the entire group of investigators.

PRELIMINARY PROTOCOL OF 1960 AND FINAL PUBLISHED PROTOCOL, JANUARY 1962. After the January (1960) meeting, the preliminary protocol[219] was modified and distributed; the final protocol,[220] including procedures regarding cerebral arteries, was published in January 1962. Major portions of the protocol were adopted by the World Health Organization at a planning conference held in March 1962, for a similar survey of atherosclerosis in Europe.

CONFERENCE, NEW ORLEANS, APRIL 1963. At the interim conference of all investigators, the dangers of generalizing from a group of autopsied cases to a living population were again emphasized.

PROBABILITY OF AUTOPSY. In order to obtain estimates of "conditional probabilities of autopsy," data were collected on all deaths and reported autopsied cases in Orleans Parish for the period January 1, 1959 to December 31, 1961. Each resident case was assigned to a census tract. These data, in combination with data from the 1960 Census of Population, provided the basis for estimating the "probability of autopsy" for residents of Orleans Parish;[290] thus that study is one attempt, under strict assumptions, to relate a group of autopsied cases, through a group of deaths, to a living population.

POPULATION, DEATHS, AND AUTOPSIED CASES

In a study such as this, three groups should be clearly distinguished within each geographic population, where population is used in the demographic sense in contrast to the statistical sense. These three groups are as follows: group 1 (G_L): the living population as of a specified instant of time, say, t_0; group 2 (G_D): those persons who belonged to the population G_L at the specified time, t_0, and who died during a specified period of elapsed time, called "deaths" for convenience; and group 3 (G_A): those cases within group G_D who happened to be necropsied.

This report is focused on only one of the three groups, namely, the third group, autopsied cases, G_A. Not the slightest effort is made to relate data from those who died, G_D, to the living population, G_L; no attempt is made to relate the demographic characteristics of these autopsied cases, G_A, to the group of dead persons, G_D. More important, no inference whatsoever is made from demographic data on the group of autopsied cases, G_A, about the living population, G_L.

Every competent investigator in the health sciences knows that, in general, autopsied cases compose a select and biased sample of deaths in many ways. Even if all dead persons were autopsied, one might err seriously in making judgments about a living population based on data obtained only from a group of dead persons.

UNITED STATES AS A FRAME OF REFERENCE

Some tentative hypotheses concerning demographic characteristics of autopsied cases in the United States follow: (1) Dead males are more likely to be autopsied than dead females. (2) The average reported age at death for autopsied cases is lower for females than for males. (3) Persons dying in the early teen-age years are least likely to be autopsied. (4) The proportion of dead persons reported autopsied declines for those dying after about age 40. (5) Persons dying at ages 75 and over have small probability of being autopsied. (6) Nonwhite persons appear to be autopsied in somewhat greater proportions than white persons. (7) The proportion of deaths autopsied in southern states is smaller than the proportions of deaths autopsied in other sections of the United States. (8) States which rank high in the percentage of the population classified as urban, high in wealth, and high in number of physicians per 100,000 population, tend to rank high in the proportion autopsied. (9) Differential autopsy rates prevail not only among states but among counties within states. (10) Autopsied cases are selective, in part, of deaths which occur in institutions. (11) There may be a tendency for autopsied cases to be selective of the more uncommon causes of death.[57, 282-286]

COL	CODE	
1-2		2. Identification No: Laboratory code
3-6		Accession no.
7		3. Source of item 1: (1) Charity (2) Coroner's Off.
8-9		4. Date of death Month (January, 01; ... December, 12)
10-11		Day (First Day, 01; ...; Last Day, 31)
12-13		Year (1958, 58; 1959, 59)
14		5. Charity adm. status: (1)LSU (4)No-admit, Charity DOA (2)Tulane (5)No-admit, other (3)Ind. (6)Charity admit, not specf. (x)Unknown
15		6. Race: (1) White (4) Indian (x) Unknown (2) Negro (5) Mestizo (3) Mulatto (6) Other
16		7. Sex: (1) Male (2) Female (x) Unknown
17-18		8. Age in years(2 digits): Less than 1 yr., 00; Unkn, xx
19-21		9. If age less than 1 yr, age in days(3 digits): Less than 24 hrs, 000; Unknown, xxx; Not applicable, 999
22		10. If age less than 24 hrs, specify: (1)Stillborn (2)Liveborn; (9)Not applicable; (x)Unknown
23		11. Autopsy permit: (0) No permit (2) Partial (1) Complt. autpsy (3) Permit, unspf (x) Unknown
24		12. Autopsy status: (0)Not performed (4)At CO on CH (1)At CH on admit no-admit (2)At CH on no-admit (5)At another for CO hosp. for CO (3)At CO on CH admit (x)Unknown
25		13. Coroner's case: (1)Yes (2) No (x) Unknown
26		14. If item 13 was yes, was autopsy performed? (1) Yes (2) No (x) Unknown (9)Not Applicable
27-28 29-32		15. Charity Hospital autopsy number or Coroner's Office case number:
33		16. Specimens collected: (0) None (2) Coronaries only (1) Aorta only (3) Aorta & coronary
34-36		17. Heart weight in grams (3 digits): Unknown, xxx

COL	CODE	
37		18. State of nutrition:Body wt............... Lgth......... (see code) Fluid...............Edema + ++ +++
38		19. Thickness of panniculus adiposus: (see code) ....mm
39-40		20. Principal Cause of Death - Clinical Diagnosis: (see code)
41-42		21. Principal Cause of Death - Provisional Anatomic Diagnosis: (see code)
43		22. Accidental death: (1) Yes (2) No (x) Unknown
44		23. If age is less than 1 yr., is there a severe congenital abnormality incompatible with life? (1) Yes (2) No (x) Unknown (9) Not applicable
45		24. Hypertension: (0) Not present (1) Benign essential hypertension (2) Malignant hypert. or nephroscl. (3) Hypertension other than (1) or(2) (9) Not applicable (x) Unknown
46		25. Diabetes mellitus: (0) Not present (1) Present, presumptive (2) Present, established (9) Not applicable (x) Unknown
47		26. Syphilitic heart disease: (0) Not present (1) Present (9) Not applicable (x) Unknown
48		27. Myocardial infarction, old or recent: "
49		28. Coronary occlusion with death, but without infarction: "
50		29. Cerebral thrombosis with cerebral infarction: "
51		30. Cerebral hemorrhage: "
52		31. Cerebral vascular disease, unclassified: "
53		32. Disabling peripheral vascular disease: "
54.		33. Other disease due to atherosclerosis: "

FIG. 1. Schedule for the collection of data on deaths and autopsied cases at Charity Hospital of Louisiana at New Orleans, 1959.

DATA

IMPRESSIONS OF THE SOURCES OF DATA

The author has visited three laboratories in which data were collected for the International Atherosclerosis Project; these are the impressions gained from these visits and from many other communications with the investigators in the various laboratories. It appears that major sources of the data were large state or municipally supported general hospitals which cared for indigent patients. Other major sources were "medicolegal laboratories"; medicolegal cases usually include not only accidental deaths, homicides, and suicides, but also natural deaths which occur "without medical care" for a specified period of time prior to death and thus become the responsibility of the coroner or medical examiner. Locations of medicolegal laboratories which contributed the overwhelming proportion of such cases are Lima, Peru; Santiago, Chile; San Juan, Puerto Rico; New Orleans; Cali, Colombia; and São Paulo, Brasil.

According to Dr. Solberg, data from Oslo, Norway, do not stem exclusively from the lowest social strata, but probably stem from a cross-section (not necessarily representative) of the population. Undoubtedly there are other exceptions regarding socioeconomic status, for example, at Roosevelt Hospital in Guatemala City and

University Hospital in Caracas, Venezuela, where some data stem from strata other than the lowest.

TABLE 1. NATIONAL ORIGIN AND MAJOR RACIAL CLASSIFICATION OF AUTOPSIED CASES[a]

Country	Dominant city	Major racial groups
Brasil	São Paulo	White, Negro, and mulatto
Colombia	Bogotá	American Indian-white and white
	Cali	American Indian-white, white, and American Indian
Costa Rica	San José	White
Guatemala	Guatemala City	American Indian and American Indian-white
Chile	Santiago	White
Jamaica	Kingston	Negro and mulatto
Mexico	Mexico City	American Indian-white
Norway	Oslo	White
Peru	Lima	American Indian and American Indian-white
Puerto Rico	San Juan	White, mulatto, and Negro
Philippines	Manila	Filipino
South Africa	Durban	Bantu and Asian Indian
United States	New Orleans	Negro and white
Venezuela	Caracas	American Indian-white, white, and American Indian

[a] In this and all subsequent tables, unless otherwise specified the data were derived from the International Atherosclerosis Project, 1960 to 1965.

RACE

Some writers make use of only three major subdivisions of man, namely, Mongoloid, Negroid, and Caucasian; however, since the epidemiologist is interested in differentials due to either biologic or social factors or both, cases in the IAP have been classified in terms of more detailed descriptive terminology. Race as used in this study refers to that category (social race) which was assigned at the time of autopsy. Racial or ethnic categories utilized were as follows: white, Negro, mulatto, American Indian, American Indian-white, Bantu, Filipino, and Asian Indian.

NATIONAL ORIGIN AND RACE

Data collected on autopsied cases were generated in 15 cities within 14 nations and involved at least eight so-called racial groups (Table 1).

AGE

This study is limited to the age group 10 to 69 inclusive, where age means the age reported at time of death. Some of the data are dependent upon records, like those of Oslo, and thus appear to be highly accurate, while some of the data seem to be estimates.

TABLE 2. NUMBER AND PERCENTAGE OF AUTOPSIED CASES BY AGE, SEX, AND RACE[a]

Age (x to $x + n$)	All classes			White			% = (cases x to $x + n$)/ (total white)		Negro and mulatto			% = (cases x to $x + n$)/ (total Negro and mulatto)		American Indian and American Indian-white			% = (cases x to $x + n$)/ (total American Indian and American Indian-white)	
	Total No.	Male	Female	Total No.	Male	Female	Male	Female	Total No.	Male	Female	Male	Female	Total No.	Male	Female	Male	Female
All ages (yr.)	21,302	13,908	7394	10,783	7326	3457			5186	3182	2004			5333	3400	1933		
10–14	603	394	209	301	206	95	1.9	0.9	118	72	46	1.4	0.9	184	116	68	2.2	1.3
15–19	1,115	669	446	601	381	220	3.5	2.0	211	113	98	2.2	1.9	303	175	128	3.3	2.4
20–24	1,579	1,012	567	804	536	268	5.0	2.5	337	219	118	4.2	2.3	438	257	181	4.8	3.4
25–29	1,638	1,055	583	799	538	261	5.0	2.4	432	270	162	5.2	3.1	407	247	160	4.6	3.0
30–34	1,868	1,208	660	919	629	290	5.8	2.7	458	293	165	5.6	3.2	491	286	205	5.4	3.8
35–39	2,086	1,337	749	1,002	682	320	6.3	3.0	563	336	227	6.5	4.4	521	319	202	6.0	3.8
40–44	1,948	1,307	641	927	648	279	6.0	2.6	541	343	198	6.6	3.8	480	316	164	5.9	3.1
45–49	1,998	1,324	674	986	677	309	6.3	2.9	533	335	198	6.5	3.8	479	312	167	5.9	3.1
50–54	2,347	1,605	742	1,181	839	342	7.8	3.2	617	386	231	7.4	4.5	549	380	169	7.1	3.2
55–59	2,058	1,421	637	1,096	774	322	7.2	3.0	511	341	170	6.6	3.3	451	306	145	5.7	2.7
60–64	2,344	1,474	870	1,192	785	407	7.3	3.8	568	315	253	6.1	4.9	584	374	210	7.0	3.9
65–69	1,718	1,102	616	975	631	344	5.9	3.2	297	159	138	3.1	2.7	446	312	134	5.9	2.5
Mean	42.9	43.2	42.5	43.4	43.4	43.2			42.9	42.7	43.2			42.1	43.0	40.6		
S.D.	15.6	15.4	15.8	15.8	15.7	16.2			14.6	14.4	15.0			15.9	15.9	15.9		
P_{10}[b]	21	21	20	21	21	20			22	23	22			20	20	19		
$Q_1 = P_{25}$	30	31	30	30	31	30			32	32	32			30	30	28		
Median = $Q_2 = P_{50}$	44	44	43	45	45	44			43	43	44			42	44	40		
$Q_3 = P_{75}$	56	56	56	57	57	58			55	55	56			56	56	55		
P_{90}	63	63	63	64	64	64			62	61	62			63	64	62		
$Q_3 - Q_1$	26	25	26	27	26	28			23	23	24			26	26	27		
$P_{90} - P_{10}$	42	42	43	43	43	44			40	38	40			43	44	43		

[a] Asian Indian and Filipino cases are not included in this table.
[b] P_{10} designates the 10th percentile and P_{90}, the 90th percentile; P_{25} refers to the 25th percentile which is obviously the first quartile, Q_1; likewise P_{75} is the 75th percentile and thus the third quartile, Q_3.

TABLE 3. NUMBER OF AUTOPSIED CASES IN 19 LOCATION-RACE GROUPS COMBINED, BY SINGLE YEARS OF AGE, AND SEX

Age	All groups combined		
	Total	Male	Female
yr.			
All ages	22,509	14,606	7,903
10	109	79	30
11	97	61	36
12	135	85	50
13	122	80	42
14	189	123	66
15	193	122	71
16	188	104	84
17	249	149	100
18	267	154	113
19	284	175	109
20	338	214	124
21	291	194	97
22	376	228	148
23	323	206	117
24	350	226	124
25	387	248	139
26	311	199	112
27	329	221	108
28	397	257	140
29	299	173	126
30	534	323	211
31	261	167	94
32	455	300	155
33	367	246	121
34	364	237	127
35	533	327	206
36	451	282	169
37	377	253	124
38	467	288	179
39	366	248	118
40	639	394	245
41	285	204	81
42	434	291	143
43	360	247	113
44	337	232	105
45	549	356	193
46	345	226	119
47	337	226	111
48	515	335	180
49	385	259	126
50	838	543	295
51	336	246	90
52	491	332	159
53	424	298	126
54	416	287	129
55	510	351	159
56	465	319	146
57	368	262	106
58	446	287	159
59	387	271	116
60	901	512	389
61	315	209	106
62	440	296	144
63	439	285	154
64	358	230	128
65	520	333	187
66	303	182	121
67	297	187	110
68	333	215	118
69	327	222	105

SEX

Sex was determined at autopsy and is assumed to contain little error.

RESULTS

Findings presented in this paper are based on varying numbers of autopsied cases, from approximately 21,000 to 23,000 cases.

THREE BROAD RACIAL GROUPS

This initial discussion refers to 21,302 autopsied cases of which approximately one-half were classified as white, one-quarter as Negro or mulatto, and one-quarter as American Indian or American Indian-white (Table 2). The reasons for these crude racial classifications are more or less obvious; however, it is worth noting that the classification Negro or mulatto does include the Bantu.

REPORTED AGE AT DEATH

Inspection of Table 2 indicates that selected percentiles, mean age at death, and measures of variability do not differ markedly among the three groups. A description of these terms will be found in an elementary statistics or biometry text.[287] The table contains data for constructing age-sex pyramids if a reader is motivated to do so.

Throughout this entire survey, analyses are made according to location-race groupings. Data for single years of age and sex have been pooled for 22,509 cases involving 19 location-race groups (Table 3). It is of interest to inspect the ages ending in zero and note the higher frequencies at these ages. For example, refer to age 50 where the frequency is more than twice as great as the frequency at either age 49 or 51; in fact, the number of females reported as dying at age 50 is more than 3 times as great as the number of females reported dying at age 51.

LOCATION-RACE GROUPS, BY AGE. It is also interesting to examine the age distribution within each location-race grouping.

Concentration Ratio at 0 and 5. In order to measure the tendency to report age at death in years ending in 5 or 0, an index was computed for each sex within each location-race grouping. If data from a life table were used, the ratio would be expected to be close to 1.00. In these data for the Project (Table 4), the concentration ratio (at 0 and 5) varies from a low of 0.86 to a high of 2.39, whereas a ratio less than 1.00 indicates that fewer deaths were reported at ages ending in 0 or 5 than was to be expected.

Concentration Ratio at 0 Only. If there is a willingness to make even heavier assumptions, concentration in the years ending in 0, namely at ages 30, 40, 50, and 60, can be "measured." In addition to the two sex groups over all location-races, 34 of 38 location-race-sex groupings (approximately 89 per cent) indicated greater concentration at years ending in 0 only than at years ending in 0 or 5.

Percentiles. Inspection of the percentiles also yields some interesting findings. For example, 10 per cent of autopsied males in Manila (Philippines), Puerto Rico, and São Paulo (white) were 18 years of age or less, while the 10th percentile for males in Oslo was 37; moreover, the

205

Table 4. Number of Autopsied Cases in Three Broad Age Groups, Measures of Central Tendency, Variability, and Concentration in Ages Ending in 0 or 5, by Sex and 19 Location-Race Groups

Broad age interval and selected statistical measures	All location-race groups M	F	Bogotá M	F	Cali M	F	Caracas M	F	Costa Rica M	F	Durban Bantu M	F	Durban Asian Indian M	F	Guatemala M	F	Jamaica M	F	Lima M	F
All ages (yr.)	14,606	7903	555	605	402	268	356	269	775	553	1101	843	369	243	1073	615	426	354	1113	228
10–22	1,768	1070	54	71	63	62	28	42	99	70	78	110	47	36	134	99	38	32	178	61
23–62	11,184	5910	425	466	310	190	284	198	537	391	980	700	294	188	768	441	323	278	791	146
63–69	1,654	923	76	68	29	16	44	29	139	92	43	33	28	19	171	75	65	44	144	21
For 23–62																				
Ages ending in 0 or 5[a]	3054	1837	150	187	101	75	64	58	152	111	396	335	112	70	237	157	91	71	307	53
Concentration ratio, 0 or 5[b]	1.37	1.55	1.76	2.01	1.63	2.26	1.13	1.46	1.42	1.42	2.02	2.39	1.90	1.86	1.54	1.78	2.01	1.41	1.94	1.82
Concentration ratio, 0 only[c]	1.58	1.93	2.09	2.49	2.00	—	—	1.97	1.62	1.87	2.89	3.46	2.35	2.50	1.77	2.29	—	1.58	2.17	1.85
Mean	43.1	42.5	46.0	43.4	39.0	36.5	46.1	41.8	45.4	45.0	42.2	40.6	42.6	42.0	45.0	41.5	47.9	46.0	40.7	34.9
S.D.	15.4	15.8	15.8	15.6	15.5	15.2	14.5	16.0	16.1	16.1	13.1	14.4	14.8	15.4	16.3	16.7	14.6	16.4	16.4	16.5
P_{10}	21	30	23	21	20	17	24	19	20	20	25	20	20	20	20	19	23	24	20	16
P_{25}	31	31	33	31	24	24	35	24	29	24	32	30	29	29	33	28	39	36	27	22
Median $= P_{50}$	44	43	50	45	38	35	49	41	47	47	42	40	45	45	48	41	52	48	40	30
P_{75}	56	56	59	57	51	50	63	56	60	60	52	50	60	60	60	57	59	58	55	45
P_{90}	63	63	64	63	60	60	69	63	65	65	60	60	60	60	65	63	63	63	60	60
$Q_3 - Q_1$	25	26	24	26	26	24	21	26	27	26	20	20	26	26	27	29	20	23	28	23
$P_{90} - P_{10}$	42	43	41	42	40	39	39	44	45	45	35	40	40	40	45	44	42	39	45	44

Broad age interval and selected statistical measures	Manila M	F	Mexico M	F	New Orleans Negro M	F	New Orleans White M	F	Oslo M	F	Puerto Rico Negro M	F	Puerto Rico White M	F	Santiago M	F	São Paulo Negro M	F	São Paulo White M	F
All ages (yr.)	329	266	356	348	931	518	975	340	725	381	384	136	897	272	2694	1163	340	153	805	348
10–22	58	36	31	37	91	38	58	30	32	25	55	12	172	45	341	180	53	21	158	63
23–62	237	208	299	286	742	385	784	243	461	222	295	102	626	181	2137	889	279	129	612	267
63–69	34	22	26	25	98	95	133	67	232	134	34	22	99	46	216	94	8	3	35	18
For 23–62																				
Ages ending in 0 or 5[a]	51	43	88	114	150	68	170	44	81	38	80	27	178	52	436	226	74	41	136	67
Concentration ratio, 0 or 5[b]	1.08	1.03	1.47	1.99	1.01	0.88	0.88	0.91	0.88	0.86	1.36	1.32	1.42	1.44	1.02	1.27	1.33	1.59	1.11	1.25
Concentration ratio, 0 only[c]	1.31	1.30	1.81	2.24	0.98	1.04	1.08	1.15	1.15	0.99	1.56	1.18	1.50	1.60	1.10	1.41	1.36	1.40	1.05	1.61
Mean	40.6	41.0	42.6	42.6	44.3	47.4	48.5	47.6	54.9	54.0	40.6	45.5	40.5	42.8	40.8	39.7	35.6	35.5	36.9	38.1
S.D.	16.2	15.2	13.4	13.9	14.8	14.8	13.4	14.8	12.8	14.4	15.9	15.9	16.6	17.2	14.6	15.2	12.6	13.3	14.7	14.8
P_{10}	18	18	29	29	23	25	28	25	37	29	18	24	18	18	21	20	20	21	18	19
P_{25}	27	29	32	32	32	37	40	40	48	48	28	34	27	28	29	28	26	25	24	26
Median $= P_{50}$	41	42	43	40	44	49	51	51	58	59	40	44	42	44	40	38	35	34	36	38
P_{75}	54	54	52	52	56	60	59	61	64	64	53	60	54	58	54	52	43	44	49	50
P_{90}	63	60	60	60	63	66	64	65	68	67	62	66	63	65	61	61	54	57	58	58
$Q_3 - Q_1$	27	18	19	22	24	23	19	23	16	19	25	25	27	30	23	24	17	19	25	24
$P_{90} - P_{10}$	45	37	37	38	40	41	36	40	31	38	44	42	45	47	40	41	34	36	40	40

[a] Explicitly, the eight ages 25, 30, 35, 40, 45, 50, 55, and 60.

[b] Concentration ratio, 0 or 5 $= \dfrac{5(X_{25} + X_{30} + X_{35} + X_{40} + X_{45} + X_{50} + X_{55} + X_{60})}{\sum\limits_{i=23}^{62} X_i}$ for $23 \leq i \leq 62$ where X = No. of autopsied cases reported at age i.

[c] Concentration ratio, 0 only $= \dfrac{10(X_{30} + X_{40} + X_{50} + X_{60})}{\sum\limits_{i=23}^{62} X_i}$ for $23 \leq i \leq 62$ where X = No. of autopsied cases reported at age i.

Age	All loca-tion-race groups	Bogotá	Cali	Caracas	Costa Rica	Durban Bantu	Durban Indian	Guate-mala	Jamaica	Lima	Manila	Mexico	New Orleans Negro	New Orleans White	Oslo	Puerto Rico Negro	Puerto Rico White	Santi-ago	São Paulo Negro	São Paulo White
yr.																				
All ages	1848	917	1500	1323	1401	1306	1518	1744	1203	4881	1236	1022	1797	2867	1902	2823	3297	2316	2222	2313
10-14	1910	944	1300	583	1313	833	3000	1379	1333	3692	1900	2000	1800	1666	1750	5333	5400	2071	3333	3454
15-19	1475	687	727	937	1571	553	842	1390	1062	2520	1583	687	1352	2454	1142	3714	2576	1946	1909	2064
20-24	1750	666	1806	714	1468	983	1352	1230	1500	2789	1269	787	3809	2052	1181	4000	4647	1782	2058	3156
25-29	1756	714	1956	1133	1727	1297	1181	1434	680	3400	850	807	3000	2187	400	3800	3181	2198	1620	2097
30-34	1798	787	1433	969	1333	1261	1631	1107	1300	4583	1172	828	2058	3705	1857	5142	3842	2244	2750	2048
35-39	1756	758	810	777	1264	1383	1272	1692	750	4739	1320	1085	1695	1941	2266	1818	3900	2575	2041	2888
40-44	1991	846	1764	2105	1060	1690	2125	1920	810	8142	900	1205	1596	2656	2842	3307	2913	2728	3750	2062
45-49	1923	783	1115	1545	1107	1552	1666	1846	1050	9200	1178	1305	1700	2891	*2368	7200	3541	2754	2875	2000
50-54	2135	1266	2611	1965	1764	1291	1882	2275	1367	500	1608	1146	1985	3434	1761	4000	3962	2680	2444	2548
55-59	2172	1346	3000	2043	1509	2036	1863	2170	1925	4933	1037	1120	2018	5117	2203	2000	3272	2217	2142	1965
60-64	1663	977	1714	1222	1211	1039	1074	1913	1018	2000	1208	827	1709	2933	2021	1458	2960	2116	1166	1950
65-69	1776	1020	1583	1687	1807	1200	1307	2408	1769	5750	1666	1055	802	1826	1698	1466	1918	2279	4000	1916

[a] Sex ratio = $\dfrac{\text{No. of males}}{\text{No. of females}} \times 1000$.

90th percentile for Oslo was highest of all the 19 location-race groupings.

SEX RATIOS

The sex ratio is sometimes defined as the number of males per 100 females; in order to avoid using a decimal point, the ratio was computed in terms of the number of males per 1,000 females. In the group of autopsied cases contributing specimens to the IAP, males predominated nearly 2 to 1; the ratio was nearly 5 to 1 in Lima, whereas slightly fewer specimens were collected from males than from females in Bogotá, Colombia.

SEX RATIOS BY AGE. For 22,509 autopsied cases, the sex ratio at any single reported age at death was invariably above 1,000; the range of the sex ratio was from 1,238 (at age 16) to 2,733 (at age 51). It was difficult to detect a consistent pattern in the sex ratios by single years of age when sex ratios were plotted on the y-axis against single years of age on the x-axis. Moreover, in contrast to most living populations, the female does not predominate among autopsied cases at the older ages examined.

In terms of 5-year age groups, the sex ratio was lowest in the 15 to 19 age group and highest in the 55 to 59 age group. In terms of decades of life, the highest sex ratio was found in the sixth decade (50 to 59) of life.

Inspection of Table 5 indicates considerable variability in the sex ratio by age and by location-race group. Further inspection indicates a preponderance of males within each location-race group, with the exception of Bogotá. In Bogotá, nine of 12 of the 5-year age groups had sex ratios less than 1,000. However, considering all 228 (12 × 19) basic cells of Table 5, less than 15 per cent (33) of all these cells yielded sex ratios of less than 1,000.

At age 50 and over, there are 76 basic "age-race" cells (four 5-year age groups combined with 19 location-race groups: 4 × 19 = 76); only four of the 76 cells had sex ratios less than 1,000 which is slightly more than 5 per cent of all basic cells among this arbitrarily designated "older age grouping."

DISCUSSION

In this demographic study, no attempt was made to relate demographic aspects of any group of autopsied cases to the corresponding group of deaths emanating from a specified living population. Even if time, money, and manpower had been available, as was hoped in accordance with original plans, it seems unlikely that the effort to utilize the usual enumerated and registered data, hospital statistics, and other such materials would have yielded evidence with a satisfactory degree of reliability. However, if demographic data had been collected on the entire "population" under study, on all deaths, and on all autopsied cases, it could at least have been determined whether the characteristics of the autopsied cases utilized in the Project were representative of demographic characteristics of the entire population, all deaths, or all autopsied cases. Even so, findings in autopsied cases might not be representative of arterial involvement in a living population.

From this paper, it is clear why each investigator refrained from presenting summary findings, and, as a minimal precaution, always considered data in terms of age-sex subgroupings. It can also be realized that the statistician had more than the usual methodologic problems. Incomplete data collection forms (unknowns) and impossible codes (coding errors), as well as zero frequencies and zero involvement, weighting by the number of cases in a subgroup, unweighted means, and ranking presented problems. The difficulties of clearly reporting averages and making analyses involving disproportionate subclasses were also present.

It is possible to describe these autopsied cases of the Project by stating that the variability of the demographic characteristics was both large and inconsistent; as was to be expected when differentials with regard to age-s-x. and race were small, the findings were often incon-

207

sistent. It appears clear, however, that the autopsy procedure used to generate specimens for this international study was selective of males. Differentials in reported age at death were slight for the three broad racial groups of white, Negro or mulatto, and American Indian or American Indian-white; in fact, age differentials by sex within these three groups were slight and inconsistent.

Obviously, in any study, the investigator must decide about which statistical population to make generalizations. This decision determines the sample which will be examined. A population survey can be conducted to collect data on each individual in order to describe a population at a specific instant of time, for example, the United States Census of Population, 1960, describing the population, say, as of 0001 hour, April 1, 1960. This international effort can likewise be considered as a survey of a specified instant of time, a snapshot, a cross-section; instead of the survey being conducted on a specified calendar date, data of the Project were collected to describe each individual at "the instant of time that death occurred." Elapsed time was involved only because time was required to accumulate cases.

Individual histories can be utilized in conducting a survey so that a population or sample is characterized over a period of elapsed time. Some writers find it convenient, as a beginning, to classify such a study as prospective when samples are selected on the basis of demographic, quasi-demographic, or other possible etiologic variables, and when the observed variable is the disease condition. Moreover, it should be noted that the prospective study involves elapsed time on an individual basis.

If groups are to be selected on the basis of the presence or absence of a disease and then the demographic or other variables are observed, the study is classified as retrospective. The labels prospective (forward) and retrospective (backward) remain somewhat nebulous, even though the merits and shortcomings of these two types of studies have been detailed by many authors; nevertheless, some aspects of this terminology are worth exploring further in the context of the IAP.

ABBREVIATED OPERATIONAL CONCEPT OF A RETROSPECTIVE STUDY. Assume that a group of persons, G_1, with a severe and obviously diseased condition Y has been selected or is available (in short, given a group of persons with disease Y): calculate the relative frequency of those persons who have a characteristic (demographic, quasi-demographic, or other) X, which is a possible etiologic factor. Also, given a comparable large group of persons, G_2, obviously without disease Y, compute the relative frequency of persons with the characteristic X in this control group. If the relative frequency of X is significantly greater among those with Y than among those without Y, then it can be speculated that an association between X and Y has been found.

OVERSIMPLIFIED OPERATIONAL CONCEPT OF A PROSPECTIVE STUDY. Select two groups: one group with the characteristic (demographic, quasi-demographic, or other) X, which is believed to be a possible etiologic factor, and

the other group without the factor X. Follow each member of the two groups for a definite period of time in order to estimate the risk of developing disease Y in the presence of X, as well as in the absence of X.

Note that the prospective method does not necessarily require waiting time since it can be utilized anytime a population can be defined as of an exact instant of time, t_0, and "follow-up" can be accomplished. However, for certain studies and estimates, the concept of "person-time interval of exposure," say, person-years of exposure to the risk of dying from heart disease, must necessarily be used.

In light of these operational concepts, suppose that the state of the art of diagnosis, excluding the autopsy procedure, permitted the classification of cases with regard to presence or absence of calcified atherosclerotic lesions. Let C denote the event presence of calcified lesions and $\overline{C}$ denote the event absence of calcified lesions. Further suppose that the study is limited to Negro and white males, born between 1900 and 1904, and that two large closed groups of live-born white and Negro males are followed from birth for 50 years in New Orleans. (Not only is this a prospective study, but it is also a cohort study since all individuals were born in a specified period.) Let W denote the event individual male selected is white, and N denote the event individual male selected is Negro.

Now consider this hypothetical 50-year prospective study, beginning at time t_0, as one which will provide the following four items of information and thus enable the computation of a ratio of relative risk (where relative frequency based on a large number of cases is treated as probability): (1) probability of calcified lesions, given that an individual is white, or $Pr(C \mid W)$; (2) probability of no calcified lesions, given that an individual is white, or $Pr(\overline{C} \mid W)$; (3) probability of calcified lesions, given that an individual is Negro, or $Pr(C \mid N)$; and (4) probability of no calcified lesions, given that an individual is Negro, or $Pr(\overline{C} \mid N)$.

Findings of this prospective study, in terms of the number of cases (frequencies, f), can be presented symbolically in Table 6.

By definition, the conditional probability of event F given event E is defined[287] by the following equation:

$$Pr(F \mid E) = \frac{Pr(F \text{ and } E)}{Pr(E)} \qquad (1)$$

In terms of Table 6, it follows that

$$Pr(C \mid W) = \frac{f_1}{f_1 + f_2},$$

$$Pr(\overline{C} \mid W) = \frac{f_2}{f_1 + f_2},$$

$$Pr(C \mid N) = \frac{f_3}{f_3 + f_4}, \quad \text{and}$$

$$Pr(\overline{C} \mid N) = \frac{f_4}{f_3 + f_4}.$$

A question of interest can be raised and answered directly from this prospective study. What is the rela-

208

| Race | Condition | | Total |
	C	$\bar{C}$	
W	f_1	f_2	$f_1 + f_2$
N	f_3	f_4	$f_3 + f_4$
Total	$f_1 + f_3$	$f_2 + f_4$	n

TABLE 7. CASES OF CALCIFIED LESIONS IN A HYPOTHETICAL
RETROSPECTIVE STUDY

Race	Condition C
W	z_1
N	z_2
Total	$z_1 + z_2$

TABLE 8. ESTIMATES OF POPULATION, BY RACE, IN HYPOTHETICAL
RETROSPECTIVE STUDY

Race	Sample
W	m_1
N	m_2
Total	$m_1 + m_2$

TABLE 9. DATA FOR ESTIMATING $Pr(W)$ AND $Pr(N)$ IN HYPO-
THETICAL RETROSPECTIVE STUDY (SPECIAL)

| Race | Condition | | Total |
	Disease	No disease	
W	d_1	t_1	$d_1 + t_1$
N	d_2	t_2	$d_2 + t_2$
Total	$d_1 + d_2$	$t_1 + t_2$	$d_1 + d_2 + t_1 + t_2$

tive risk of white males developing calcified lesions as compared to Negro males developing calcified lesions? An estimate of this relative risk can be obtained from the ratio $R_{(pros)}$, where

$$R_{(pros)} = \frac{Pr(C \mid W)}{Pr(C \mid N)} = \frac{\dfrac{f_1}{f_1 + f_2}}{\dfrac{f_3}{f_3 + f_4}}.$$

OVERSIMPLIFIED OPERATIONAL CONCEPT OF A RET-ROSPECTIVE STUDY. Now consider a retrospective study (of the same disease) at time t_{50}. Since it is customary to begin a retrospective study with cases of a disease, in this instance cases with calcified atherosclerotic lesions, Tables 7 and 8 can be inspected in order to see clearly what additional data are required in order to estimate relative risk. From the cases with calcified lesions, z_1 and z_2 (Table 7) can be obtained, and estimates of the $Pr(W \mid C)$ and the $Pr(N \mid C)$ can be computed. Clearly,

the investigator must have additional data to estimate relative risk. The additional data needed are the probabilities (or at least estimates) of selecting an individual possessing the etiologic characteristic in the general population; in this case, the investigator requires the $Pr(W)$ and the $Pr(N)$ in the general population. It may be possible to obtain these probabilities from some independent source. If the investigator does not have, or cannot obtain, this information on the general population, an attempt to make estimates based on a sample will probably be made; another group will be selected which it is hoped will be "representative" of W and N in the general population. In other words, an attempt is made to obtain m_1 and m_2 of Table 8. Then estimates could be made as follows:

$$Pr(W) = \frac{m_1}{m_1 + m_2} \quad \text{and}$$

$$Pr(N) = \frac{m_2}{m_1 + m_2} .$$

In Very Special Circumstances. If a disease condition is very rare, that is, if the group without disease is very large compared to the group with disease, then the investigator might hope to obtain estimates of the approximate $Pr(W)$ with $(d_1 + t_1)/(d_1 + d_2 + t_1 + t_2)$ and the $Pr(N)$ with $(d_2 + t_2)/(d_1 + d_2 + t_1 + t_2)$ as shown in Table 9.

Summing up to this point, given the following four items of information, relative risk from a retrospective study can be estimated: (1) probability that an individual is white, given that he has calcified lesions, or $Pr(W \mid C)$; (2) probability that an individual selected at random in the control population is white, or $Pr(W)$; (3) probability that an individual is Negro, given that he has calcified lesions, or $Pr(N \mid C)$; and (4) probability that an individual selected at random in the control population is Negro, or $Pr(N)$.

Now other details of computing relative risk from retrospective data can be outlined. Explicitly, begin by rearranging Equation 1 so that $Pr(F$ and $E) = Pr(E) \cdot Pr(F \mid E)$; hence, by substitution, the probability that an individual is white and has calcified lesions is

$$Pr(W \text{ and } C) = Pr(C) \cdot Pr(W \mid C). \quad (2)$$

Order being unimportant, the $Pr(W$ and $C)$ is the same as the $Pr(C$ and $W)$,

$$Pr(C \text{ and } W) = Pr(W) \cdot Pr(C \mid W). \quad (3)$$

It follows in a similar manner that

$$Pr(N \text{ and } C) = Pr(C) \cdot Pr(N \mid C), \quad (4)$$

and

$$Pr(C \text{ and } N) = Pr(N) \cdot Pr(C \mid N). \quad (5)$$

Clearly then, the right side of Equation 2 is equal to the right side of Equation 3, or

$$Pr(C) \cdot Pr(W \mid C) = Pr(W) \cdot Pr(C \mid W), \quad (6)$$

and the right side of Equation 4 is equal to the right side of Equation 5, so

$$Pr(C) \cdot Pr(N \mid C) = Pr(N) \cdot Pr(C \mid N). \qquad (7)$$

Now the relative risk of developing calcified lesions among the group of white males, as compared to the group of Negro males, can be calculated from Equations 6 and 7 by simply recalling that if $a = b$ and $c = d$, then $(a/c) = (b/d)$; hence,

$$\frac{Pr(C) \cdot Pr(W \mid C)}{Pr(C) \cdot Pr(N \mid C)} = \frac{Pr(W) \cdot Pr(C \mid W)}{Pr(N) \cdot Pr(C \mid N)} .$$

Canceling on the left and transposing,

$$\frac{Pr(W) \cdot Pr(C \mid W)}{Pr(N) \cdot Pr(C \mid N)} = \frac{Pr(W \mid C)}{Pr(N \mid C)} .$$

Dividing both sides by $Pr(W)/Pr(N)$, the ratio of relative risk for this retrospective study is

$$R_{(retro)} = \frac{Pr(C \mid W)}{Pr(C \mid N)} = \frac{Pr(W \mid C) \cdot Pr(N)}{Pr(N \mid C) \cdot Pr(W)} . \qquad (8)$$

The right side of Equation 8 can be obtained from a retrospective study, provided a "representative" control group is used, or that data are available to compute the $Pr(N)$ and the $Pr(W)$ in the general population. (*Note.* Clearly, from the point of view of mathematical statistics, any such ratio of relative risk is a complex index since it involves the ratio of two ratios.)

A Note from the "Theoretical": A Provocative (Unjustified) Example Involving Data on Autopsied Cases. Now for a few paragraphs of fantasy to vex some collaborating colleagues who are "convinced" that the risk of developing calcified arterial lesions is greater among white males than among Negro males in New Orleans. If this be true, under certain assumptions, a retrospective ratio, such as shown in Equation 8, would be expected to be greater than 1.00; in short,

$$R_{(retro)} = \frac{Pr(C \mid W)}{Pr(C \mid N)} > 1.00 .$$

To illustrate a use of this retrospective ratio, suppose that focus is centered on making an unjustified inference about New Orleans males aged 45 to 54. Assume that the Project's data are retrospective, and that it is not only appropriate to use data from the 1960 Census of Population, but also that these data provide sound estimates. Further assume that the classification of non-white implies essentially Negro in New Orleans.

In 1960, there were 36,054 males aged 45 to 54 enumerated in Orleans Parish; in terms of race, there were 24,790 white (W) males and 11,264 nonwhite (N) males. Now suppose that there were data for each male; assuming random sampling,

$$Pr(W) = \frac{24,790}{36,054} \approx 0.688,$$

$$Pr(N) = \frac{11,264}{36,054} \approx 0.312.$$

Data from the Project regarding calcified lesions of the abdominal aorta for New Orleans males aged 45 to 54 are available on 500 cases, as shown in Table 10. From

TABLE 10. DATA ON CALCIFIED LESIONS IN THE ABDOMINAL AORTA IN 500 NEW ORLEANS MALES

Race	Condition		Total
	C	$\bar{C}$	
W	180	85	265
N	92	143	235
Total	272	228	500

TABLE 11. SYMBOLIC RESULTS BASED ON AUTOPSIED CASES

Race	Condition identified		Total
	C	$\bar{C}$	
W	a_1	a_2	$a_1 + a_2$
N	a_3	a_4	$a_3 + a_4$
Total	$a_1 + a_3$	$a_2 + a_4$	$\sum a$

the column labeled C, the following probabilities can be computed:

$$Pr(W \mid C) = \frac{180}{272} \approx 0.662,$$

$$Pr(N \mid C) = \frac{92}{272} \approx 0.338.$$

Then substituting in Equation 8,

$$R_{(retro)} = \frac{Pr(W \mid C)}{Pr(C \mid N)} = \frac{(0.662)(0.312)}{(0.338)(0.688)} ,$$

$$= \frac{0.206544}{0.232544} ,$$

$$R_{(retro)} = \frac{Pr(C \mid W)}{Pr(C \mid N)} \approx 0.888.$$

The conclusion is that, clearly, this is not the result (stated previously) which was expected to be found. Under the explicitly stated assumptions, these particular data might lead to the conclusion that the risk of developing calcified lesions is less among white males than among Negro males in New Orleans. This finding contrasts sharply with results reported elsewhere in this series of reports.

How is it possible to obtain a ratio with a value less than 1.00 when $180/265$ or 68 per cent of the necropsied white males had calcified lesions while only 39 per cent ($92/235$) of necropsied Negro males had calcified lesions? Is there a flaw in the logic here? Or, is this an example, *par excellence*, of the underlying thesis of this entire paper?

Returning to the paragraph regarding very special circumstances explicitly stated earlier, in terms of Table 9, computation of the retrospective ratio of Equation 8 could imply a comparison of $d_1/(d_1 + t_1)$ with $d_2/(d_2 + t_2)$.

Theoretical considerations might be sharpened even further by considering data collection and data analysis separately, in terms of the labels of prospective and retrospective. Moreover, in a large study both approaches might be used. However interesting these distinctions may be found, when reality is faced the present state of the art of diagnosis of degree of involvement with atherosclerotic lesions requires an autopsy. All items of the foregoing relating to the diagnosis of calcified lesions depend upon the autopsy being performed, and the probability of autopsy is unknown (recalling that neither the probability of autopsy nor the probability of race within the 500 autopsied cases was used in the foregoing illustrative example). In terms of the format of Tables 6 to 10, findings based on autopsied cases alone in the Project can be presented as in Table 11. Beyond question, the autopsy procedure generated (selected) the sample from which the data were obtained; any estimated probabilities apply only to the group of autopsied cases. Clearly, these data must be used with caution in the search for association between a possible etiologic characteristic and degree of atherosclerotic involvement, both present at the "same instant of time in this cross-sectional study."

In summary, if this study had been limited to populations in which morbidity, enumeration, and registration data were of high quality, in which special surveys could have been conducted well and inexpensively, and in which all deaths came to autopsy, a "purist" would be correct in warning against generalizing to living populations. 'Even though this study was conducted forward from a "cut-on date" to a "cut-off date," the data collected are neither retrospective nor prospective in nature; moreover, from a rigorous point of view, findings of this study, which may indicate differential arterial involvement by age, should not be interpreted as age changes unless it is inconceivable that such results could be accounted for in any other way (and the "principle of inconceivability" is explicitly stated). This statement holds even though it probably could be demonstrated, by the use of overlapping 5-year age groups and moving averages, that arterial involvement is closely associated with age.

CONCLUDING STATEMENT: A CHALLENGE

The International Atherosclerosis Project was carefully designed, and considerable demographic data were collected; the specimens themselves were well collected and errors in evaluation estimated. It is reasonable, therefore, to assert that results (including all implicit and explicit biases) regarding involvement with arterial lesions may suggest some sound, as well as testable, hypotheses for future research—in spite of the many limitations imposed by the very nature of this study. Moreover, this section on demography is concluded by asking the "purist" (including the author) the following questions: What positive suggestions can be set forth for overcoming the limitations which have been explicitly stated? Are there research findings which indicate that the hypotheses generated by this Project are unsound? Are there unimpeachable data which support the current assertions and which can be brought to bear on the problems outlined here?

211

Diabetes Mellitus in Eskimos

George J. Mouratoff, MD, Nicholas V. Carroll, PhD, and Edward M. Scott, PhD

Clinical experience has long suggested that diabetes mellitus is rare in Alaskan Eskimos. A study in 1957[1] based on death certificates, hospital records, and screening of adult Eskimos confirmed the infrequent occurrence of the disease. At that time, with the use of strict criteria to define diabetes, only one Eskimo with diabetes was known in Alaska. Since that time, seven others have been discovered (Table 1). A similar rarity has been reported in Eskimos in Greenland.[2]

In the present study the response of an Eskimo population to challenge with a glucose load or to tolbutamide was determined. The results were analyzed in terms of age, sex, body weight, and pregnancy status, and compared to responses recently reported in other populations.[3-6]

Population Studied

The Eskimos studied lived in ten villages with a total population (1960 census) of 2,167, all within 40 miles of Bethel, Alaska. The age distribution by five-year intervals of the population studied is shown in Fig 1. By comparison with the US population (1960), there was a distinct shortage of women and of all persons more than 55 years old.

Table 1.—Eskimos Known to Have Clinical Diabetes Mellitus

Sex	Present Age, yr	Year Case Discovered	Residence
F	56	1953	Nome
F	40	1960	Savoonga
M	66	1960	Selawik
M	66	1960	Kiana
F	63	1962	Nome
F*	49	1962	Napaskiak
F	50	1963	Mountain village
F	45	1964	Golovin

*Discovered in present study.

On the other hand, there was an excess of persons under 35. At least 95% of those studied were full Eskimos, with the rest having one white ancestor.

Dietary studies, made in three of these villages,[7] have shown that less than 50% of the total calories comes from foods gathered from local sources. From Table 2, it is apparent that this diet is high in protein, moderate in fat, and lower in carbohydrates than the average diet in the United States.

Methods

All residents aged 20 or more were interviewed and given a brief physical examination to detect abnormalities of lungs, heart, liver, kidney, and joints. Height and weight were measured, the pregnancy status of women ascertained, and a fundoscopic examination made. The weight of each Eskimo was compared to the mean weight of whites of the same sex, age, and height.[8] The difference so calculated is designated here as "differential" weight.

A simplified glucose tolerance test, consisting of measurement of the fasting level of glucose in blood and of the glucose level two hours after oral administration of 100 gm of glucose was given to 535 persons. A complete glucose tolerance test with measurements at 0, ½, 1, 1½, and 2 hours was performed on 46 persons. In 124 additional persons, the response of blood glucose to tolbutamide was measured.[9] In this test, after a sample of blood was taken for the fasting level of glucose, 1 gm of tolbutamide was given intravenously, and the glucose level was measured after 20 minutes and again at 30 minutes. The response of plasma insulin to glucose was measured in 30 subjects. A summary of the screening schedule is presented in Table 3. Of those persons not tested, a considerable number aged 20 to 24 years were away from the village at school.

For retesting, all persons who had glucose levels in excess of 140 mg/100 ml after two hours and those with glucose levels in excess of 82% of the fasting level 20 minutes after tolbutamide administration, or in excess of 77% thirty minutes after receiving tolbutamide, were given a complete test

Table 2.—Average Daily Food Intake and Source of Food of Adult Eskimos in Winter									
	Akiak			Kasigluk			Napaskiak		
Calories	Men 2,650	Women 2,408	Local.* % 46	Men 2,979	Women 2,407	Local.* % 47	Men 2,194	Women 1,977	Local.* % 37
Protein, gm	169	170	80	280	244	88	150	165	86
Carbohydrate, gm	201	174	1	216	158	<1	180	152	<1
Fat, gm	133	118	51	108	88	41	97	82	31

*Percentage of food nutrient obtained from local sources.

Table 3.—Numbers of Eskimos Screened for Abnormalities of Glucose Metabolism

Groups	Men		Women	
Persons Tested				
Glucose tolerance, complete	29	} 379	17	} 326
Glucose tolerance, 2 hr	291		244	
Response to tolbutamide	59		65	
Not Tested				
Invalids, incapacitated	10	} 105	18	} 75
Absent from village	33		7	
Unknown reason	54		37	
Date incomplete, loss of sample, etc	8		13	
Total		484		401
% Tested		78		81

Table 4.—Selection for Retesting and Results

	Glucose Tolerance		Tolbutamide Response	
	Men	Women	Men	Women
Persons in original test	320	261	59	65
Selected for retesting				
Retested; found positive	1 } 2	10 } 14	1 } 10	3 } 12
Retested; found negative	1	3	8	6
Unavailable, moved	0	1	0	2
Refused	0	0	1	1

of glucose tolerance. After retesting, those persons with glucose levels more than 200 mg/100 ml at one hour or more than 140 mg/100 ml at two hours were admitted to the Alaska Native Medical Center, Anchorage, for a complete clinical and laboratory evaluation.

Glucose was determined on an automatic analyzer by the method of Hoffman,[10] the results are believed to be comparable to those found with the Nelson-Somogyi method.[11] Plasma insulin was measured by the double-antibody method.[12] Student's t test was used to determine statistical significance with the 5% level adopted as a criterion.

Results

Sixteen persons were selected for retesting because of glucose levels of more than 140 mg/ml two hours after a glucose load, and 22 persons were selected from the response to tolbutamide (Table 4). Three of the 14 women selected for retesting by glucose tolerance were pregnant during the first screening, but were not at the time of retesting; all again showed elevated glucose levels. One woman (patient 2, Table 5) selected by tolbutamide response was not pregnant originally, but at retesting was pregnant and had elevated glucose levels. Four persons showed normal glucose tolerance on retesting; they may have eaten during the original two-hour test. One woman and one man (patients 10 and 14, Table 5) selected by response to tolbutamide had glucose levels at one hour in excess of 200 mg/100 ml but less than 140 mg/100 ml at two hours; these two would have been considered normal if screened by two-hour glucose levels alone. Only one person (patient 13, Table 5) had a high fasting level of glucose.

One woman (patient 6, Table 5), the daughter of patient 13, was included in the study because of an error in birthdate; she was only 18 years old at the time of the original test. Four persons found to be abnormal on retesting were related, as shown in Fig 2. In addition, patient 2 was a half-cousin of patient 3 (Table 5).

The results of clinical and laboratory evaluation of the 15 persons finally selected are summarized in Table 5. Only patient 2 had normal tolerance to glucose; she had shown abnormal tolerance previously while pregnant. Glucose tolerance curves of the other 14 were similar to those obtained on the retest a year earlier. Several clinical aberrations were found in these persons, but in no case was there an obvious cause

1. Comparison of age distribution of United States and Eskimo population. Inner cross-hatched area represents Eskimos tested, while the outer area are those not treated. Solid line is distribution expected from US Census, 1960.

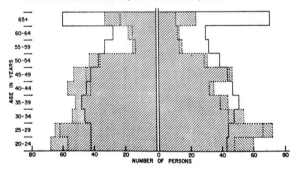

213

for abnormal tolerance to glucose. Patient 13 was the only person with obvious clinical diabetes.

Test results related to liver function were within limits of normal in all subjects. Electrophoresis of serum proteins and glycoproteins gave normal patterns. Serum electrolytes and 17-ketosteroid excretion were within limits of normal. Evidence of impairment of kidney function was found in several

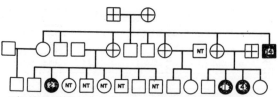

2. Family relationship of four Eskimos (patients 1, 2, 4, and 14) selected for abnormal glucose tolerance. Only persons over 20 years of age are in diagram. Squares = males; circles = females; crossed symbols = deceased; open symbols = normal glucose tolerance; solid symbols = abnormal glucose tolerance; NT = not tested.

subjects, but did not appear to be related to the degree of abnormality of glucose metabolism. Kidney biopsy was performed on patients 1, 9, and 13 (Table 5), and evidence of nephrosclerosis was found in each instance. Neuropathy and retinopathy were not found in any of these persons.

Glucose Tolerance of the Eskimo Population.—The complete glucose tolerance of 46 normal adult Eskimos is shown in Fig 3. Fasting glucose levels were the same in men and women, but all other levels averaged 15 mg/100 ml higher in women than in men. From this data, it is apparent that many more women than men would be selected if a single high level of blood glucose were chosen as a criterion.

The fasting and two-hour levels of glucose obtained on all subjects are summarized in Table 6 and Fig 4. Fasting levels approximated a normal frequency distribution and were no different in men, women, or pregnant women. Fasting levels increased with age, with correlation coefficients of 0.19 for males and 0.25 for females.

The distribution of levels two hours after glucose administration was skewed, so that the standard deviations shown must be used with caution. The expected difference between men and women was found, but the levels in pregnant women were no higher than those in the others. The two-hour levels increased with age, with correlation coefficients of 0.16 for men and 0.06 for women (the latter is not significant).

Height, Weight, and Glucose Tolerance.—Eskimos are short in stature (Table 7) and younger adults are taller than older persons. Eskimos weighed slightly more than whites of the same age, sex, and height (Table 8). The dependence of weight on age was the same in the two populations and thus "differential weight" was not correlated with age in the Eskimos. The dependence of weight on height was greater in Eskimos.

Fasting levels of glucose increased with excess weight in women but not significantly so in men. The correlation coefficients of "differential weight" and fasting glucose levels were 0.20 in women and 0.08 in men. The two-hour levels of glucose showed no correlation with differential weight.

Other Tests.—The response of blood glucose to tolbutamide is shown in Fig 5. The difference be-

Table 5.—Laboratory and Clinical Results on 15 Eskimos With Abnormal Tolerance to Glucose

Patient No.	Sex/ Age	Height, cm (in)	Weight, kg (lb)	Glucose Tolerance, mg/100 ml				Average Glucose Excretion,* gm/day	PSP† Excretion, %		No. of Pregnancies	Remarks
				Fasting	1 hr	2 hr	3 hr		15 min	2 hr		
1	F/32	157.5 (62)	53.1 (117)	77	216	200	180	0	7	22	6	Pregnant 3 mo; history of schizophrenia
2	F/36	153.7 (60.5)	49.4 (110)	81	107	98	90	0	...	79	8	
3	F/29	146.1 (57.5)	52.1 (115)	69	250	285	130	0.7	50	76	7	Pregnant 4 mo; PBI 11.0 mg/ 100 ml; Hgb 9.6 gm/100 ml
4	F/37	156.2 (61.5)	54.9 (121)	85	285	228	180	0	18	69	9	
5	F/58	151.1 (59.5)	55.3 (122)	87	239	216	200	0.5	30	61	5	
6	F/20	151.1	50.3 (111)	77	198	164	150	0	20	39	2	Rheumatoid arthritis
7	F/46	146.1	46.7 (103)	68	184	200	158	0.6	33	68	11	Pregnant 7 mo; benign nodular goiter; arteriosclerosis
8	F/42	151.1	52.1	86	186	118	77	0	38	68	8	BP 170/90 mm Hg
9	F/28	154.9 (61)	54.0 (119)	77	193	124	92	0	42	60	5	History of schizophrenia
10	F/32	156.2	74.4 (164)	93	191	129	70	0.7	30	66	4	
11	F/57	143.5 (56.5)	47.2 (104)	90	237	131	95	0	9	38	4	Rheumatoid arthritis; arteriosclerosis; history of renal tubular acidosis; Hgb 10.2 gm/ 100 ml; BUN 34.5 mg/100 ml
12	F/48	147.3 (58)	44.9 (99)	83	242	252	166	0	...	61	12	
13	F/48	149.9 (59)	58.5 (129)	170	300	350	200	7.1	38	68	8	Myocardial damage; mammary carcinoma; diabetes controlled with tolbutamide
14	M/53	165.1 (65)	69.4 (153)	90	215	67	70	0	...	52	...	
15	M/52	157.5 (62)	68.9 (152)	94	200	204	150	0	...	77	...	

*Average of three days; diet contained 220 gm of carbohydrate per day.
†Phenosulfonphthalein.

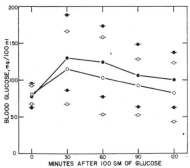

Age, yr	Number Tested†		Glucose, mg/100 ml			
			Fasting Level		Two-Hour Level	
	Men	Women	Men	Women	Men	Women
20-29	105 (82)	108 (83)	75.9 ± 9.7	73.9 ± 8.2	73.5 ± 16.3	86.3 ± 26.5
30-39	92 (73)	80 (62)	77.2 ± 9.4	75.7 ± 10.0	76.0 ± 21.5	95.0 ± 31.9
40-49	82 (72)	74 (53)	78.1 ± 9.7	78.4 ± 15.0	72.1 ± 15.9	89.1 ± 29.4
50-59	46 (38)	41 (29)	80.0 ± 9.8	81.2 ± 11.9	83.3 ± 25.9	92.6 ± 24.1
60+	33 (26)	20 (17)	81.7 ± 9.8	80.9 ± 7.3	87.8 ± 18.8	92.7 ± 26.9
All subjects	358 (291)	323 (244)	77.8 ± 9.8	76.8 ± 11.3	76.3 ± 19.2	90.3 ± 28.6
Pregnant women		37 (31)	...	70.6 ± 7.5	...	94.4 ± 34.5
Correlation coefficient of age and glucose level			0.19	0.25	0.20	0.06

Table 6.—Fasting Levels of Blood Glucose and Two-Hour Levels After Administration of 100 Gm of Glucose* (Means and Standard Deviations)

*Administered orally.
†Figures in parentheses are number of two-hour determinations.

3. Average results of tolerance to glucose in Eskimos. Open symbols are males and solid symbols, females. Averages are connected by lines. Unconnected symbols are average plus or minus two standard deviations.

Age Group, yr	Men		Women	
	Number	Inches	Number	Inches
20-29	117	64.5 ± 2.6	112	59.6 ± 2.5
30-39	93	63.7 ± 2.8	77	59.4 ± 2.6
40-49	86	63.4 ± 2.3	77	59.1 ± 2.4
50-59	48	62.7 ± 2.3	41	58.9 ± 2.3
60+	35	61.9 ± 2.3	21	58.0 ± 2.0
Total	379	63.6 ± 2.6	328	59.2 ± 2.5
Correlation coefficient of age and height		−0.31		−0.19

Table 7.—Height of Eskimos (Means and Standard Deviations)

Men	Weight, lb*	Women	Weight, lb*
All men	5.1 ± 0.7	All women	2.6 ± 1.2
Men 149.8 cm (59 in) tall†	0.5	Women 137.1 cm (54 in) tall†	−6.0
Men 175.3 cm (69 in) tall†	10.4	Women 162 6 cm (64 in) tall†	15.4

Table 8.—Average Differences in Weight Between an Eskimo and a White Population of the Same Age, Height, and Sex

*A positive value indicates Eskimos weigh more than whites; mean and standard error of the mean.
†Calculated from the regression of weight on height.

tween levels of men and women at 20 minutes was barely significant at the 5% level, and there was no difference at 30 minutes. The response to tolbutamide was unimodal in both men and women. Average levels of insulin in plasma in response to 100 gm of glucose administered orally (Fig 6) were not unusual.

Comment

The principal difficulty in determining the prevalence of diabetes mellitus in a population has always been one of definition of the disease. No clearly defined point exists between normal and abnormal glucose metabolism or between abnormal glucose metabolism and clinical diabetes, where one can divide the population into diabetic and nondiabetic classes. The estimation of prevalence of diabetes by division of a population into arbitrary classes has nevertheless been used.[9] The most valid application appears to be one in which the criteria for diabetes are strict, including abnormal glucose metabolism, high fasting levels of blood glucose, significant glucosuria, and clinical evidence of diabetes.

To avoid such arbitrary classification, attempts have been made to determine the response of a segment of a population to a glucose load,[9-6] as a descriptive measure of diabetes. An advantage of this method is that no subjective decisions need be made; a disadvantage is that the response to glucose may not necessarily be related to the prevalence of clinical diabetes mellitus.

All recent studies of response of a population to glucose were started at about the same time, but the methodology used differed (Table 9). In the present study, the amount of glucose given was larger, a fasting level of glucose was obtained, and we were able to follow-up all suspected diabetic persons. The results of similar studies are compared in Table 10.

From these results, the following conclusions can be drawn: (1) The distribution of glucose levels two hours after challenge is in all cases unimodal regardless of whether diabetes is frequent or rare. There is no rational cut-off point to divide the population into diabetic and nondiabetic classes. (2) The differences in these populations consist primarily of differences in the proportion of persons in the upper tail of the distribution curve. Neither the 25th nor 50th percentile levels appear to be related in any way to the higher percentiles.

(3) Qualitative differences may occur in the distribution curve. Thus, a comparison of Malaysian men and women shows that the average level of glucose in women was higher than that in men below the 90th percentile, but was lower above that point.

The unimodal distribution of the results from glucose tolerance suggests that there is no simple biochemical lesion associated with impaired glucose metabolism in adults, although this may be the case in juvenile diabetes, where insulin is clearly deficient.

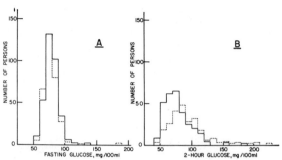

4. Fasting levels of glucose in Eskimos and levels two hours after 100 gm of glucose administered orally. Solid lines represent males and dotted lines, females.

Diabetes in Eskimos.—The present study confirms the rarity of diabetes in Eskimos. Eight Alaskan Eskimos are now known to have diabetes (Table 1), and all are being treated with hypoglycemic agents. Four of these were studied intensively at the Alaska Native Medical Center and were found to have typical diabetes mellitus of the adult type, with various complications. Juvenile diabetes is unknown in Eskimos.

The reason for rarity of diabetes in Eskimos is still open for speculation. Although obesity was

5. Effect of tolbutamide on glucose levels in Eskimos. Open circles represent men and solid circles, women. Averages are connected by solid lines. Dotted lines represent averages plus or minus two standard deviations.

less common in this group than in those Eskimos studied previously, lack of it does not appear adequate as an explanation for rarity of diabetes. Both the low prevalence of abnormal glucose tolerance and the rarity of diabetes may be due in part to the relative lack of older people in the Eskimo population.

In comparing our results with others, no effect of diet on prevalence of imparied glucose tolerance was evident. The diet in Uruguay is stated to be similar to that in the United States,[6] and abnormal glucose tolerance is relatively common. Abnormal tolerance is much less frequent in both East Pakistan[6] and in Eskimos, but the diets in these two groups are very different. The protein intake in Eskimos is higher than in Uruguay, but it is much lower in Pakistan. Carbohydrate consumption is lower in Eskimos than in Uruguay, but it is higher in Pakistan. Fat intake is highest in Eskimos, next highest in Uruguay, and lowest in East Pakistan.

6. Effect of glucose on levels of insulin in plasma.

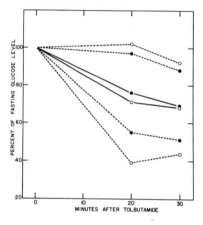

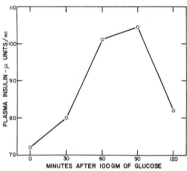

216

Table 9.—Methodology in Studies of Response of Populations to Glucose

Study Population	Duration of Fasting, hr	Glucose Given, Gm	Time of Testing, hr	Age Group, yr	Follow-up
Bedford, England[3]	None	50	2	20+	None
United States[2]	None	50	1	18+	None
Cherokee Indians[4]	2-8	1*	2	35+	None
Venezuela Uruguay, East Pakistan, Malaya[6]	2-14	1*	2	35+	None
Eskimos (Alaska)	>7	100	0,2	20+	Complete

*Per kilogram of body weight.

Table 10.—Percentile Levels of Glucose Two Hours After a Glucose Load

Population	Sex	Percentile					% of Values >190 mg/ml
		25	50	75	90	95	
Glucose, 50 gm Bedford, England	Both	77	99	113	128	149	(1.5)†
Glucose, 1 gm/kg* East Pakistan	M	63	77	87	98	106	0.6
East Pakistan	F	65	77	88	100	115	2.4
Malaya	F	75	85	100	115	128	0.8
Venezuela	M	68	79	92	115	139	1.5
Malaya	M	69	83	97	113	144	3.0
Uruguay	M	65	80	98	138	180	4.2
Venezuela	F	78	93	111	146	196	4.7
Uruguay	F	71	86	103	128	212	5.5
Cherokee Indians		72	96	123	165	>200	(7.0)†
Glucose, 100 gm Eskimo	M	61	71	82	101	114	0
Eskimo	F	73	86	103	124	146	1.3

*Per kilogram of body weight.
†Interpolated values.

One important way in which Eskimo men differ from white men is that they are physically much more active. It was noted previously that such men are well-muscled[13] and that physical activity and fitness is maintained until age 60 or older. The physical fitness of Eskimo women has not been defined. The numerous pregnancies of Eskimo women have not resulted in a high prevalence of diabetes.

This investigation was supported in part by Public Health Service research grant A-5929.

Rita Hausknecht, California State Department of Health, provided statistical assistance. Streeter Shining, MD, and M. Walter Johnson, MD, Alaska Native Medical Center, assisted in clinical studies. SP 4 Richard Cohen, Sgt Mary Lyons, Philip Cranz, and Nicholas Cavalancia, Letterman General Hospital, gave field and laboratory assistance.

The tolbutamide used in this investigation was supplied as Orinase by the Upjohn Co., and the glucose solution was supplied by Biological Research, Inc.

Generic and Trade Names of Drug

Tolbutamide—*Orinase*.

References

1. Scott, E.M., and Griffith, I.V.: Diabetes Mellitus in Eskimos, *Metabolism* 6:320-325 (July) 1957.

2. Sagild, U., et al: Epidemiological Studied in Greenland, 1962-1964: I. Diabetes Mellitus in Eskimos, *Acta Med Scand* 179:29-39 (Jan) 1966.

3. Gordon, T.: Glucose Tolerance of Adults, United States, 1960-1962, US Public Health Service publication 1000, series 11, No. 2, US Government Printing Office, May 1964.

4. Sharp, C.L.; Butterfield, W.J.H.; and Keen, H.: Diabetes Survey in Bedford 1962, *Proc Roy Soc Med* 57:193-202 (March) 1964.

5. Stein, J.H., et al: The High Prevalence of Abnormal Glucose Tolerance in the Cherokee Indians of North Carolina, *Arch Intern Med* 116:842-845 (Dec) 1965.

6. West, K.M., and Kalbfleisch, J.M.: Glucose Tolerance, Nutrition, and Diabetes in Uruguay, Venezuela, Malaya, and East Pakistan, *Diabetes* 15:9-18 (Jan) 1966.

7. Heller, C.A.: The Diet of Some Alaskan Eskimos and Indians, *J Amer Diet Assoc* 45:425-428 (Nov) 1964.

8. *Medicoactuarial Mortality Investigations*, Association of Life Insurance Medical Directors and the Actuarial Society of America, New York, vol 1, 1912.

9. Unger, R.H., and Madison, L.L.: Comparison of Response to Intravenously Administered Sodium Tolbutamide in Mild Diabetic and Non-Diabetic Subjects, *J Clin Invest* 37:627-630 (May) 1958.

10. Hoffman, W.S.: A Rapid Photoelectric Method for Determination of Glucose in Blood and Urine, *J Biol Chem* 120:51-55 (Aug) 1937.

11. Nelson, N.: A Photometric Adaptation of the Somogyi Method for the Determination of Glucose, *J Biol Chem* 153:375-380 (May) 1944.

12. Morgan, C.R., and Lazarow, A.: Immunoassay of Insulin: Two Antibody System: Plasma Insulin Levels of Normal, Subdiabetic and Diabetic Rats, *Diabetes* 12:115-126 (March-April) 1963.

13. Mann, G.V., et al: The Health and Nutritional Status of Alaskan Eskimos, *Amer J Clin Nutr* 11:31-76 (July) 1962.

Peyote Cult, Mescaline Hallucinations, and Model Psychosis

LOUIS PELNER, M.D., F.A.C.A.

THE PEYOTE CULT is a ritual of the Native American Church whose parishioners include American Indians of many tribes. Under the influence of peyote or mescal buttons, the participants in this ritual may develop unusual hallucinations. These hallucinations have some resemblance to hallucinations reported by patients with schizophrenia, although there are significant differences. Thus psychiatrists and psychologists have known for many years a number of substances, including peyote, capable of producing temporary psychotic-like states. It is impossible to determine by direct methods if animals develop hallucinations when treated with a drug. Peyote and one of its alkaloids, mescaline, has therefore been given to human beings by psychologic laboratories to produce a model psychosis. Klüver[1] believes that the chief value of the drug lies in its effectiveness as a research tool in the solution of some fundamental problems of biologic psychology and psychiatry.

Peyote cult

The use of peyote was originally associated with the rites of the pre-Columbian Mexican Indians and more recently in this country with the American Indian. Peyote consists of the hairy buttons on top of the carrot-shaped cactus, Lophophora williamsii, which is grown principally in Mexico and along the Rio Grande River in Texas. In this country peyote in the form of these dried buttons is used in the services of the Native American Church which has numerous members in many American Indian tribes. The ritual differs somewhat with each tribe and is under direction of the peyote priest. The members congregate in small groups around an altar and ingest these peyote buttons which have a disagreeable taste and are extremely nauseating. A fire is usually started and kept burning a short distance away. This setting results in deep introspection and autohypnosis on the part of the participant and is climaxed by visual hallucinations in color which appear in several hours. In some tribes, Christian elements are added to the supernaturalism of the indigenous culture. This may include Bible readings. In the Osage tribe three officials are said to represent the Trinity. Peyotism is clearly involved with symbolism, both pagan and Christian.

Mescaline, one of the eight alkaloids of peyote, reproduces nearly all of the effects of the crude peyote buttons. It is a close chemical relative of amphetamine. If the structural formula is written another way, it has an indole-like nucleus. This alkaloid is given in 200- to 500-mg. doses. It produces visual and occasionally auditory hallucinations, illusions, depersonalization, and depressive symptoms. The cerebral effects of mescaline are somewhat similar to those observed with 50 to 100 mg. of LSD (lysergic acid diethylamide), a drug which has an indole nucleus. An acquired tolerance for peyote is developed by the peyote priests, but there appears to be no emotional dependence or significant harm to the participants from this substance.[2,3]

The leaders of the Native American Church of North America, disturbed by a controversy over their ritual concerned with the use of peyote, invited Dr. J. S. Slotkin, a well-known anthropologist, to live among them and to comment on his findings. According to Slotkin,[4] peyote helps the Indians to maintain themselves in that larger grouping that is non-Indian.

The peyote service, in which the most important part is the eating of the mescal buttons, is accompanied by song, prayer, and contemplation. According to Slotkin, the peyote-eating Indians say "The peyote religion is the only thing left to us." "Peyote is always teaching you something new." It is Slotkin's opinion that the peyote religion is "an Indian defense against the consequences of white domination," in which, so to speak, a small, beaten, but proud group accommodates itself to a larger victorious group without full sublimation of their own culture. Other methods were tried by the Indians: resistance, submission, and adaptation. Only peyotism has proved its value to them.[4]

I do not question the reasons given by this distinguished anthropologist, Dr. Slotkin, but I feel that there is another reason why some American Indian tribes indulge in the peyote ritual. North American Indians attached great importance to visions or hallucinations in the conduct of their daily lives.[3] Perhaps the auditory hallucinations, where the Indian heard voices telling him how to handle the particular problem, were even more frequent than the visual hallucinations. Many of the plains Indian tribes taught their children how to experience these hallucinations at an early age, but even where this instruction was not practiced, the growing child quickly learned the value of the visions. The Indians usually had some strong emotional impulse to experience the vision such as serious illness or death in the family, revenge for real or fancied insults, loss of his property, or other great problem. He would go into seclusion in a comfortable wooded spot, he would fast and not drink water for four days, and then he would beg the "spirits" to help him. In some tribes this was accompanied by self-mortification, for example, cutting off a joint of the left little finger. He would usually receive his hallucination on the fourth day. The number four had a magical connotation for the Indians of the plains.[3]

The hallucination was usually in conformity with the visionary patterns of the tribe. Naturally, anything that the Indian heard or imagined was interpreted in this context. We do not have to assume any fabrication on the Indian's part in talking of his visions. He would naturally fill in any obscure areas in his recollection according to the established myths of his tribe. Again, many of the subjects would have the same hallucination. A vision retold by several Crow Indians was of a battle between several spirit horsemen and the surrounding rocks and trees that suddenly became their enemies. In this vision, the horsemen triumphed against all odds, and the visionary presumably would conquer also. The similarity of these visions was certainly based on tribal folklore.

A visionary would accumulate a "medicine bundle" which consisted of articles suggested by the hallucination and which would presumably later remind the Indian of the vision. These objects were venerated as almost sacred. Only among some tribes such as the Pawnee was a standard religious system created with a supreme sky-dwelling creator. What of that poor unfortunate who could not experience an hallucination? He could purchase a copy of the "medicine bundle" from a more successful Indian.[3]

Thus the peyote ritual enables the Indian to successfully pursue an established aim of the Indian culture, to achieve the visionary experience.

Peyote and mescaline hallucinations

One of the early experimenters with peyote was Havelock Ellis[5] who wrote an article called "Mescal, A New Artificial Paradise." He writes about beautiful hallucinations which he calls living arabesques, in which in image after image numerous polished facets appeared over a large part of the field. Then a large number of jewel-like flowers appeared all over the field of vision. After watching the visions in the dark for some hours, he turned on a gas jet and he found an entirely new series of visual phenomena. The gas jet seemed to burn with great brilliance sending out waves of light which expanded and contracted in an exaggerated manner. This was an illusion. Throughout all the sensations his mind remained perfectly clear, and he believed he had an unusual lucidity. Ellis concluded that for a healthy person to be once or twice admitted to the likes of mescal is not only an unforgettable delight but an educational influence of no mean value.

Klüver[1] deals with the nature and character of the hallucinations induced by peyote and tries to catalogue them. Even though the hallucinations have a high degree of individuality, various form constants recur repeatedly in various subjects: spirals, cones, latticework, fretwork, arabesques, stripes, and cobweb-like forms, usually in colors. There may be sudden developing micropsia or macropsia, that is, a decrease or increase in the size of the object viewed.[1] The phenomenon of synesthesia was often noted: hallucinations in two different sensory systems, for example, hearing noises and seeing colors at the same time.[1] Besides the development of hallucinations and illusions in the mescal state, strong doses of mescal produce abnormal emotional states. Many of the subjects described euphoria with much inappropriate laughter, talkativeness, and jocularity or, alternatively, sometimes depression.[1]

R. C. Zaehner,[6] Professor of Eastern Religions and Ethics at the University of Oxford, became the subject of an experiment with mescaline on December, 3, 1955. It seems strange for this observer of various types of religious experience to have attained no great religious experience following mescaline. He mentions that there were various periods of uncontrollable laughter during the experiment. He also describes an interesting illusion in which the stained glass sections in the various churches that he visited seemed to move, that is, each piece of stained glass, even though imprisoned in the lead surrounding it, still moved. Zaehner felt that his experience was in a sense antireligious; by this he meant that it was not conformable with a religious experience. All things were equally funny to him. The quality of the funniness and incongruity had swallowed up all others. He also stated that he would not take the drug again based entirely on moral grounds. To him mescaline was quite unable to reproduce the natural mystical experience that he himself had described elsewhere, although he said that he half hoped that it would. Once the drug started working and he was plunged into a "universe of farce," he realized the religious experience was not to be. The reticence on the part of Dr. Zaehner may have made it impossible for him to

have had the religious experience that he "half hoped" he would have. I think the word "half hoped" is very expressive and probably indicates his subconscious antagonism to the experience.[6]

The subjective experiences of time may undergo profound distortions. In some subjects this is the predominant effect that was noted.[1] Christopher Mayhew,[7] a member of Parliament of Britain, was contacted by two Canadian scientists, H. Osmond, M.D., and J. Smythies, M.D., and he agreed to serve as a volunteer in an experiment with mescaline. Dr. Osmond was the person who administered mescaline to Aldous Huxley who described his fascinating experiment in the Doors of Perception. Mayhew was given 400 mg. of mescaline hydrochloride. In about an hour he developed the extraordinary visual hallucinations like those described by Huxley in the Doors of Perception and by many others. However, thereafter, peculiar events occurred in which there was disorganization of the time sense. He was not experiencing events in the normal sequence of time. The events that were experienced by Mayhew were not in the familiar sequence of "clock time" but in a different capricious sequence that was outside his control. He described it as somewhat like the flash backs that occur in films, in which events of the year 1956 are suddenly interrupted by events of 1939. Mayhew experienced another time phenomenon in which at regular intervals he became aware of his surroundings and in which he stated he enjoyed complete bliss for a tremendous length of time. However, to the experimenters, these events lasted no time at all. The experimenters felt that these events could not have happened because there was not time for them to have happened. The whole interview was filmed, and the films show Mayhew going off on these excursions and coming back, but allow no time for any kind of experience in between, and certainly left no time for the large areas of bliss which he claimed to have enjoyed. Mayhew believes that these experiences may have been subjective, produced subconsciously by himself. He had been studying religious experiences and even had hinted in a recent book that some such experience "outside of time" would be theoretically possible and he believed that

220

mescaline merely enabled him to experience what he was predisposed to.[7] This may be what the Indians in the Native American Church experienced but could not express so well as Mayhew.

Klüver[1] stated that it was worth stressing that variability and inconstancies characterize hallucinations and other subjective phenomena and that they share these characteristics with olfactory, emotional, and sexual phenomena. Klüver believes that the temporal rhinencephalon plays a dominant role in shifts, inconstancies, and fluctuations in symptoms, and this area is probably the part of the brain involved in hallucinations.[1]

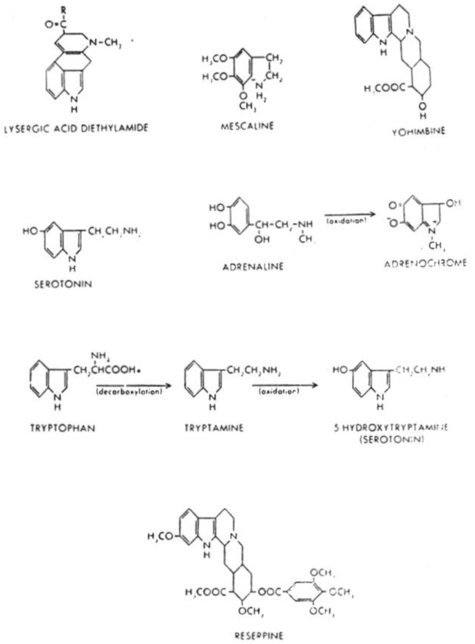

Model psychosis

The reawakened interest in psychopharmacology has stimulated an intense amount of research into the basic nature of schizophrenia. Since the pathlogist cannot find either microscopic or macroscopic histologic lesions in the brain after death in this disease, the possibility exists that this disease may be caused by a deviation from the normal at the molecular or biochemical level. Recently two biologically active amines, serotonin and norepinephrine, were found to be present in an uneven distribution in brain tissue. The amount of these substances in brain and their interrelationships are thought to be important determinants of psychiatric symptoms.[8] Serotonin is antagonized by LSD, yohimbine, and ergotamine, all of which contain the indole nucleus. Mescaline also antagonizes serotonin but has an indole-like nucleus (Fig. 1).[9] Woolley and Campbell[8] suggested that the mental changes caused by these drugs are the result of induced deficiency of serotonin in the brain. They also believed that schizophrenia whose mental symptoms are mimicked by these drugs is caused by a cerebral serotonin deficiency, arising from a metabolic defect. Also, many of the psychotherapeutic drugs have been shown to influence the action of serotonin, while producing a favorable effect on mental symptoms. Norepinephrine has been found to be present in some quantity in the brain, especially in certain areas of the brain such as the hypothalamus which is concerned with autonomic regulation. Experimen-

FIGURE 1. Chemical substances that cause personality changes. All these substances have indole nucleus except mescaline which has indole-like nucleus.[9]

tally, adrenochrome and adrenolutin, both degradation products of epinephrine, have been found to be psychosomimetic.[10] One of the patients of Hoffer, Osmond, and Smythies[10] recalled having hallucinatory experiences while taking epinephrine for asthma. Deteriorated epinephrine, which contains adrenochrome, has been known to cause psychologic disturbances.[10] It is generally admitted, but not proved so far, that both serotonin and norepinephrine have a neurohumoral role and both can be considered as neurohumors or neurohormones. By neurohormones we mean either a transmitter substance or one that enhances or inhibits (modulates) the action of the actual transmitter. However, the most decisive type of evidence, the collection and identification of either substance after stimulation of nerve tissue, has not yet been obtained.[11] Hess[12] suggested a subcortical system whose function is to integrate autonomic, psychic, and somatic functions. Chemical mediators released by nerve impulses cause the production of either serotonin or norepinephrine with serotonin acting on the cholinergic center and norepinephrine acting on the adrenergic center, in either case producing the appropriate action on the specific organ. In this system, drugs may also block the action of serotonin and norepinephrine.[12]

Psychomotor epilepsy consists of an attack involving twisting or writhing movements of the extremities or trunk, smacking movements of the lips, incoherent speech, and involuntary performance of apparently purposeful activities, after which the patient has a complete amnesia for the entire attack. Patterns similar to those observed in psychomotor epilepsy have been reported following stimulation of the hippocampal area in cats.[13] In experimental animals a suggestive counterpart of catatonic schizophrenia has been provoked during hippocampal seizures.[13] The hippocampal area is part of the limbic lobe which is the modern name for what used to be called the rhinencephalon. As indicated earlier, it is thought that this area of the brain is involved in hallucinations.

While it is impossible to verify the presence of hallucinations in animals, one can sometimes suspect that they have occurred. The following quotation from MacLean[13] seems to implement this suspicion.

MacLean induced a propagating hippocampal seizure by unipolar stimulation of the hippocampus in a cat which allowed him to observe behavioral changes thought to be due to a functional ablation of the limbic system.

> With the onset of the afterdischarge produced by electrical stimulation of the superior hippocampus, the pupils usually dilate and any turning movements that were present during the initial stimulation appear to reverse themselves. Purring, if previously present, may cease and be replaced by occasional meows or yowls. Concurrently the animal assumes attitudes that strike one at first as being rapt attention or fearful alerting for the unexpected. Further examination indicates, however, that it is poorly in contact with its environment. Although the pupils react to light, the animal will not avoid the light, nor will it cringe when one pretends to strike the face. If one forcefully blows smoke at it, it will withdraw a little, but not persist in avoiding the smoke. Occasionally, an animal will show a reduced threshold to anger on receiving a noxious stimulus of moderate intensity . . . . Intense noxious stimulation, however, results in changes that are remarkably dramatic because of their suddenness and violence. Momentarily touch the cat's nose

with a lighted cigaret and the animal will suddenly jump a distance of several feet, and will just as suddenly assume a catatoniclike stance that will be maintained for several seconds. A prolonged hard pinch of the tail may elicit violent struggling and rage. Usually, it impresses one as being sham rage because of the animal's apparent inability to direct and prosecute its attack. When the stimulus is terminated, the animal temporarily assumes a catatoniclike stance in which it appears as in a trance . . . .[13]

The limbic system consists of the limbic lobe together with its subcortical cell stations. The limbic lobe is essentially the anatomic area formerly called the rhinencephalon. This system is strategically located for receiving and associating oral, visceral, sexual, and basic sensory sensations, such as ocular and auditory, and then discharging them through multiple hypothalamic connections. All surrounding brain areas, that is, the visual, parietal, auditory, temporal, and olfactory, relay transcortical impressions to the hippocampal gyrus. The limbic system connects the hypothalamus, the head ganglion of the autonomic nervous system, with the other structures of the brain stem.[14]

Thus far we have shown that certain drugs and the stimulation of certain parts of the brain can produce a psychosis-like state in human beings and animals. But how closely does this psychosis-like state resemble an actual psychosis such as schizophrenia? Hollister[15] believes that the symptoms in drug-induced states and in schizophrenia display important differences.

For example, schizophrenic patients withdraw from personal contacts, while drug subjects prefer someone to talk to. Schizophrenic patients are preoccupied with bodily functions but blame the difficulty on some impossible antagonist like the devil, while drug subjects blame the abnormality of bodily function on the drug situation. Schizophrenic patients and drug subjects have difficulty expressing thoughts. In schizophrenia the words are symbolic and have no relation to reality, and the patient has no concern with the failure to communicate to others. Drug subjects make incoherent remarks, but they are related to reality, and they are greatly concerned about the failure to communicate. Both schizophrenic patients and drug subjects have daydreaming states. Schizophrenic patients and drug subjects both have hallucinations, but these are usually auditory in type in schizophrenic patients and visual in drug subjects. A schizophrenic patient considers his hallucinations as real, while a drug subject considers them unreal. In schizophrenic patients, delusions are common and usually are of a paranoid or grandiose nature, while delusions are rare in drug subjects. Bizarre mannerisms and attitudes are common in schizophrenia but are rare in drug subjects.

However, after all is said and done, it would seem unrealistic to require that a drug-induced state be exactly like the natural psychosis, because even if we say that both are chemically induced, the chemicals may be different. Perhaps another drug to be discovered in the future may induce a model psychosis that would more satisfactorily simulate a real one.

References

1. Klüver, H.: Mescal and Mechanisms of Hallucinations, Chicago, University of Chicago Press, 1966.

2. Seevers, M. H.: Drug addictions, in Drill V. A., Ed.: Pharmacology in Medicine. A Collaborative Textbook, New York, Blakiston Division, McGraw-Hill Book Co., Inc., 1958, p. 249.

3. Lowie, R. H.: Indians of the Plains!, Garden City, New York, Natural History Press, 1963, pp. 199, 170.

4. Slotkin, J. S.: Menomini peyotism, transactions of the American Philosophical Society, 42, part 4, page 1, 1952, partially reprinted in Ebin, D.: The Drug Experience, New York, Grove Press, Inc., 1961, p. 237.

5. Ellis, H.: Mescal: a new artificial paradise, Contemporary Review, January, 1898, reprinted in ibid., p. 225.

6. Zaehner, R. C.: Mysticism, sacred and profane: an inquiry into some varieties of the religious experiences, partially reprinted in ibid., p. 276.

7. Mayhew, C.: An excursion out of time, London Observer, Oct. 28, 1956, reprinted in ibid., p. 294.

8. Woolley, D. W., and Campbell, N. K.: Exploration of the central nervous system serotonin in humans, Ann. New York Acad. Sc. 96: 108 (1962).

9. Pelner, L.: Host-tumor antagonism. VIII. The psychologic component involved in the host resistance to cancer, J. Am. Geriatrics Soc. 5: 857 (1957).

10. Hoffer, A., Osmond, H., and Smythies, J.: Schizophrenia; a new approach. II. Result of a year's research, J. Ment. Sc. 100: 29 (1954).

11. Costa, E., et al.: On current status of serotonin as a brain neurohormone and in action of reserpinelike drugs, Ann. New York Acad. Sc. 96: 118 (1962).

12. Hess, W. R.: Diencephalon-Automatic and Extrapyramidal Functions, New York, Grune & Stratton, Inc., 1954.

13. MacLean, P. D.: The limbic system (visceral brain) in relation to central gray and reticulum of the brain stem; evidence of interdependence in emotional processes, Psychosom. Med. 17: 355 (1955).

14. Idem: Contrasting functions of limbic and neocortical systems of the brain and their relevance to psychophysiological aspects of medicine, Am. J. Med. 25: 611 (1958).

15. Hollister, L. E.: Drug-induced psychoses and schizophrenic reactions: a critical comparison, Ann. New York. Acad. Sc. 96: 80 (1962).

UNTREATED CONGENITAL HIP DISEASE

A STUDY OF THE EPIDEMIOLOGY, NATURAL HISTORY, AND SOCIAL ASPECTS OF THE DISEASE IN A NAVAJO POPULATION

David L. Rabin, M.D., M.P.H.; Clifford R. Barnett, Ph.D.; William D. Arnold, M.D.; Robert H. Freiberger, M.D.; and Gyla Brooks, R.N., M.P.H.

CONGENITAL dislocation and dysplasia of the hip joint is a disorder of relatively low occurrence in most of the United States, with a frequency of 1.3 per 1,000 live births in New York City.[26] Whenever it is diagnosed, appropriate treatment is prescribed to prevent or lessen future disability, and therefore, the natural history of the disease is not well known. Mindful of this hiatus in knowledge, the authors of this report took advantage of an unusual opportunity to study the occurrence and natural evolution of congenital hip disease among an untreated population in the United States which had, according to preliminary estimates, a prevalence rate of 10.9 per 1,000 population.

The population studied was the approximately 2,300 Navajo Indians living at Many Farms, Ariz., within the 700 square mile district studied and served by the Navajo-Cornell Research Station. The study district was located near the geographic center of the 24,000 square mile reservation and was selected as representative of the reservation as a whole in topography, economics, population structure, and culture.[25]

The people live in scattered groupings of extended families and have retained much of their traditional way of life, including elaborate curing rituals. Their economy is based upon a combination of agriculture, sheep-herding, welfare, and seasonal wage work. The terrain consists of mesas and canyons interspersed with vast sweeps of flat, semiarid, unfenced plain. The climate is rigorous, with hot, dry summers and bitterly cold winters.

The research station was staffed with social scientists, as well as physicians and nurses, which permitted intensive study of the cultural and social correlates of disease. For study purposes, the station provided health services to the population for six years, 1956-1962. Health services had been available to the Navajo of Many Farms in the past, but the facilities had been remote and transportation rudimentary, so that only emergencies were routinely seen by the physicians. As a result, chronic disorders often were not brought to the attention of the physicians and there were no organized programs for early detection of children with congenital hip disease.

Congenital hip dislocation, which produces a characteristic limp or rolling gait in the child or adult, was described by Hippocrates and recognized by him as a congenital disorder. The exact nature of the abnormality, however, is still a subject of controversy.[1,14] Radiographs of the newborn, for example, do not show clearly the relationship of the femur to the acetabulum because the major portion of both these elements is formed in cartilage and cannot be visualized on the radiograph. Radiographs of affected older infants show either frank dislocation, or a deformity of the acetabulum and some degree of underdevelopment of the femur without complete dislocation of the femoral head from the acetabular fossa. This latter condition is called hip dysplasia.[15] Both conditions are considered to be manifestations of the same disease, but their relationship and the primacy of either condition has not been fully determined.

Until recently, it was believed that *hip dysplasia* was the primary abnormality.[13,14,23,30] According to this theory, dislocation occurred after the neonatal period because the sloping acetabular roof provided insufficient support for the femur. The stress of motion and finally, weight-bearing, were believed to produce dislocation.

The contemporary concept of the disease states that the basic abnormality is *hip dislocation* which is present at the time of birth.[1-3,5,7,29] Hip dislocation in the neonatal infant is easily reduced and can be demonstrated by skillful clinical examination.[1,27] The diagnosis can also be confirmed by radiographic procedures.[2,3] In addition to these clear-cut cases, a number of newborns (approximately 1.5 per cent) show an abnormal degree of hip joint laxity in which, by manipulation, it is possible to produce a hip dislocation and reduction.[2,3,5] In the majority of both groups of infants, the hip joint becomes stable and normal within the first few weeks of life; only a small percentage of those found initially with dislocated hips retain a complete dislocation or show radiographic evidence of hip dysplasia. According to current concepts, hip dysplasia, characterized by a shallow acetabulum, increased slope of the acetabular roof and late development of the proximal femoral epiphysis, is secondary to and represents a recovery stage of hip dislocation.[4,21] In many cases this recovery proceeds to normal, while in others, the patient retains the stigmata of hip dysplasia.

The concepts of pathogenesis and course expressed above do not pertain to teratologic dislocations which occur early in fetal life and are combined with other congenital anomalies. These have been excluded from this study along with the various forms of hip dislocation caused by neuromuscular disorders or obvious abnormalities of connective tissues, as in Ehlers-Danlos disease.

The study reported here had three objectives: (1) to supply an accurate picture of the prevalence of the disease by radiographic examination; (2) to investigate genetic and environmental factors which might be associated with the expected high prevalence of congenital hip disease; and (3) to ascertain the natural history of the disease.

The sporadic pattern of occurrence in widely varying populations, such as the Lapps[11] in the far North and the Italians of the South Tyrol,[33] led to postulation of a genetic factor peculiar to these populations. Familial clustering and simple hereditary transmission of the disease have been reported by a number of investigators, but no agreement has emerged regarding the mode or extent of genetic causation.[9,10,17] It was anticipated that the presence of a stable population in the Many Farms area and the accumulation of demographic and kinship data before the present study was initiated would facilitate investigation of the hereditary transmission of the disease.

Epidemiologic studies also have implicated certain environmental factors. It has been noted, for example, that children in the high prevalence populations are tightly swaddled after birth and the enforced adduction position has been postulated as a causative or contributory factor in the expression of the disease.[29,31] Preliminary observations at Many Farms corroborated statements in the anthropological literature that the Navajo still kept their children swaddled on cradle boards; this factor was one of a number of environmental conditions that was of interest in this study.

With regard to the natural progression of the disease, it has long been believed that infants with radiographic and physical signs of hip dysplasia might progress to dislocation if treatment were not instituted. But as early as 1925, Hilgenreiner[15] discussed several cases illustrative of spontaneous improvement. More recent studies have shown that some hips appearing abnormal by physical examination and radiograph will become normal in appearance and stability if left untreated.[5,21,35] In most studies, however, treatment has modified the prognosis of the cases under consideration.[19,24] The medical history of the Many Farms population indicated that treatment for congenital hip disease had not been available to the adult population and, therefore, we believed they could provide information on the untreated course of the disease.

Methods and Materials

Selection of the Population

The hip disease investigation had the advantage of utilizing the exact demographic data gathered in a series of census counts obtained as part of the larger research program of the research station. According to the last census (as of December 31, 1961) there were 2,299 Navajos residing in the district. The research staff also attempted to assess the degree of non-Navajo mixture in the population and as far as could be determined, the population was remarkably homogeneous.

Marriage records showed there had been little outmarriage with representatives of other groups. In the contemporary population there were several children fathered by whites, and three marriages with non-Navajos were known to have occurred two or three generations ago. Historically, there was mixture with the Pueblo peoples, with the Spanish, and with the Apaches, but it is impossible to derive any quantitative measure of the mixing that occurred historically.

Blood grouping determinations were made on a sample of 258 area residents seen in the clinic (Table 1). The results are comparable to a similar series taken at Ramah, N. M., among a Navajo population where little outmarriage has been known to occur. The small percentage of AB blood types in the Many Farms population is indicative of some other mixture, as these Indians have no B.[6]

The study district had long been settled by Navajos, even before their confinement at Fort Sumner in 1864. The area reached its economic peak at the turn of the century with a combination of herding and agriculture. As the range became rapidly depleted, the community came to rely more on flood farming. Nevertheless, the population seems to have been fairly stable until 1943 when the government completed construction of a reservoir and ditch system. The system brought an influx of people into the valley section of the district, but according to local accounts, most of the people came from within or on the immediate borders of the present area. These accounts were corroborated in the course of tracing pedigrees over six generations. The pedigrees did not take us far afield from the district.

The research design called for the simultaneous study of adults and children in the community. It was believed that, given the stability and homogeneity of the population (and the absence of diagnosis and treatment in the past), findings on the adults would reflect the unmodified course of the disease as well as provide a prognosis for children who might be untreated. The adults also would provide a measure of the frequency of the presumed sequelae of the disease, such as osteoarthritis.

Ideally, it would have been worth while to screen the entire population, but this was not possible because of their dispersal over an area of 700 square

Table 1—Navajo Blood Groups, Many Farms and Ramah*

Group	Many Farms		Ramah	
	No.	%	No.	%
O	177	68.6	277	76.7
A	78	30.2	84	23.3
AB	3	1.2	0	—
B	0	—	0	—
Total	258	100.0	361	100.0

All bloods at Many Farms and at Ramah were Rh positive.
* Boyd.[6]

Table 2—Number and Percentage of Population Radiographed

Prevalence Group	Birth Year	Total*	No. Radiographed	% Radiographed
I	1910–1930	357	270	76
II	1955–1961	628	548	87
—	All other years	1,327	298	23
Total	—	2,312	1,116	Av. 48

* Population adjusted to reflect number of individuals available for radiograph during study period, 1957-1962.

miles which lacked paved roads. Therefore, two segments of the population were selected for intensive study. Group I consisted of adults born in the years 1910-1930, thus making them between 30 and 50 years old in 1961. Group II consisted of all children born in the years 1955-1961. The children in Group II were born recently enough for us to rely upon their parents' recall of birth order and birth circumstances. Approximately 40 per cent of these births occurred at home and in the absence of adequate official records recency was a prime factor in obtaining valid information. Such information could not be obtained for the adults in Group I.

In addition to the two prevalence groups, radiographs were taken of all first degree relatives and siblings of those found to have congenital hip disease. Additional roentgenograms were taken of any individual who came to the clinic with symptoms referable to congenital hip disease. Films also were taken of all lineal and collateral relatives in several family groups selected for genetic study because of the high prevalence of the disease.

Most radiographs were taken when patients came to the clinic for medical attention. During the last year of the study, however, patients were specifically invited in and transportation was provided. In this manner, 76 per cent of the Group I population (adults) and 87 per cent of the Group II population (children) were radiographed (Table 2). The two groups consisted of 985 individuals of whom 818 were examined radiographically.

The picture is quite different for the other 298 individuals outside of Groups I and II who were radiographed. Because of the high degree of selectivity, (these patients were radiographed because they either showed some clinical evidence of the disease or were related to affected individuals), and the small percentage examined, findings pertaining to these individuals are not utilized except where specifically noted in the attitudes, treatment, and genetics portions of the paper.

Diagnosis

The radiographs were sent to New York accompanied only by name, birth date, and identification number. They were read, without benefit of history or knowledge of findings from previous physical and radiographic examinations, by an orthopedist (W.D.A.) and a radiologist (R.H.F.). Readings were returned to Many Farms where follow-up was initiated on abnormal cases.

The findings are not subject to the well known deficiencies inherent in radiographic diagnosis of congenital hip disease in the newborn.[7] By the age of six months, the radiographic evidence of the disease is sufficiently obvious to permit diagnosis in the absence of special pelvic films or a physical examination. Intensive examination of the children did not begin until 1960, and radiographs were taken usually during a clinic visit. Therefore, most of the films (80 per cent) were taken on children over the age of six months (Table 3). Only 6 per cent of all the radiographs taken were of children under one month of age at the time of first examination. The statistics then are not based upon neonatal examinations, such as those of Barlow,[5] Andrén,[1-3] and others.

For screening purposes, we relied upon a single A-P radiographic examination of the pelvis, with the patient's legs extended in an approximately neutral position. The abnormalities disclosed by these films were separated into two groups. The first, *frank dislocation,* implied complete displacement of the femoral head from the acetabulum. The second group, termed *dysplasia,* consisted of abnormal hips in which frank, complete dislocation of the femoral head was not present at the time of the radiographic examination.

The radiographic criteria used in determining the presence of hip dysplasia are essentially those described by Hilgenreiner in 1925[15]:

1. Displacement of the femoral head within the acetabulum.
2. Alteration in the shape of the acetabulum, as reflected in the ossification center of the acetabular roof formed by the body of the ilium.
3. Delayed appearance and decreased size of the ossification center of the femoral head.

In a child below the age of two years, at least two of these abnormalities had to be present before the hip joint was classified as dysplastic. The acetabular angle[20] was recorded for comparison with other series, but in no case was this used as a sole criterion for diagnosing a hip dysplasia. Above the age of three, the diagnosis of hip dysplasia rested to a greater extent upon the abnormal shape of the acetabulum.

The orthopedic co-author of this paper (W.D.A.) also visited the project and saw a large number of the affected children. Most diagnosed cases were examined and appropriate treatment was prescribed by a visiting Public Health Service orthopedist at the Chinle Clinic, 15 miles from Many Farms. Altogether, some 90 per cent of the children were examined by an orthopedist. In no in-

Table 3—Age at Radiograph of Group II Population

Age in Months	% Radiographed	% of Total Radiographed (545)	Cumulative %
0–5	109	20	20
6–11	72	13	33
12–17	35	6	39
18–23	35	6	45
24–29	48	9	54
30–35	39	7	61
36–41	28	5	66
42–47	31	6	72
48 and over	148	27	99
Total	545*	99	

* Three individuals not included because age at radiograph could not be determined.

Table 4—Dislocation and Dysplasia Rates by Prevalence Groups

Prevalance Group	Born:	Total Population	No. Radiographed	% Radiographed	Dysplasias No.	Dysplasias % of Radiographed	Dislocations No.	Dislocations % of Radiographed
I	1910–1930	357	270	76	2	0.7	7	2.6
II	1955–1961	628	548	87	18	3.3	4	0.7
Total		985	818	83	20	—	11	—

stance, however, did the results of the clinical examination alter the classification established by the radiographic examination.

Treatment and Follow-up

When the intensive study of congenital hip disease was started in 1960, treatment had been prescribed for some children as described above. By early 1961, it became evident to the physician and anthropologist at Many Farms that some of the children at least were not following prescribed treatment, yet reading of serial films returned from New York indicated that some of the children showed improvement. Therefore, an attempt was made to obtain serial radiographs of all affected children and the clinic files were searched for usable films of these children that might have been taken from the time the clinic was established in 1957.

Affected children were taken back to Chinle Clinic when the orthopedist returned to the area. Patients and their families were interviewed, either in the clinic or at their homes, by the anthropologist (C.R.B.) who collected data on place of birth, birth practices, cradle boarding, attitudes toward the disease, faithfulness with which prescribed treatment was followed, and on native healing practices.

Available records at the clinic and in the regional Public Health Service and missionary hospitals were reviewed by the nurse to corroborate field evidence and to yield information on the non-afflicted population who served as the comparison group. These records provided information on birth order, birth location, date of birth, and the name and ages of parents of affected children. Extensive use was made of the basic demographic and kinship material gathered by the project staff over a six-year period. This material was utilized as a base to trace the pedigrees of all affected individuals and was supplemented by field interviews conducted by the anthropologist.

Observations

Prevalence and Factors of Conceivable Relevance

Prevalence

The findings indicate that the Navajo study population has an exceedingly high prevalence of congenital hip disease (Table 4). A total of 31 abnormal hips were uncovered in the two prevalence groups, producing an over-all rate of 3.8 per cent. The combined prevalence of dysplasia and dislocation among adults (Group I) is 3.3 per cent. The comparable rate for the children (Group II) is 4 per cent, and given the small numbers in each group the difference is not significant.

There is a striking difference, however, in the type of abnormality that

Table 5—Dislocations and Dysplasias by Prevalence Group and Sex

Sex	Group I (1910–1930) Total X-Rayed	Group I Dislocations No.	%	Group I Dysplasias No.	%	Group II (1955–1961) Total X-Rayed	Group II Dislocations No.	%	Group II Dysplasias No.	%	Total Dislocations No.	%	Total Dysplasias No.	%	Combined No.	%
Males	113	1	14	0	—	282	1	25	4	22	2	18	4	20	6	19
Females	157	6	86	2	100	266	3	75	14	78	9	82	16	80	25	81
Total	270	7	100	2	100	548	4	100	18	100	11	100	20	100	31	100

Table 6—Affected Side by Prevalence Groups

Affected Side	Group I (1910–1930) Dislocations No.	%	Group I Dysplasias No.	%	Group II (1955–1961) Dislocations No.	%	Group II Dysplasias No.	%	Total Dislocations No.	%	Total Dysplasias No.	%	Combined No.	%
Left Only	1	14	0	—	2	50	7	39	3	27	7	35	10	32
Right Only	4	57	2	100	2	50	7	39	6	55	9	45	15	48
Bilateral	2	29	0	—	0	—	4	22	2	18	4	20	6	19
Total	7	100	2	100	4	100	18	100	11	100	20	100	31	99

Table 7—Comparison of Acetabular Angles of Many Farms Normals (Group II) with New York City Series*

	Right Angle					Left Angle		
	Many Farms			N.Y.C. Series		Many Farms		N.Y.C. Series
Age	No.†	Range	Mean	No.†	Mean	Range	Mean	Mean
Under 1 month	32	38–18	25.8	344	27 (Neonatal)	35–18	26.7	28.2 (Neonatal)
1 mo–3 mo	44	34–15	24.7			33–9	24.1	
4 mo–6 mo	43	34–12	22.6	290	20.8 (6 mo)	34–11	21.6	22.2 (6 mo)
7 mo–9 mo	37	31–10	20.1			32–10	19.8	
10 mo–12 mo	20	28–11	20.1	279	19.8 (12 mo)	29–12	19.3	21.3 (12 mo)
13 mo–18 mo	25	29–12	19.6			30–10	19.2	
19 mo–24 mo	37	33–10	17.9			28–11	18.4	

* Values obtained for white infants by Caffey.[7]
† Number for both right and left sides are the same.

Table 8—Group II, Normals and Abnormals by Birth Order

	Total X-Rayed		Abnormals	
Birth Order	No.	% (548)	No.	% (22)
1	69	12.6	2	9.1
2	66	12.0	4	18.2
3	64	11.7	4	18.2
4	64	11.7	3	13.6
5	64	11.7	2	9.1
6	56	10.2	0	—
7	42	7.7	2	9.1
8	43	7.9	2	9.1
9	32	5.8	2	9.1
10 and over	48	8.8	1	4.6
Total	548	100.1	22	100.1

occurs in each of the prevalence groups. The percentage with dysplasia in Group I (adults) is 0.7 compared with the rate of 3.3 per cent for the children in Group II. Similarly, the dislocation rate of 2.6 per cent in Group I differs sharply from the rate of 0.7 in Group II. All of these differences are significant at the 0.01 level. Dysplasias then are nearly five times as common among children born between 1955 and 1961 than they are among adults in the 30-50 age group. Among the latter group, dislocations occur at a rate nearly three times that in the children. An interpretation of these differences will be found in the discussion.

An additional 18 abnormal hips were diagnosed in patients outside of the two prevalence groups. Seventeen of these patients (ten with dislocations and seven with dysplasias) were born between 1931 and 1954, and one individual with a dislocation was born before 1900. The biased selection of these cases has excluded them from our analysis.

Sex, Side, and Pelvic Structure

Particular attention was directed toward determining the correspondence between the disease characteristics of those affected here as compared to those seen in other populations. In regard to occurrence by sex (Table 5), the disease occurs predominantly in females. Sorting by prevalence group and type of abnormality, the ratio is never less than one male to three females and the overall ratio is a little over four to one. This ratio is less than the seven to one reported for low incidence populations but it is typical of that reported in other high incidence populations.[2]

The condition was found to be bilateral in six (19 per cent) of the cases (Table 6) and to involve the right hip somewhat more than the left (15 to 10). In two of the cases in Group I (both women) there was a dislocation on one side and a dysplasia on the other. In one case the dislocation is on the right and in the other it is on the left. Both of these cases were counted once each in Tables 5 and 6 as dislocations.

It was considered a possibility that the pelvis of the normal Navajo differs in shape from that of the non-Navajo population and that a primary abnormality of the shape of the pelvis and acetabulum could be responsible for the high incidence of hip dislocation and dysplasia. In order to investigate this possibility, the acetabular angles of the children considered to be normal were recorded and their values compared with a series of comparable age obtained by Caffey, et al., in New York City.[7] It was postulated that if there were a primary difference in pelvic structure there would be an increase in the values of the acetabular angles in the Navajo, as compared with the normals in New York City. The comparison shows, however, that the range of measurements falls well within the limits of normal for each age group and the mean values are practically identical to those found by Caffey (Table 7). Pelvic films of adult Navajos also were reviewed and showed no recognizable difference in size and shape from normal, non-Navajo pelves.

Birth Order and Parents' Age

Previous studies have suggested that early birth order and advanced maternal age are associated with higher incidence of this disorder.[31,37] Data were obtained to test this relationship for the Group II population at Many Farms. The normal controls were the 526 children radiographed in Group II. While the prevalence figures are high for this population, the total population and the number of abnormals is extremely small. None of the small differences observed are significant (Table 8).

A similar difficulty is evident upon examination of the relationship of the disease with parents' age (Tables 9 and 10). None of the differences observed are significant.

Table 9—Group II, Normals and Abnormals by Mother's Age at Birth of Child

Age of Mother	Total X-Rayed		Abnormals	
	No.	% (548)	No.	% (22)
15–19	53	9.7	2	9.1
20–24	145	26.5	8	36.4
25–29	144	26.3	4	18.2
30–34	108	19.7	5	22.7
35–39	68	12.5	1	4.6
40+	30	5.5	2	9.1
Total	548	100.2	22	100.1

Table 10—Group II, Normals and Abnormals by Father's Age at Birth of Child

Age of Father	Total X-Rayed		Abnormals	
	No.	% (523)	No.	% (21)
14–19	5	1.0	0	—
20–24	73	14.0	4	19.1
25–29	127	24.2	4	19.1
30–34	116	22.2	3	14.3
35–39	65	12.4	2	9.5
40–44	57	10.9	1	4.8
45+	80	15.3	7	33.3
Total	523	100.0	21	100.3
Unknown	25	—	1	—

Birth Circumstances and Complications

Two-fifths of the births in Group II occurred at home, under very primitive conditions, without benefit of a physician in attendance. Despite these circumstances there was no significant difference between the abnormal and normal children in regard to the presence of a physician at the time of birth (Table 11).

Navajo women are generally aware whether a birth presentation is cephalic or breech. If a woman experiences difficulty giving birth at home, an experienced relative or native practitioner may be called in. The practitioner will determine the position of the fetus and, if necessary, will attempt to rotate the child in utero by means of external manipulation. Internal manipulation of the fetus is reported in the anthropological literature for the Navajo,[4] but at Many Farms only external rotation was reported by a few women.

None of the 22 abnormal children in Group II were subject to this procedure. All the births were cephalic presentations without complications or prolonged labor. For the seven cases born at home, the definition of prolonged labor rests with the mother or other relatives who attended her. The data are believed to be reliable and are congruent with information obtained on the hospital-born children and with the general known birth experience of the population.

The results differ from previous reports[2,31] which indicate some association of the disease with breech deliveries. These studies showed the association most markedly in males, but the Many Farms population is much smaller and had, as noted, very few affected males.

Seasonal Variation

The seasonal distribution of the birth of abnormal children was compared with the seasonal distribution of births in the Group II population. The small number of cases again complicates the analysis (Table 12). The coldest months of the year (with which the disease has been associated in other studies) are November, December, January, and February.[28,31] The mean temperature for these months in the winter of 1960-1961 was 34.6° F with the maximum average monthly low of 12.7° in January and a high of 58.5° in November. No significant relationship is indicated between the season of birth and the occurrence of congenital hip disease.

Cradle Board Usage

It has long been postulated that tight wrapping of the infant during the period

234

of early rapid growth of the hip joint could produce an abnormal joint or exacerbate a congenitally abnormal joint. The straight-legged adduction position enforced by swaddling tends to pull the head of the femur away from its resting place in the acetabulum and is the obverse of the position enforced in conservative management of the disease. High incidence of the disease has been reported in portions of northern Italy where swaddling is common and the rate is high among the Apaches,[18,36] relatives of the Navajo who also raise their children on cradle boards. Cradle board usage by this Navajo population then was of particular interest as a possible etiologic factor in the occurrence of congenital hip disease.

The Navajo cradle board (Figure 1) is made of two boards of yellow pine, laced together in the rear with leather thongs. A footrest often is laced to the bottom and a thin piece of wood is bowed and lashed in position across the top of the board to serve as a support for the covering which is used to shield the baby from the sun or dust.

Each part of the cradle has symbolic meaning for the Navajo, derived from the origin story of the first cradle ever made.[12] Nevertheless, changes in usage have occurred; most notably the introduction of diapers which force the legs into a more abducted position. Previously, the cradle was lined with the bark of the cliff rose and urine simply ran out the back of the cradle through a hole in a single-board cradle or through the slit in the now exclusively utilized two-board type. Diapers have been widely used since 1958 when the Navajo Tribe began to distribute free layettes to mothers who appeared at a clinic for post-partum and well-baby examinations, and registered their child with the tribe. Diapers were known and used sporadically before 1958, but certainly were rare from 30 to 50 years ago.

Observation of the wrapping procedure suggested that the diapered child was not wrapped so tightly as to preclude abduction. This observation was confirmed by physical and radiographic examination of a child on the cradle board (Figure 2). The film reveals that the cradle does not maintain the legs in firm adduction and the child can partially abduct his lower limbs.

Cradle board information was obtained from the parents of all abnormal children in Group II. In addition, a survey was made of a 40 per cent sample of the parents of children born in 1960 and 1961, stratified by residence area, to determine the nature of usage in the community as a whole. All 18 of the children with dysplastic hips were raised on cradle boards as well as two of the four children with dislocations. In all, 91 per cent of the abnormal children had been kept on the cradle board for

Table 11—Group II, Normals and Abnormals by Birth Circumstance

	Total X-Rayed		Abnormals	
	No.	% (529)	No.	% (21)
Physician attended	319	60.0	14	67.0
Nonphysician attended	210	40.0	7	33.0
Total	529	100.0	21	100.0
Unknown	19	—	1	—

Figure 1—Wrapping a Child on a Cradle Board

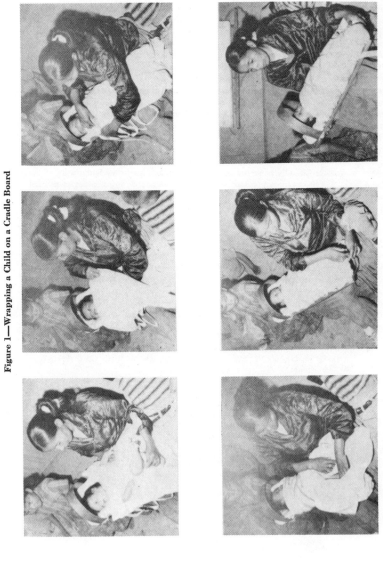

The child is diapered and wrapped in a blanket with his arms inside the wrapping and held straight along his sides. He is then lashed onto the board with a long, thin strip of leather or ribbon which is criss-crossed as it runs through loops attached to the sides of the board.

236

varying periods of time. These findings were similar to those obtained from the community survey, wherein 85 per cent of the children used the cradle board.

According to the literature on the Navajo, the child is not placed on the board until he is a month old because usually the cradle board for a first child is not prepared until after birth.[4] Unless a child dies while using the cradle, in which case it is disposed of, other siblings will use the same cradle. In the Many Farms community, however, 40 per cent of the children were placed on the cradle in the first week of life, 19 per cent in the second week, and 11 per cent in the third week. Only some 30 per cent of the children were kept off the cradle until they were a month of age. These findings also pertain to the abnormal children.

There is no cultural prescription specifying when the child should be taken off the board, and no ceremony is recorded or mentioned for this event. The only work to deal with cradle board practice among the Navajo in recent times is that of Bailey[4] and the consensus among her informants was that a child was kept on for about a year. At Many Farms the children are taken off the board for increasing periods of time during the day starting around the fifth month. By the tenth month, some 40 per cent of the normal and abnormal children are off the board completely and do not use it even to sleep. By the end of the first year, 70 per cent are permanently off the board. A few children, however, sleep on the board at night until they are about two years old. The two children with dislocated hips who were raised on the board were not taken off for protracted periods until the first year and they continued to sleep on the board until two years of age.

In summary, the great majority of the normal and abnormal population utilized

Figure 2—Radiograph of a Normal Child on a Cradle Board

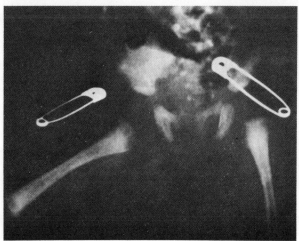

The child is wearing a single diaper. Note that the cradle board allows partial abduction.

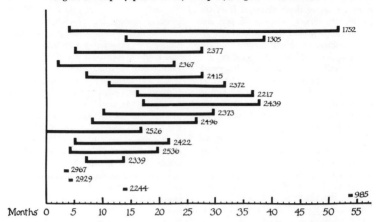

Figure 3—Hip Dysplasia Cases, Group II, Length of Observation

Figure 4—Case No. 1, Female, B.Y., No. 2377

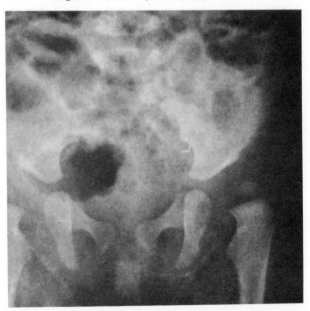

Figure 4A—Age 5 months. Severe bilateral hip dysplasia.

the cradle and in the same manner. In contrast to what has been previously reported for the Navajo, many children were placed on the board during the first month of life, at a time when it might have a maximum effect on development. The child's limbs are not immobilized by the board, but movement is restricted. The cradle board often is propped in a vertical position so that the child can observe activities around him. Thus, his feet may rest against the bottom of the board or the ground and his joint may be weight bearing at an early age. It was not possible, however, to determine the frequency and the age at which this weight bearing occurred.

Natural History

Investigation of the natural history of the disease led to an unexpected finding. We were able to demonstrate marked, spontaneous improvement to normal or near normal in nearly three-quarters of the dysplastic cases.

As previously noted, 18 cases of hip dysplasia were discovered among the Group II children (born 1955-1961). Seventeen of these children were first examined radiographically under the age of 15 months (Figure 3). Fourteen of the 18 cases were followed by physical and radiographic examination over an average period of two and a half years to a maximum of five years. The frequency of examination varied with the accessibility of the child and the presence in the area of an orthopedist to observe the clinical appearance of the joint.

Of the 14 cases followed, ten demonstrated improvement to near normal or to a condition indistinguishable from normal. Three cases showed improve-

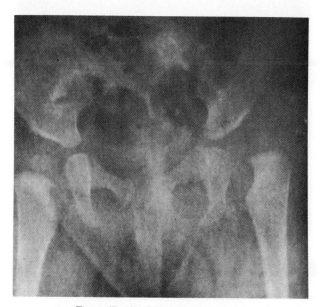

Figure 4B—Age 10 months. Improved.

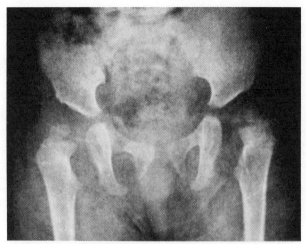

Figure 4C—Age 16 months. Further improvement.

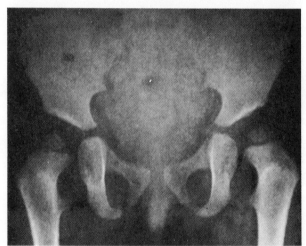

Figure 4D—Age 28 months. Mild dysplasia persists.

ment, although still presenting some stigmata of dysplasia, and one case showed no change. In no case was any increase of deformity noted nor was any progression to frank dislocation found.

The following case histories and radiographs are illustrative of the observations made.

Case No. 1, Female, B.Y., No. 2377. This child was first seen at five months of age with

Figure 5—Case No. 2, Female, C.T., No. 2373

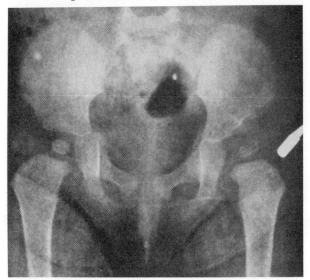

Figure 5A—Age 10 months. Left hip dysplasia.

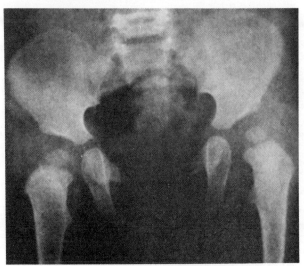

Figure 5B—Age 15 months. Improved.

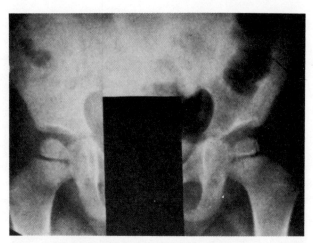

Figure 5C—Age 30 months. Further improvement.

bilateral dysplasia (Figure 4A). At that time she had been on the cradle board for approximately four months. Subsequent films were obtained at 10, 16, 21, and 28 months of age. At the age of ten months a modified Frejka apron, (a splinted diaper to hold the legs in abduction), was prescribed. The family continued to use the cradle board until the age of 15 months and the apron was used erratically until the age of 14 months. At the time of the last examination (Figure 4D), clinically the hips were entirely normal, although some irregularity of the acetabulum still persisted on the left side.

Case No. 2, Female, C.T., No. 2373. The first film of this child was obtained at ten months of age at which time the left hip was dysplastic (Figure 5A). The child was raised on a cradle board from the first month of life and the cradle board was continued until about the twelfth month. A modified Frejka apron was prescribed eight days after the first film, but the family never used it. Subsequent radiographs at 15, 22, and 30 months of age demonstrated improvement, and at the latest date the legs were normal both clinically and by radiographic examination (Figure 5C).

Case No. 3, Female, M.T., No. 2422. At age five months, this child presented instability of the hip, somewhat more on the right side where a soft click could be demonstrated. This was not, however, an Ortolani's click of reduction and dislocation. The film revealed a dysplastic hip on the right side (Figure 6A). A modified Frejka apron was prescribed at the age of nine and a half months, but the family refused to use it. The child was kept on a cradle board until 12 months of age. Subsequent films taken at 14 and 22 months of age (Figures 6B, 6C) revealed improvement to normal. At the later date, physical examination of the hips was entirely normal.

Case No. 4, Male, J.T., No. 2415. The first film at seven months of age revealed bilateral dysplastic hips, with the dysplasia more marked on the right (Figure 7A). Shortly thereafter, physical examination revealed restriction of abduction but no other abnormalities. At age eight and a half months, a modified Frejka apron was prescribed but was not used. The child was kept on a cradle board, particularly for sleeping, until age 12 months. Serial films were obtained at 12, 17, and 20 months, and demonstrated improvement to essentially normal (Figures 7B-7D). At age 17 months, the clinical examination was entirely normal.

Case No. 5, Female, L.T., No. 2367. The infant was first examined at two months of age. The left hip was believed to be dysplastic, subluxed and possibly dislocated at the time (Figure 8A). At the age of six months (Figure 8B) the child was examined by the orthopedic consultant of the Public Health Service and a pelvic osteotomy recommended. The parents refused to authorize the procedure. The child continued to use the cradle board for sleeping

242

Figure 6—Case No. 3, Female, M.T., No. 2422

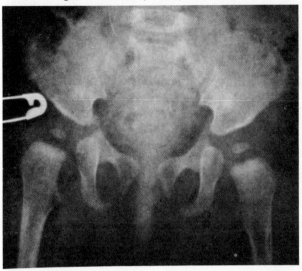

Figure 6A—Age 5 months. Minimal hip dysplasia on right side.

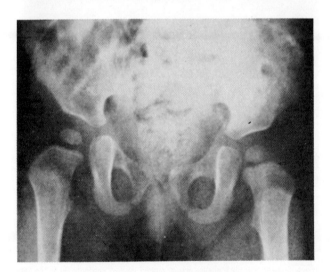

Figure 6B—Age 14 months. Nearly normal with slightly smaller right femoral capital epiphysis.

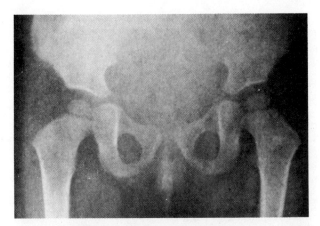

Figure 6C—Age 22 months. Normal hip.

Figure 7—Case No. 4, Male, J.T., No. 2415

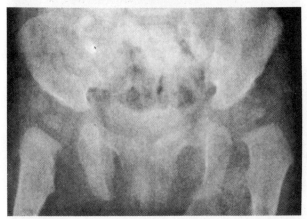

Figure 7A—Age 7 months. Bilateral hip dysplasia, more severe on left.

until 16 months of age. Radiographs were taken at 16, 21, and 23 months (Figures 8C-8E). At the time of the last examination the film indicated an irregularity of the acetabulum, although much improved from the appearance at two months. On physical examination there was a slight, soft click elicited by manipulation of the left hip but it was not a true Ortolani's sign. The hip was stable and the child walked well without a limp.

Case No. 6, Male, R.T., No. 2372. The first film at 11 months revealed dysplasia of the right hip (Figure 9A). Subsequent films at 16, 27, and 32 months (Figures 9B-9D) demonstrated marked improvement in the appearance of the hip. The cradle board was used until

244

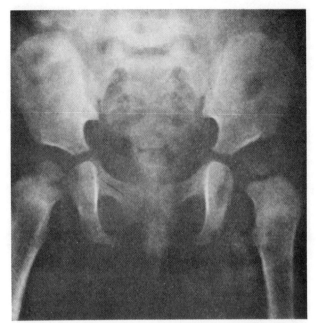

Figure 7B—Age 12 months. Right hip near normal, left improved.

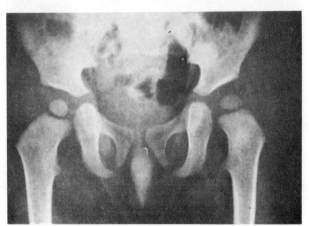

Figure 7C—Age 17 months. Marked improvement.

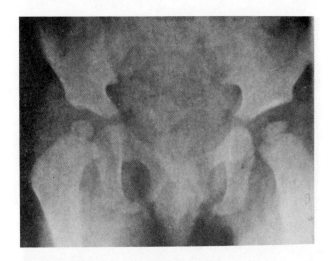

Figure 7D—Age 20 months. Continued improvement.

Figure 8—Case No. 5, Female, L.T., No. 2367

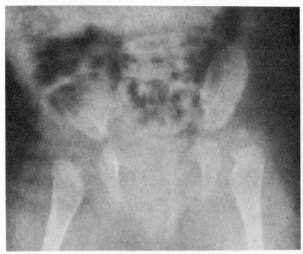

Figure 8A—Age 2 months. Severe dysplasia on the left.

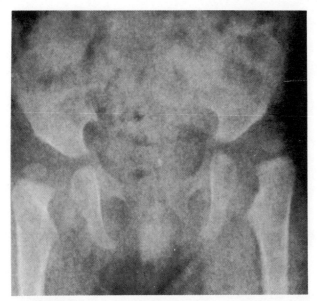

Figure 8B—Age 6 months. Still severe dysplasia on the left.

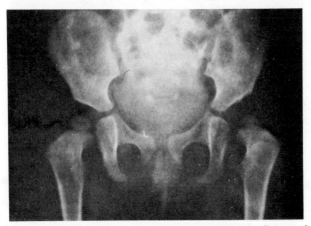

Figure 8C—Age 16 months. Some improvement, but persisting dysplasia on the left.

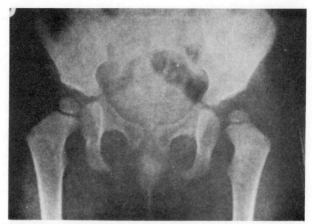

Figure 8D—Age 21 months. Further improvement, mild dysplasia persists.

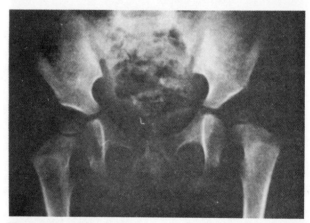

Figure 8E—Age 23 months. No change since age 21 months. Marked improvement from age 6 months.

the child started to walk at about one year of age. At no time had there been a limp noted or complaints of hip pain. No treatment had been prescribed. At the age of three and a half years the child was observed walking over rough ground helping herd the family's sheep.

None of the ten cases which progressed to normal or near normal, underwent any treatment. A modified Frejka apron was prescribed for four of the children but the parents refused to use it. Frejka aprons also were prescribed for two of the three children who showed improvement short of normal, but only one child wore the apron somewhat erratically and for a very short time.

Not all dysplastic hips progressed to normal. Three cases of dysplasia (not associated with a dislocation on the other side) were detected in adults in Prevalence Group I. In addition, seven other dysplasias were found in individuals who

Figure 9—Case No. 6, Male, R.T., No. 2372

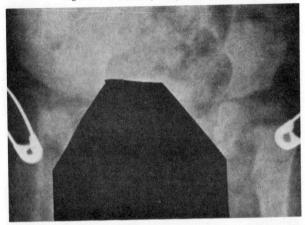

Figure 9A—Age 11 months. Technically poor radiograph, right hip dysplasia.

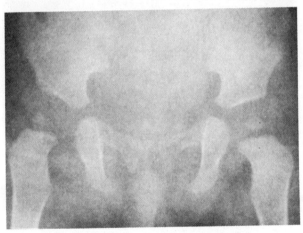

Figure 9B—Age 16 months. Still right hip dysplasia.

249

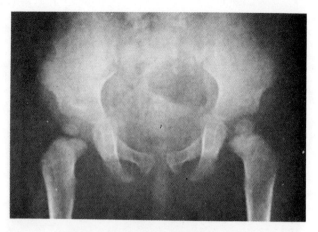

Figure 9C—Age 27 months. Improvement.

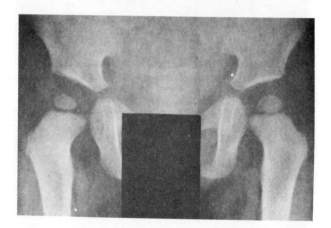

Figure 9D—Age 32 months. Near normal.

fell outside both prevalence groups (Figures 10, 11).

Later life hip disease has been attributed to a mild, unrecognized acetabular dysplasia.[13,38] In particular, this has been considered a possible etiology of osteoarthritis developing in adults between the ages of 30 and 50. Given the high rate of dysplasia in the children at Many Farms, we anticipated finding an equally high rate of dysplasia and arthritis of the hip in adults. This was not the case. The dysplasia rate was lower for the adults, as was previously noted, and only four individuals in the population were discovered to have osteoarthritis. Three of the four cases had obvious, severely dysplastic hips (Figure 12) and the fourth case had an associated dislocation. The findings suggest a relationship between dislocation or severe dysplasia and osteoarthritis, as we would expect, but the small number of adults with osteoarthritis of the hip precludes any statement regarding the relationship between unrecognized ace-

Figure 10—Right Hip Dysplasia with Minimal Osteoarthritis, Navajo Girl, Age 18

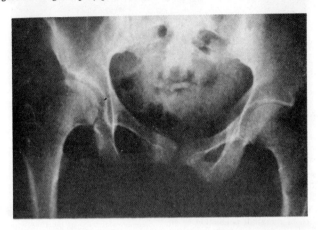

Figure 11—Left Hip Dysplasia, Navajo Girl, Age 9

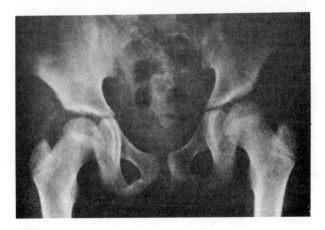

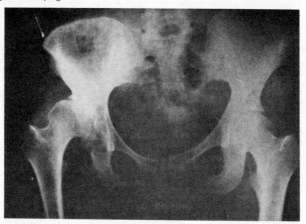

tabular dysplasia and the production of osteoarthritis of the hip.

Navajo Attitudes Toward the Disease and Its Treatment

The initial study design called for examination of the adult population as an untreated control group. Therefore, it was necessary to investigate the history of the adult patients and determine the extent and nature of medical and native treatment. This area of investigation took on greater importance in the light of the emerging findings regarding the natural history of the disease in the children. Systematic investigation was initiated to corroborate the early observations of the research station staff that parents of affected children rejected both conservative and surgical treatment of the condition.

Traditional Beliefs

A general statement of Navajo attitudes toward physical deformity was made by the Leightons in 1944:

> In general Navahos have an uneasy feeling about people who show some physical de-formity. . . . Their fear is probably in part due to feeling that since the deformed are out of harmony with the forces of nature, contact with them may bring disharmony to one's life, according to the general principles of contagious magic. . . . Their uneasiness is doubtless also linked with their admiration of physical perfection, a point of view said to have been dictated by the Holy Beings.[22]

This finding is based upon the work of many others, such as the physician-anthropologist, Hrdlicka, who in 1908 reported that "No deformed or monstrous child . . . is allowed to live."[16]

When the congenital hip study was initiated, the reaction of our Navajo staff seemed to confirm the cited literature. They stated that they did not want to talk about the disease with the people in the community. Careful inquiry, however, revealed that their sensitivity concerned treatment and treatment failure, not discussion of the disease itself. Two Navajo staff members put forth the idea that according to Navajo belief the disease represented a small family imperfection and since such imperfections were inevitable, a negligible disability like congenital hip disease was preferred to a more disabling imperfection. This concept was probed in the community, but no Navajo said he had heard of such a belief.

These preliminary findings affected our methodology. When the anthropologist began field work in June, 1961, he obtained an interpreter who had been unconnected with the research station and who felt no reluctance about interviewing members of the community about the disease. Because preliminary experience had indicated that the area of sensitivity was associated with surgical treatment of the condition, each interview was prefaced with the statement that we would not pressure affected respondents or their parents to undergo treatment. We indicated that treatment was available and advisable, but our purpose was to explore the nature of the disease, how people felt about it, and what they did for it.

In order to increase the number of respondents, interviews were not restricted to the 31 cases in the two prevalence groups, but were extended to all 49 cases discovered in the Many Farms population. Interviews were conducted with 25 of the 27 adults diagnosed as having congenital hip disease; with parents and other relatives of 21 of the 22 affected children; and with 40 of the medicine men in the district. It was believed that the medicine men could provide esoteric information about the disease and its treatment in the native medical system.

None of the medicine men or older Navajos with a knowledge of ceremonial lore and mythology knew of any myth or origin story to explain the disease or link it to any of the Navajo pantheon of supernaturals. Undefined lameness figures in the stories of two Navajo curing chants,[32] Night Chant and Bead Chant, but the medicine men emphatically stated that the reference was not to the type of limping associated with congenital hip disease.

The most striking finding obtained was that the disease is not considered particularly incapacitating or, in the absence of pain, even worth treating. "There are many who limp and get along" summed up the reaction of all but one of the parents of an abnormal child. "Getting along" includes marrying, having children, performing household tasks, and living as long as anyone else. So long as the individual can function within Navajo society, none of the feelings of uneasiness or abhorrence associated with radically deformed individuals are applied to patients affected by congenital hip disease.

In so far as possible, these attitudes were checked with measures of actual behavior. There were eight women with dislocated hips in the first prevalence group. The average age of a normal woman in this prevalence group was 20 at the birth of her first child. The average age of an abnormal woman at birth of her first child was 19 years. The normal women had an average of six children and the abnormal women an average of four. Thus, as far as can be ascertained, there is no discrimination against or social selection involving affected women, and this is in accord with the expressed attitudes of the population. Further, based upon interviews and observations, children with congenital hip disease did not suffer from neglect or differential treatment in the family.

The Navajo term for the condition is *na'nlxwod*, which translates literally as "he is lame," or "he is limping about." The same term may be applied to anyone who is crippled, to a horse with a splinter in its hoof, or humorously, to a man who has stepped into feces. The Navajo concept of the disease then indicates an awareness only of individuals who are symptomatic, i.e., those with unilateral or bilateral dislocations. Similarly, ideas regarding etiology do not apply to asymptomatic dysplasia.

Navajos recognize that children are born with congenital defects but have no one term to distinguish congenital diseases from other types of conditions. With congenital hip disease, on occasion, a dislocation will be noted before a child starts to walk, particularly if there is sufficient displacement of the femoral head to noticeably shorten the leg. In such a case, the condition is recognized as a congenital defect. Such recognition is enhanced if the family is aware of other relatives with this condition or has noticed a similar condition in their sheep.

If the disease is recognized as congenital, there are a variety of explanations that can be offered within the Navajo system of thought. The pregnant woman may have butchered an animal (women generally do the butchering) and cut the animal's joints; or, her husband may have twisted the legs of a horse in order to immobilize it while castrating or branding it. These causes are part of the whole pattern of explanation for all congenital anomalies. A six-fingered child, for example, may be produced if the mother or father made a six-pronged weaving comb during the course of the pregnancy. If the dislocated hip is believed to have been caused by injury to an animal, then recourse may be had to a short ceremony which involves "remaking" an image of the animal. None of the 22 people with dislocations reported having such a ceremony.

Generally, dislocations were not recognized by the parents until the child began to walk. At that point, the parents usually attempted to trace the defect to some specific accident in the recent past, such as a fall, pressure from the saddlehorn while carrying the baby on horseback, and so forth. If the condition was attributed to an accident and the child seemed to be in pain, then resort was had to Navajo ceremonies, particularly to the Flintway, which is the ceremony associated with internal injuries. This ceremony, like all others mentioned or utilized for congenital hip disease, does not involve any manipulation of the joint.

Modern Treatment

Given the Navajo attitude toward the disease, it is evident that they do not feel any pressing need to correct a condition which does not physically or socially handicap them. There is a more negative feeling toward treatment, however, which is related to the procedures offered.

At the time the Navajo-Cornell Research Clinic was introduced into the community, only one individual (and he was outside of the prevalence groups) had undergone surgical treatment for a dislocated hip. The operation performed had been a hip fusion procedure which produced a strong but nonflexible joint. This type of joint is acceptable in our society, but for the Navajo it creates a severe handicap. The individual so treated cannot sit on the ground with his family during meal times, he cannot ride horseback, nor can he walk easily over uneven ground. In the Navajo view, the operation produced a disability where none had existed before.

The U. S. Public Health Service was aware of this problem and after 1956 supported the development of a hip reconstruction procedure, i.e., pelvic osteotomy, the purpose of which was to provide a stable, freely movable hip joint. Unfortunately, however, the first child in the Many Farms district to be treated this way had an unsatisfactory result. Further, cast immobilization or surgery requires that the Navajo child be separated from his family for a period of several months, hundreds of miles away, perhaps among people who do not speak his language.

Of the 22 cases of dislocation discovered in the population (half of them in the two prevalence groups), medical records for seven indicate that surgery had been recommended. An additional five adults, outside of the prevalence

254

groups, recalled that sometime in their youth surgery had been advised but refused. Altogether, of the 12 cases for which surgery had been recommended, only three had accepted. Surgery also was recommended for three children with dysplasia but all refused. A hip cast was applied to one child with a dysplastic hip in Group II, and no serial films are available for her. This negative reaction to surgery is specific to congenital hip disease. When surgery is required for other conditions, such as tuberculosis, appendicitis, or cholelithiasis, there is seldom, if ever, any objection.

In regard to the three acceptances of surgical treatment, one case was a boy, with bilateral dislocation and some muscle atrophy who was operated on at the age of 11. According to the patient and his family, he had some pain and was handicapped. The family left the final decision up to the child, a common Navajo practice. The two other cases for which operative permission was granted involved younger children, first cousins, one of whose parents was highly acculturated and they helped to influence the other child's parents. The motivation of the parents in the latter two cases was the result of the statement by the physician that pain would ensue if the operation were not performed.

Parental resistance also was noted to the use of a modified Frejka apron which was prescribed for five of our dysplastic cases. Four did not use the apron at all, and one used it very erratically over a short period of time. There are a number of reasons for this failure to follow a prescribed conservative procedure.

First, use of a therapeutic apron requires that the child be taken off the traditional cradle board. Mothers are loath to give up the cradle. Its use is sanctioned not only by custom; it is of great practical benefit in a hogan which has a hot stove or open fire but ordinarily lacks a crib or playpen.

Second, institution of conservative treatment requires a great deal of parent education. The individual who limps because of a dislocated hip has an obvious physical symptom of which he and his parents are aware. Conservative treatment, however, must be instituted before the child is weight bearing. The child, therefore, has no observable symptoms and the parents must first be convinced that their child is abnormal before they will consider the need for treatment to prevent a condition which may develop sometime in the future. In summary, there was conclusive evidence based both on interviews and observation that the Navajo study population rejected both surgical and conservative treatment of congenital hip disease; it was this refusal that made it possible to observe the natural history of the disease.

Table 12—Group II, Normals and Abnormals by Season of Birth

| | Total X-Rayed | | Abnormals | |
	No.	% (546)	No.	% (22)
Winter (Nov., Dec., Jan., Feb.)	186	34.0	10	45.0
Other	360	66.0	12	55.0
Total	546	100.0	22	100.0
Unknown	2	—	0	—

Table 13—Father's Clan of Prevalence Group II

Clan	Total X-Rayed		Abnormals	
	No.	% (508)	No.	% (21)
Ashiihi	76	15	3	14.5
T'aaschi'i	48	9	2	9.5
To'Aheedliinii	43	8	2	9.5
Tachii'nii	40	8	0	—
Honaghaahnii	40	8	2	9.5
Subtotal	247	49	9	43.0
All other clans	261	51	12	57.0
Total	508	100	21	100.0
Unknown	40	7.3	1	4.5

Hereditary Transmission

Genetic studies among the Navajo were facilitated greatly by the Navajo's own understanding of and interest in tracing descent, kinship relationships and clan identification. The first line of inquiry when two Navajos meet is to trace their family lines and clan membership to determine whether they are related. This process was also engaged in by the interpreter when we visited families unknown to him in the field.

Clans

Navajos are born into social units, termed clans, which among other functions, regulate marriage. In relationship to congenital hip disease, it was hypothesized that if the disease was transmitted as a simple recessive or dominant trait and members of particular clans were more likely to intermarry with each other than with members of other clan groupings, then the incidence of the disease would be higher in certain clans. An alternate environmental hypothesis explanatory of the same findings would be the presence of some environmental factor operative for certain clans and not for others. Such an environmental factor might be a different clan tradition for handling the birth process.

Every Navajo child is "born into" and bears the clan name of his mother. Clan members address others of the same clan with kin terms as "mother's relatives," according to relative age and sex. The child is "born for" the father's clan and uses the appropriate forms of address for "father's relatives" when dealing with other members of the father's clan. As is evident from the kin terms used between members born into the same clan, blood relationship is assumed and, therefore, marriage between members of the same clan is considered to be an incestuous union. This restriction is observed in the Many Farms district: of 338 marriages recorded, not one was between people born into the same clan.

Marriage with someone in the father's or paternal grandfather's clan is preferred in some areas of the reservation,[34] but in the study area such marriages were prohibited. On the other hand, we were unable to ascertain with certainty the father's clan of 8 per cent of the study population (Table 13) and one of the partners in 2 per cent of the recorded marriages took a partner from his father's clan.

Twenty-seven clans are represented in the district and members of 26 of them were radiographically examined. Each clan is believed to be closely linked to four or five other clans and the ban on intraclan marriages extends to members of linked clans. Two of the Many Farms clans do not have linked clan members in the area while the others form six groups consisting of from two to five linked clans. There were a few marriages between members of linked clans (5 out of 338) but these occurred between clans where intermarriage is now generally acceptable.

The total number of abnormal cases in Prevalence Group II (i.e., 22) would have been too small to analyze their distribution meaningfully among 26 clans. They were distributed, however, among 14 of the 26 clans and therefore grouping was possible. The first four clans listed in Table 14 constitute 265 children or 49 per cent of the Group II population radiographed. The same four clans account for 50 per cent (or 11) of the abnormal cases. Similarly, if the father's clans are listed by their order of representation in the population (Table 13), they constitute 49 per cent of the radiographed population and 43 per cent of the abnormal cases. It is clear that clan membership is not a factor in the etiology or epidemiology of the disease and that study of hereditary transmission in this population must be investigated in terms of familial lines.

Familial Incidence

As noted earlier, radiographs were taken of parents and siblings of all propositi (affected individuals in the two prevalence groups). As a result of this procedure, a small number of cases were discovered outside the two prevalence groups. In addition, radiographs were taken of all individuals seen in the clinic with symptoms indicative of congenital hip disease. A total of 18 cases were discovered in this manner, in addition to the 31 found in Groups I and II. It should be emphasized that all of these cases were diagnosed by radiographic examination.

In order to trace pedigrees, a history was taken if individuals were deceased or otherwise unavailable for examination or x-ray. A history will uncover a dislocation but will not reveal a dysplasia unless it is symptomatic. The histories obtained from the Navajo are handicapped by the great amount of tuberculosis present in the population. Many adults two and three generations ago suffered from tuberculosis of the hip which sometimes was treated by a fusion operation. Particular care was observed when taking a history to attempt to distinguish between such a condition and congenital hip disease, but this was not always possible. Any error inherent from this confusion, however, would weight

Table 14—Mother's Clan of Prevalence Group II

Clan	Total X-Rayed		Abnormals	
	No.	% (541)	No.	% (22)
Tachii'nii	93	17	6	27.5
Todich'ii'nii	68	13	1	4.5
Ashiihi	53	10	3	13.5
To'Aheedliinii	51	9	1	4.5
Subtotal	265	49	11	50.0
All other clans	276	51	11	50.0
Total	541	100	22	100.0
Unknown	7	1.3	—	—

257

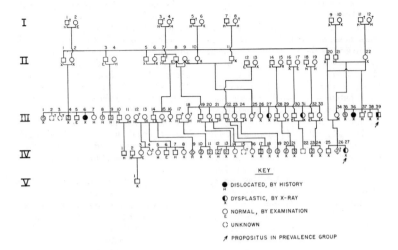

KEY

● DISLOCATED, BY HISTORY

◑ DYSPLASTIC, BY X-RAY

○ NORMAL, BY EXAMINATION

◌ UNKNOWN

⤴ PROPOSITUS IN PREVALENCE GROUP

the findings in favor of showing a high familial incidence. Every attempt was made to authenticate a diagnosis through a description of all the known circumstances. Limping due to no known accident or illness was the prime diagnostic feature when taking a history. If a child died before he started to walk, his condition on the pedigree was recorded as unknown.

Radiographs were obtained from 68 per cent of the parents of the propositi (Table 15). In no case did a propositus have a parent with a disease. There were two pedigrees (Nos. 2 and 4), however, which show such a relationship. In Pedigree 2, the paternal grandfather and great grandfather of IV-12 (not a propositus) both reportedly limped. The great grandfather was deceased and the grandfather could not be located. Both had lived outside the study area. In Pedigree 4, the mother (I-3) of II-10 was reported to have a dislocated hip by history. Neither of these two women was

a propositus and they both resided outside the study district.

Offspring of propositi also were traced and are shown on Pedigrees 1, 3, 4, 5, 7, and 24. The average age at which both women and men in the population first bear or father offspring is 19.5 years. Only 15 of 49 cases (2 men and 13 women) had attained this age by 1961. Of this group, ten women and one man had a total of 51 children (Table 16). A radiograph or history was obtained from

Table 15—Parents of Propositi

	No.	% (83)
Propositi	49	
Parents of propositi	83	
Normal parents, by radiograph	56	68
Normal parents, by examination	12	14
Normal parents, by history	15	18
Total normal	83	100

258

Table 16—Offspring of Propositi

	No.	% (51)
Propositi with offspring	11	
Total offspring	51	
Normal offspring, by radiograph	18	35
Normal offspring, by examination	16	31
Normal offspring, by history	11	22
Unknown	6	12
Total	51	100

88 per cent of these offspring and none were found to be abnormal. All of the unknown cases consist of children who died before they walked; therefore no determination of their condition could be made.

There was only one twin propositus (Pedigree 2). The dislocated female (IV-7) had a normal fraternal male twin. These twins also had dizygotic twin first cousins (IV-18 and 19), both of whom were normal.

Six families had two or more affected full siblings (Pedigrees 1, 2, 3, 8, 13, and 19). One of these families had three affected siblings and the rest two. Where familial incidence seemed to be high, great effort was made to obtain information on all collateral relatives, as illustrated in the first five pedigrees. Pedigree 1 illustrates the type of pattern that occurred in all such extended pedigrees, demonstrating as well some of the complexities of Navajo marriage and kinship.

The propositus first screened in Prevalence Group II, was the dysplastic male, III-39. Films taken on other siblings revealed a sister, (III-36), with a dislocation. These children also had an affected step-sister or niece (IV-27), depending upon the way the relationship is calculated. The step-sister with a dysplastic hip (IV-27) has a father (II-20) in common with III-36 and 39. But the mother of IV-27 is the child of II-22 by a previous husband (II-21). The mother of III-34 later married III-20 and he in turn polygymously married her daughter (III-34).

The mother of the children III-34 to 39 had no known siblings. The father of these children (II-20), however, had normal siblings indicated at II-10, 5, 3, and 1. Some of these siblings also had experienced multiple mar-

PEDIGREE NO. 2

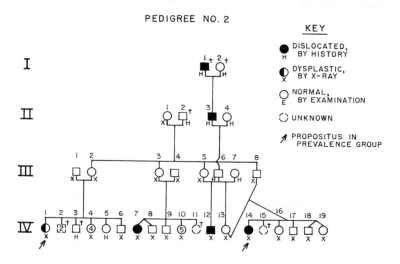

KEY

● DISLOCATED, BY HISTORY

◐ DYSPLASTIC, BY X-RAY

○ NORMAL, BY EXAMINATION

◌ UNKNOWN

↗ PROPOSITUS IN PREVALENCE GROUP

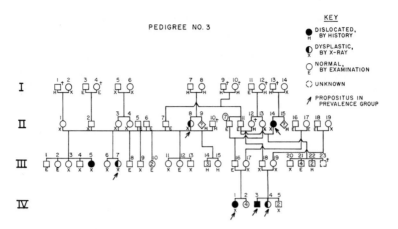

riages and as a result of one such marriage, one sibling (II-10), produced two children with dysplastic hips, (III-27 and 31). Another married sibling (II-1) produced one child with a dislocation (III-6). Other siblings produced a number of children via multiple marriages but no abnormal children were noted.

Similar multiple marriages and the crossing of generation lines are evident in the other pedigrees presented here. Siblings, and to some extent cousins, tend to produce some family aggregations of abnormal cases, but there is almost no indication of transmission through generations. Of the total of 49 cases, 18 were related as siblings or half siblings. The numbers are too small to assess the probability of older or younger siblings being affected.

There are five first cousin groupings of propositi illustrated in Pedigrees 1, 2, 5, 8, and 14, and second cousin groupings in Pedigree 3. In these groupings there does not seem to be any tendency to favor the maternal over the paternal line.

In summary, these pedigrees taken as a whole do not conform to a simple dominant or recessive gene hypothesis. They are compatible, however, with a hypothesis suggesting dominant single

or multigene factors with a variable degree of manifestation. The findings, however, must be evaluated against the tendency demonstrated in this paper for the condition to improve spontaneously. If a propositus was diagnosed as dysplastic, he was so indicated on the appropriate pedigree even though later radiographs may have shown progression to normal or near normal. But for individuals over the age of four years at the time the first film was taken there is no way of knowing how many would have been dysplastic if radiographed at an earlier stage of development. Therefore, many affected individuals may have been lost and a clear-cut pattern of transmission may thereby have been masked.

Discussion

The prevalence findings raised a most difficult problem of interpretation and understanding. The disease rate in both prevalence groups was essentially the same, but the nature of the disease was markedly different. The children in Group II had a prevalence of dysplasia of 3.3 per cent, while the adults, in Group I, had a rate of 0.7 per cent.

Similarly, the rate of dislocation was reversed between the two groups, with the children manifesting a rate of 0.7 per cent and the adults a rate of 2.6 per cent. The key to an understanding of these differences is to be found in the natural history of the disease as observed in this population.

Findings regarding the natural history of the disease are unique only in numbers, not in the phenomena observed. Spontaneous improvement of hip dysplasias has been noted by several investigators[5,13,15,21,23,30] but they have never been reported with such frequency for a given population. In large measure, this is the result of the nature of the research situation. No other study has had a large number of untreated dysplasias available for observation over a period of several years. Only the reluctance of this Navajo population to accept treatment enabled us to follow untreated cases.

Any judgment regarding the extent to which findings relating to the natural

PEDIGREE NO. 4

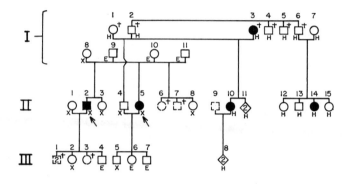

PEDIGREE NO. 5

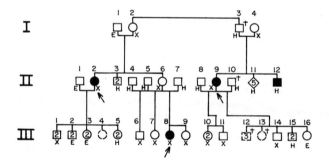

261

PEDIGREE NO. 6

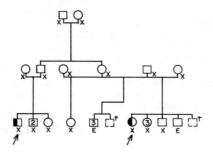

PEDIGREE NO. 7

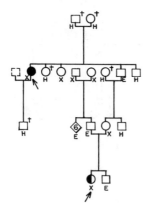

PEDIGREE NO. 8

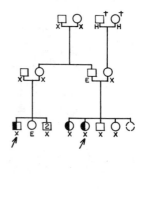

history of the disease may be generalized to other populations, rests in part on the presence of evidence that the disease described here exhibits characteristics typical of congenital hip disease. The dysplasias presented appear indistinguishable from similar conditions seen in non-Indians which are considered abnormal and treated vigorously. Certainly, there is a gradient from clearly normal to distinctly abnormal. The proper point of separation is difficult to establish and to some degree will vary with the individual interpreter. The criteria of abnormality for postneonatal infants utilized in this study, however, have been described and are conservative. They are in general use among orthopedists and radiologists today.

The findings are consistent with previous reports relating to the sex ratio for a high incidence population, and the comparison of the acetabular angles of normal Navajo children with children in

New York City demonstrates that there is nothing unique about Navajo pelvic structure.

An independent verification of the observations was found possible. If the spontaneous reduction demonstrated here is a natural process, occurring not only in the cases which were followed, but in all cases of dysplasia in the population, then the prevalence of hip dysplasia should vary inversely with the age of the child at the time a radiograph was taken. In the study population, children born in 1955 and 1956 were not examined radiographically until they were at least four years old. By that time, most of the dysplasias which might have been evident in the first or second year of life should have disappeared. The prediction can be made that the dysplasia rate for children in the upper age limits of Group II would be lower than the rate for children in the early years of life.

As may be seen in Table 17, this is indeed the case. The older the children at the time the radiograph was taken, the lower the dysplasia rate. Only one case of dysplasia occurred in the age group over 23 months of age. This result is not a by-product of the number of radio-

Table 17—Incidence of Dysplasia by Age of Child at First Radiograph

Age of Child at Radiograph	No.	Dysplasias	
		No.	%
Under 1 year	181	13	7.2
12–23 mo	70	4	5.7
24–35 mo	87	0	—
36–47 mo	59	0	—
48 months and over	148	1	0.7
Total	545*	18	—

* Excludes three normal children whose age at radiograph could not be determined.

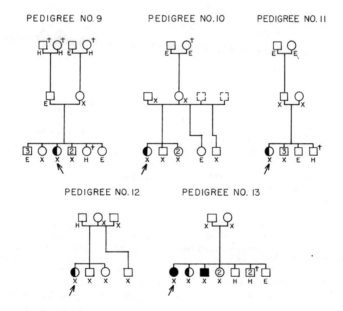

PEDIGREE NO. 9   PEDIGREE NO. 10   PEDIGREE NO. 11

PEDIGREE NO. 12   PEDIGREE NO. 13

263

PEDIGREE NO. 14

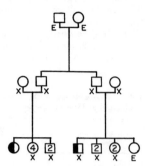

PEDIGREE NO. 15

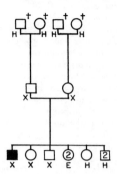

PEDIGREE NO. 16

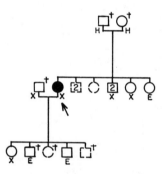

PEDIGREE NO. 17

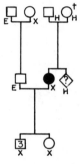

graphs taken, as 54 per cent of those so examined in Group II were in the older age category. The only known fact to account for this phenomenon is the demonstrated tendency for most dysplasias to improve spontaneously.

The tendency for dysplastic hips to improve has been documented and we believe that these observations account for the low percentage of dysplastic hips in older children and adults in the two prevalence groups. No such ready explanation is available to account for the substantially larger numbers of dislocated hips to be found in the adults.

In no instance did a hip once classified as dysplastic, later, when followed, become dislocated. Therefore, we can discard this hypothesis as an explanation for these figures.

Two hypotheses are proposed to account for the larger percentage of dislocated hips in the older Indian population. One or both may explain the phenomenon; neither can be proved. The first hypothesis assumes that the adults born with dysplastic hips in the period of 1910-1930 underwent the same process of spontaneous improvement observed in the children born 1955-1961. It further assumes, based upon observations of the children, that the dislocation rate remained constant, i.e., the number of dislocations found in the adults (seven) was the same at the time they were born. It follows then that the over-all incidence of congenital hip disease was considerably higher among the newborns in the period 1910-1930, and may have affected 14 per cent of the population. This rate is derived by applying the ratio of dislocations to dysplasias found in the children (4 to 18) to the adults (7 to 31.5), producing a dysplasia rate of 11.6 per cent. Given the natural history of the disease, however, some 90 per cent of the 31.5 cases could be expected to have undergone spontaneous improvement, leaving three cases of dysplasia (two of which were actually found). The assumption that the same natural course

of the disease found in the children was operative in the adults then leads to the conclusion that in the last 30 to 50 years there was an unexplained decrease of more than 70 per cent in the over-all incidence of congenital hip disease.

An alternative hypothesis is preferred because it does not imply an inordinate change in the occurrence of the disease and is more in keeping with the modern concepts of congenital hip disease.[1-3,5,7,21] According to this theory, children with dysplastic hips have had at birth, or shortly thereafter, hips that were dislocated or dislocatable with manipulation. Dysplasia is recognized simply as the healing stage of a previously dislocated hip. The transformation of a dislocated or dislocatable hip, without treatment, into what we have termed a dysplasia, is the result of natural forces con-

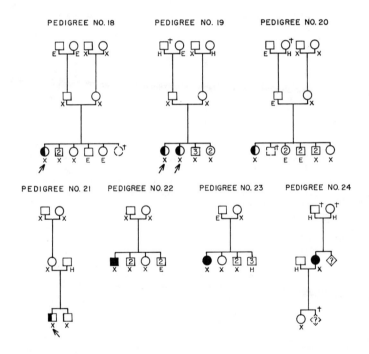

ditioned to some extent by environmental factors, such as positioning of the infant. This hypothesis suggests that there may have been no difference in the hip disease rate of the adult population if we had examined them as infants 30 to 50 years ago. Rather, something acting in the environment 30 to 50 years ago, and not so acting today, prevented the neonatal dislocated hip from becoming dysplastic and then improving further to normal.

There have been many environmental changes affecting the Navajo in the past 30 to 50 years. One change, which may be significant, is the general introduction of diapers. Without diapers the infant's legs might have been held in more constant adduction on the cradle board than at present.

The cradle board itself has long been thought to be implicated in the disease since it produced some adduction and partially immobilized the infant's legs. Our findings demonstrate that for this Navajo group the cradle board is not implicated directly in the etiology of the disease. Nine of the 13 cases which spontaneously improved, showed that improvement while on the cradle board. Two of the children with dislocations were never kept on cradle boards. This is a community, however, in which most children (85 per cent) are brought up on cradle boards and the practice may affect some children and not others. Cradle board usage (without diapers) might have been closer to 100 per cent 30 to 50 years ago, but there is no quantitative evidence for this.

In order to compare our findings with those from another, environmentally different, Navajo population a survey was carried out at Ft. Defiance, Ariz. This is a highly acculturated community, 106 miles from Many Farms. Radiographs were obtained on 148 children, born between 1955 and 1961, to make them comparable to the Group II children at Many Farms. The children were selected because at least one parent was a gov-

ernment employee which entitled them to live in housing with internal temperature control and connected to municipal water and sewage—all conditions which were absent at Many Farms.

The parents of all children were interviewed at home by two Navajo residents of the community. Information was obtained comparable to that at Many Farms on circumstances, location and type of birth, season of birth, birth order, parents' age, and cradle boarding practices. Blood grouping data was obtained to assure that there had been no appreciable intermarriage with other ethnic groups and direct information was recorded on the ancestry of children through the F2 generation. The Ft. Defiance and Many Farms children proved to be markedly different in regard to location of birth (all were hospital-born at Ft. Defiance), birth order, parents' age, and cradle boarding practices. In contrast to widespread usage at Many Farms, only 11 per cent of the children in the Ft. Defiance study group had been raised on cradle boards. The attitude of parents toward the disease also was markedly different. The highly educated Navajo parents at Ft. Defiance were as concerned over the possibility of their children having the disease as are parents in New York City.

Of the 148 children examined, none had dysplastic or dislocated hips. In the light of our natural history findings, however, the two groups cannot be considered strictly comparable. In contrast to the Many Farms study, which was carried out over a period of four years, the survey at Ft. Defiance was completed in a period of six weeks. As a consequence, only 20 per cent of the population was under the age of two years at the time they were radiographed, as compared to 46 per cent under the age of two at Many Farms. Therefore, the much lower disease rate found for the older children at Many Farms must be applied to the Ft. Defiance data. Because of the low rate, combined with the small number of children examined, the lack of dysplasias and dislocations at Ft. Defiance is not significant.

The evident deficiency in the Ft. Defiance data could be remedied by instituting a long-term study, not only at Ft. Defiance, but at other communities on the Navajo reservation. Similar studies could be extended fruitfully to other Indian groups who also have a high incidence of the disease. In this manner, varying environmental factors could be studied in relationship to varied rates of the disease.

The findings raise the question as to whether hip dysplasia detected after the neonatal period should be treated. Treatment for dysplasia of the hip with an abduction splint in early infancy is simple and apparently free from complications. We believe it should be recommended for use in the young Navajo infant, since a few dysplastic hips do persist to adult life and become symptomatic.

The rejection of such recommendations by the Navajos of Many Farms, documented here, is an excellent lesson in the basic principle that what constitutes a "disease" in one culture does not necessarily constitute a "disease" in another culture. The affected individual can function freely in traditional Navajo society. But as the culture changes Navajo parents will come to recognize, as have the parents at Ft. Defiance, that the affected individual is handicapped for full participation in life off the reservation, and, therefore, treatment is desirable even before symptoms appear.

Summary

The prevalence, natural history, and environmental factors associated with congenital hip disease were investigated among a population of Navajo Indians with a high incidence of the disease. Treatment for the condition had been unavailable to the adults, and was rejected by Navajo parents for their children. The research conditions permitted not only comparison of the adult and the child populations but study of the untreated course of the disease in the children.

The population was divided into two groups: children born between 1955 and 1961 and adults born between 1910 and 1930. Diagnosis was made by radiographic examination utilizing conservative diagnostic criteria. The dysplasia rate established for the children was 3.3 per cent and for the adults 0.7 per cent. Dislocations were diagnosed in 0.7 per cent of the children and in 2.6 per cent of the adults. Osteoarthritis associated with hip dysplasia was noted in a few adults, but findings were inconclusive regarding the relationship between mild or unrecognized acetabular dysplasia and arthritis.

The sex ratio, acetabular angles, and other observed characteristics were typical of the disease as described in other populations. Fourteen of 18 children with hip dysplasia were followed with serial films over an average period of two and a half years. In the absence of treatment, ten progressed to normal or to a condition indistinguishable from normal. In the absence of treatment, three others showed marked improvement. These findings led to the correct prediction that the dysplasia rate would be inversely related to age at first radiographic examination. A decreased prevalence of dysplasia was shown with an increase in age.

Findings suggest multigenetic factors in the etiology of the disease, with expressivity greatly influenced by undetermined environmental factors. Genetic findings, however, are highly tentative because dysplasias in the older population may have been lost due to spontaneous improvement.

Two hypotheses are suggested to account for the higher rate of dislocation in the adults as compared to the children. The first hypothesis suggests that the over-all rate of the disease was much higher 30 to 50 years ago in this population. The dysplasias tended to disappear without treatment leaving only the dislocations. The second, and preferred, hypothesis suggests that environmental conditions over the past 30 to 50 years have changed, so that today they favor the natural improvement of dislocations to a state of dysplasia, and in many, normality. One environmental change known to have occurred which might have produced this result relates to the positioning of infants on the Navajo cradle board due to the introduction of diapers. We believe that our findings, and their interpretation in the latter hypothesis, are consonant with modern concepts of hip disease that view the primary abnormality in the disease as a dislocation which under suitable environmental conditions may progress through the secondary changes of osseous dysplasia to normality.

REFERENCES

1. Andrén, L. Modern Concept of Congenital Dislocation of the Hip. Cereb. Palsy Bull. 3:167, 1961.
2. ————. Pelvic Instability in Newborns. Acta radiol. scandinav. Suppl. 212, 1962.
3. Andrén, L., and von Rosen, S. The Diagnosis of Dislocation of the Hip in Newborns and the Primary Results of Immediate Treatment. Acta radiol. Suppl. 49, 1958.
4. Bailey, F. Some Sex Beliefs and Practices in a Navajo Community. Cambridge: Papers of the Peabody Mus. of Am. Arch. & Ethn. XL, No. 2, 1949.
5. Barlow, T. G. Early Diagnosis and Treatment of Congenital Dislocation of the Hip. J. Bone & Joint Surg. 44-B:292, 1962.
6. Boyd, W. C., and Boyd, L. G. The Blood Groups and Types of the Ramah Navajo. Am. J. Phys. Anthropol. 7:569, 1949.
7. Caffey, J.; Ames, R.; Silverman, W.; Ryder, C.; and Hough, G. Contradiction of the Congenital Dysplasia-Predislocation Hypothesis of Congenital Dislocation of the Hip Through a Study of the Normal Variation in Acetabular Angles at Succesive Periods in Infancy. Pediatrics 17:632, 1956.
8. Corrigan, C., and Segal, S. The Incidence of Congenital Dislocation of the Hip at Island Lake, Manitoba. Canad. M.A.J. 62:535, 1950.
9. Faber, A. Erbbiologische Untersuchungen über die Anlage zur "angeborenen" Hüftverrenkung. Zeit. f. orth. 66:140, 1937.
10. ————. Untersuchungen über die Atiologie und Pathogenese der angeborenen Hüftverrenkung. Liepzig, Germany: Thieme Verlag, 1938.
11. Getz, B. The Hip Joint in Lapps, and Its Bearing on the Problem of Congenital Dislocation. Acta orthop. scandinav. Suppl. 186, 1955.
12. Goddard, E. P. Navajo Texts. New York Anthro. Papers A.M.N.H. Vol. 34, pt. 1, 1933, pp. 148–149.
13. Hart, V. Congenital Dysplasia of the Hip Joint and Sequelae. Springfield, Ill.: Thomas, 1952.
14. Hass, J. Can Congenital Disease of the Hip Be Prevented. New York J. Med. 58:847, 1958.
15. Hilgenreiner, H. Zur Frühdiagnose und Frühbehandlung der angeborenen Hüftgelenkverrenkung. Med. Klin. 21:1385–1388, 1425–1429, 1925.
16. Hrdlicka, A. Physiological and Medical Observations Among the Indians of Southwestern U. S. and Northern Mexico. Washington, D. C.: Smithsonian Institute, B.A.E., 1958, pp. 165–166.
17. Idleberger, K. Die Erbpathologie der sogenannten angeborenen Hüftverrenkung. Munchen and Berlin, Germany: Urban & Schwarzenberg, 1951.
18. Kraus, B., and Schwartzmann, J. Congenital Dislocation of the Fort Apache Indians. J. Bone & Joint Surg. 39-A:448, 1957.
19. Larson, R. L.; Newman, R. F.; and Meredith, D. C. Congenital Subluxation and Dislocation of the Hip. J.A.M.A. 178:14, 1961.
20. Laurenson, R. The Acetabular Index. J. Bone & Joint Surg. 41-B:702, 1959.
21. Leffman, R. Congenital Dysplasia of the Hip with Special Reference to Congenital Subluxation of "Preluxation." Ibid. 41-B:689, 1959.
22. Leighton, A., and Leighton, D. The Navajo Door. Cambridge, Mass.: Harvard University Press, 1944, p. 61.
23. Lorenz, A. Die sogenannte angeborenen Hüftverrenkung: Ihre Pathologie und Therapie. Stuttgart, Germany: Ferdinand Enke, 1920.
24. MacKenzie, I. G.; Seddon, H. J.; and Trevor, D. Congenital Dislocation of the Hip. J. Bone & Joint Surg. 42-B:689, 1960.
25. McDermott, W.; Deuschle, K.; Adair, J.; Fulmer, H.; and Loughlin, B. Introducing Modern Medicine in a Navajo Community. Science 131:197–205, 280–287, 1960.
26. McIntosh, R.; Merritt, K.; Richards, M.; Samuels, M.; and Bellows, M. The Incidence of Congenital Malformations: A Study of 5,964 Pregnancies. Pediatrics 14:505, 1954.
27. Ortolani, M. La lussazione congenita dell'anca. Bologna, Italy: Capelli, Editore, 1948.
28. Nagura, S. Einfluss der Jahreszeiten auf die Hänfigkeit der angeborenen Hüftverrenkung. Zentralbl. f. Chir. 30:1249, 1957.
29. Palmén, K. Preluxation of the Hip Joint. Acta paediat. Suppl. 129, 1961.
30. Putti, V. Early Treatment of Congenital Dislocation of the Hip. J. Bone & Joint Surg. 15:16, 1933.
31. Record, R., and Edwards, J. Environmental Influences Related to the Aetiology of Congenital Dislocation of the Hip. Brit. J. Prev. & Social Med. 12:8, 1958.
32. Reichard, G. Navaho Religion: A Study of Symbolism. New York, N. Y.: Pantheon, Vol. 1, 1950, pp. 94–95.
33. Scaglietti, O. A Clinical-Statistical Study of Cases of Congenital Dislocation of the Hip Seen at the Rizzoli Orthopedic Institute in the Period from 1899 to 1921. Chir. Org. movimento 17:225, 1932.
34. Spencer, K.; Carr, M.; and Wooley, D. Navaho Clans and Marriage at Pueblo Alto. Am. Anthrop. 41:245, 1939.
35. Ueda, F.; Ueke, T.; Okuda, H.; Tanaka, H.; Suda, M.; Suzuki, Y.; and Ando, Y. X-Ray Study of So-Called Spontaneous Healing in Congenital Dislocation of the Hip Joint. Nagoya Med. J. 8:5, 1962.
36. U. S. Department of Health, Education, and Welfare. Health Services for American Indians. Washington, D. C.: Gov. Ptg. Office, PHS Publ. 531, 1957, p. 77.
37. von Rosen, S. Early Diagnosis and Early Treatment of Congenital Hip Luxation. Acta orthop. scandinav. 29:164, 1959.
38. Wiberg, G. Studies on Dysplastic Acetabula and Congenital Subluxation of the Hip Joint. Acta chir. scandinav. Suppl. 58, 1939.

Disease Patterns Among Southwestern Indians

MAURICE L. SIEVERS, M.D.

SOUTHWESTERN AMERICAN Indians often differ significantly from the white population in the frequency, distribution, and manifestations of disease. Either hereditary or environmental influences may be responsible. Several aspects of these variations are discussed in this report, which includes reviews of numerous investigations conducted by others and by me. Most of the observations were made during studies at the Phoenix Public Health Service Indian Hospital during the 8-year period 1957–64. In this period, there were 14,161 admissions and 116,993 outpatient visits to this hospital. Statements which are not referenced are based upon unpublished results of my investigations.

Health Care of American Indians

In 1955, the Division of Indian Health of the Public Health Service was delegated responsibility for the health care of most American Indians and Alaskan Natives. Seven Indian health areas were established. The Phoenix area includes all Indian reservations—except those of the Navajo—which are within Arizona, California, Nevada, and Utah (fig. 1). Ten Indian hospitals, 5 Indian health centers, and 25 Indian health stations are in the Phoenix area.

The Phoenix Public Health Service Indian Hospital serves as a special referral center for all of the other Indian health facilities within the four States. The Phoenix Indian health area has an Indian population in excess of 48,000. Some Indians from other areas also are admitted to this hospital, the largest number being from the Navajo tribe. The 1957–64 tribal distribution of inpatients was as follows: Pima—35.1 percent, Apache—21.3 percent, Navajo—10.2 percent, Papago—8.0 percent, Hopi—6.3 percent, other southwestern Indians (Maricopa, Yavapai, Cocopah, Yuma, Hualapai, Chemehuevi, Mohave, Shoshone, Ute, Paiute, and Washoe)—15.9 percent, and non-southwestern Indians—3.2 percent.

The majority of southwestern Indian families have very low incomes and reside in substandard housing on isolated reservations in desert areas (fig. 2), in mountainous terrain (fig. 3), or within canyons (frontispiece). In addition, ritualistic healing practices persist in many tribes. The Indian medicine man may become a strong ally, however, in motivating the tribal acceptance of modern medical practices if physicians and other workers exhibit an understanding, cooperative attitude toward the established Indian customs (fig. 4).

Disease Patterns

The various studies included in this report were primarily prospective, based on clinical evaluations, laboratory and X-ray examinations, and autopsy observations. Although some tribal variations in the occurrence of a few conditions are stressed, most of the comments concern the differences between the southwestern Indians and the general population in disease distribution. These observations are presented by disease category.

Duodenal ulcer. In an 8-year study of gastric secretory diseases, only three Indians were discovered with duodenal ulcer, and all three were from nonsouthwestern tribes (*1*). Gastrointestinal X–ray examinations were performed on southwestern Indian patients who had symptoms suggesting possible gastrointestinal dysfunction (fig. 5). Gastric cancer was found in 19 patients, pernicious anemia in 6, and benign gastric ulcer in 5. Laparotomy for acute abdominal disease was performed on 554 patients, but there was no evidence of duodenal ulcer. Although each of the common complications of duodenal ulcer—intestinal perforation, obstruction, or hemorrhage—occurred, all were due to other causes than duodenal ulcer.

Study of autopsy reports revealed 10 deaths

Figure 1. Federal Indian reservations and health facilities in the Phoenix area (Arizona, California, Nevada, and Utah)

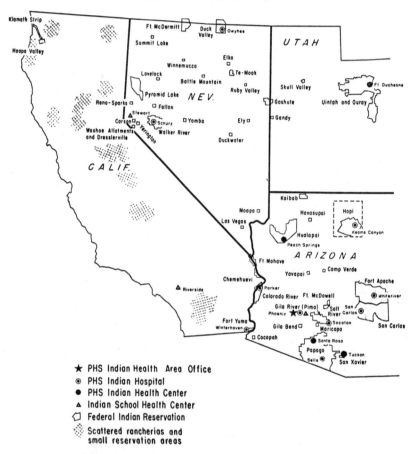

★ PHS Indian Health Area Office
⊚ PHS Indian Hospital
● PHS Indian Health Center
▲ Indian School Health Center
◁ Federal Indian Reservation
⠿ Scattered rancherias and
small reservation areas

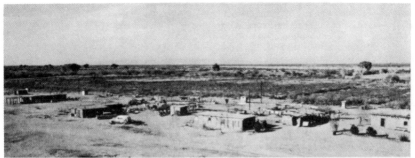

Figure 2. A Pima Reservation Indian community in an isolated desert area. The adobe dwellings—"sandwich houses"—are typical for this tribe

from massive gastrointestinal hemorrhage; portal cirrhosis was present in 8 of these patients, while the other 2 evidenced trauma and azotemia. Healed gastric ulcer was found in 1 of 194 postmortem examinations of adults; no evidence of duodenal ulcer was noted. In contrast, approximately 10 percent of the white population have signs of peptic ulcer at necropsy.

Both hereditary and environmental influences may relate to the deficit of duodenal ulcer among the Indians of the Southwest. To explore these possibilities further, I conducted a study of gastric secretory function among 982 southwestern Indians (2). An increased incidence of achlorhydria was noted compared with that for white persons, but not compared with that for Negroes. Comparison of these results with other published studies for the white population also suggested that achlorhydria occurs more frequently among the Indians. There was no evidence that ethnic tribal origin, diabetes mellitus, or ABO blood groups—all reflections of heredity—were related to the increased frequency of achlorhydria among Indians of the Southwest. Environmental factors such as dietary insufficiency and alcoholic ingestion may contribute to gastric secretory dysfunction. An excess of achlorhydria may be one of the basic reasons for the infrequency of duodenal ulcer among these Indians. Further investigation is needed, however, to delineate other possible factors which protect southwestern Indians from developing duodenal ulcer.

Biliary disease. The incidence of gallbladder disease in most Indian tribes exceeds the rate in the white population. Data supporting that conclusion have been presented previously for the Sioux (3), the Navajo (4), and Pima (5) tribes. Hesse (5) estimated that 2.3 percent of the Pima Indians over 15 years old are hospitalized each year for cholecystitis. In a recent study (6) we did at the Phoenix Public Health Service Indian Hospital, 32 percent of the adult Indians had gallstones at autopsy, in contrast with a reported occurrence of 6 percent among white persons (7). During the 8-year study period 1954–61, 414 patients had cholecystectomies performed, while only 115 had surgery for acute appendicitis (6). Cholelithiasis occurs more often in the Indians at a younger age than in the white population. The female-to-male ratio for occurrence of the disease is approximately 7 to 1 for southwestern tribes (5, 6) and 3 to 1 for white persons (7). About 2 percent of the Indians with biliary calculi also have carcinoma of the gallbladder. Kirshbaum and Kozell found malignancies in 3 percent of the general U.S. population with calculous gallbladders (8).

Since peptic ulcer is uncommon among southwestern Indians, most severe gastrointestinal symptoms are due to cholecystitis, and laparotomy is performed most often for biliary disease. Early and frequent childbearing, recurrent enteric infections, and obesity may relate to the high frequency of pathologic gallbladder among Indians. Since tribes differ in the prevalence of obesity, a comparative study of tribal incidence of cholelithiasis is desirable. Although 90 percent of gallstones are comprised of cholesterol (9), the relationship of steroid metabolism to biliary calculi is obscure. Study results vary, but most authors suggest that southwestern Indians have blood cholesterol levels similar to (10), or somewhat lower (reference 11 and unpublished data of mine for 1965) than those of white people.

Hepatic disease. Dietary deficiencies and alcoholism are frequent on most reservations and probably contribute to the prevalence of portal cirrhosis. Sporadic epidemics of infectious hepatitis also occur, perhaps as a result of deficiencies in sanitation and water supply. Fatty liver is a common postmortem observation. Laennec's cirrhosis occurs more often at a younger age and more frequently among females than it does in the white population. Esophageal varices are overwhelmingly the most frequent cause of major gastrointestinal bleeding in the Indian population.

Diabetes mellitus. Among American Indians, the prevalence of diabetes mellitus varies considerably, but it is far more frequent in the southwestern tribes whose members tend to be obese than in the general U.S. population. , In 1954, Kraus (12) estimated that diabetes was least frequent in the Navajo and Apache tribes and most frequent in the Papago and Pima tribes. Among adult patients admitted to the medical service of the Phoenix Public Health Service Indian Hospital, 26 percent are diabetic (males—21 percent and females—30 percent). Major tribal rates are as follows: Pima—45 percent, Colorado River tribes—33 percent, Papago—32 percent, Hualapai and Supai—28 percent, Colorado River tribes—33 percent, Hopi—9 percent, Apache—7 percent, and Navajo—about 1 percent.

In a 1963 survey of 85 percent of the Pima

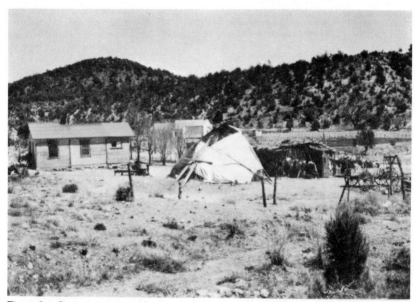

Figure 3. Contrast in types of housing on Whiteriver Apache Reservation. These mountain-dwelling Indians continue to use extensively the traditional wickiup, shown in the foreground

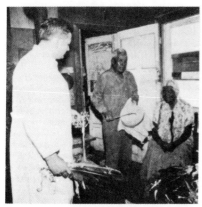

Figure 4. An Apache Indian medicine man with drum performing a traditional ceremony for an ill Indian woman while a Public Health Service Indian Health physician, maintaining a respectful attitude, holds bells and feathers

Indians of the Sacaton Service Unit, Division of Indian Health, who were over 30 years old, postprandial hyperglycemia was reported among 31.3 percent—25.7 percent of the males and 36.4 percent of the females (personal communication from Dr. W. L. Nash, now director of the Indian Health Service Unit, Public Health Service Indian Hospital, Cherokee, N.C., and Dr. S. O. Foster, department of medicine, San Francisco Medical Center, San Francisco, Calif., dated May 16, 1963). A subsequent study (*13*) revealed that 49 percent of the Pimas over 30 years of age had true blood sugar levels greater than 160 mg. per 100 cc. 2 hours after ingestion of 75 grams of glucose. These observations suggest that the incidence of diabetes mellitus among the Pimas—one of the highest ever reported—is about 15 times that for the general population.

Characteristically, diabetes mellitus is the fairly stable "adult" type. A very high blood sugar level is apparently a less ominous finding in southwestern Indians than in white people, as acidosis is infrequent among them, and no deaths directly attributable to diabetic coma have been encountered. An elevated renal threshold for glucose is common enough in these Indians that tests for glycosuria are of limited usefulness for diabetes detection or for assessing treatment results.

One of the bizarre observations about Indians with diabetes mellitus who develop gangrene in a lower extremity is that bounding pedal pulses are present in most cases. Presumably these persist because only the more distal arterioles are seriously involved.

Enteric infections. Diarrhea and gastroenteritis have been a major cause of Indian infant mortality and adult morbidity. A bacterial origin is common. Typhoid fever, salmonellosis, shigellosis, and amebiasis are not unusual, and the specific diagnosis needs to be sought in every appropriate situation. Typhoid carriers are occasionally discovered on some reservations. Deaths from fulminant amebiasis still occur.

Tuberculosis and coccidioidomycosis. Tuberculosis continues to plague the southwestern Indians far more than the general population. The presence of the disease, however, is sometimes inapparent. In particular, extrapulmonary tuberculosis often has the unrecognized capacity to mimic other diseases. Therefore I have suggested that tuberculosis be referred to as "the second great imitator" (*14*) and be given foremost consideration as the cause of obscure illness in Indians.

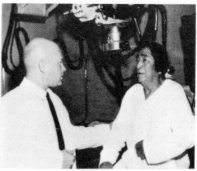

Figure 5. A Hopi Indian man being prepared by the radiologist of the Phoenix Public Health Service Indian Hospital for gastrointestinal X-ray examination.

273

Coccidioidomycosis infection originates in the Lower Sonoran life zone (*15*), a biogeographic area which is comprised of the most southerly portions of the arid areas of the western United States and central Mexico. Therefore, only those reservation Indians residing in these limited regions (the various Colorado River tribes and the Pimas, Papagos, and San Carlos Apaches) or Indians who visit these areas develop the disease (*16*). Direct transmission from an infected human being does not occur; only spore-bearing dust is a source of infection (*17*). The regions where *Coccidioides immitis* inhabits the soil closely approximate the area where the creosote bush flourishes, as stressed by Maddy (*15*). In my recent study of southwestern tribes (*16*), the San Carlos Apache reservation had the highest rate of coccidioidin skin reactivity and the greatest frequency of disseminated coccidioidomycosis.

Primary glaucoma and trachoma. Primary open-angle glaucoma is probably the most frequent cause of blindness in white adults. Several ophthalmologists, however, who have had extensive experience with southwestern Indians report that they have never seen this condition among them (personal communications to author from Dr. Phillips Thygeson, clinical professor of ophthalmology, University of California School of Medicine, San Francisco, Calif., and Dr. R. O. Schultz, department of ophthalmology, Marquette University School of Medicine, Milwaukee, Wis., dated February 8, 1963; from Dr. D. K. Powers, area consultant to the Phoenix Indian Health Area Office, and Dr. S. Davidson of Phoenix, dated September 11, 1964). The explanation for the deficit of glaucoma is obscure, but further study is proposed.

Trachoma has become rare in the white population of the United States, but it continues to occur in members of all southwestern Indian tribes at all ages. It is a major cause of entropion, irreversible blindness, and significant ocular disability in Indians. Preventive programs are underway (fig. 6).

Malignancy. Despite the widespread opinion that Indians seldom develop cancer, few valid data have been assembled on cancer among Indians. A recent analysis of autopsy data revealed no age-adjusted deficit of malignant disease among southwestern American Indians, although distribution of malignancy by organ site differed significantly from that of the general population (personal communication from Dr. D. D. Reichenbach, department of pathology, University of Washington, Seattle, May 26, 1965). These data confirm an earlier study of mine at the Phoenix Public Health Service Indian Hospital (*18*), which revealed a striking absence of bronchogenic cancer. Whether heredity or environment contributes to this deficit is uncertain. The air of Indian reservations, however, is not contaminated by industrial fumes, and Indians smoke infrequently and seldom extensively.

Gastric cancer is the malignancy most often encountered among the southwestern Indians (*1*, *6*, *18*). A possible increased incidence of achlorhydria over that of the white population (*2*) may be pertinent. The significant frequency of cervical carcinoma (*1*, *6*, *18*) among southwestern Indian women may relate to their high rate of childbearing and to deficiencies in the hygiene of the male and female genitals. The marked prevalence of gallstones among these Indians may have an etiological relationship (*8*) to an apparently greatly increased rate of malignancy of the gallbladder and bile duct as compared with the rate for the white population (*6*), although this association is not universally accepted (*19*).

There is a relative deficit of breast cancer (*1*, *6*, *18*) among southwestern Indians. Smith and associates (*20*) also noted this deficit in their study of death certificates of Navajos. Among white women, the breast is the site of most malignancies (*21*). The lower rate of breast cancer in these Indians may relate to factors known to be associated with decreased incidence—gestation, lactation, and multiparity (*21*)—all of which are more frequent in Indian women than in white.

Atherosclerosis and hypertension. Atherosclerosis among southwestern Indians is less frequent than in the white population (*4, 5, 11, 22, 23*). Some evidence (reference 11 and unpublished data of mine for 1965) suggests that southwestern Indians also have lower blood cholesterol levels than the white population.

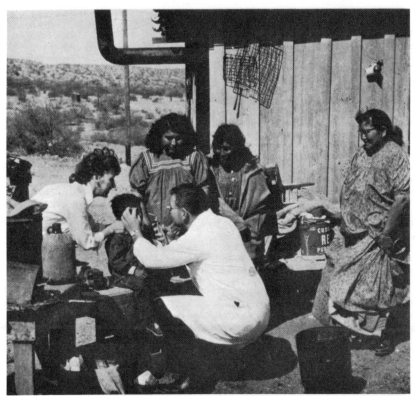

Figure 6. Examination and treatment for trachoma often requires the Public Health Service Indian Health physician to visit Indian homes such as this one in the community of Bylas on the San Carlos Apache Reservation

Although many have suspected that atherosclerosis is related to diet, these Indians use lard almost exclusively and seldom consume unsaturated fats (5). Coronary heart disease does occur occasionally, although angina pectoris is very infrequent. Over a 10-year period (fiscal years 1957–66), an autopsy or electrocardiographic diagnosis of myocardial infarction was established for 138 Indians, but only 56 of these had a history of an acute infarction. Most coronary thrombosis or severe atherosclerosis among the southwestern Indians is associated with well-known precipitating causes such as diabetes mellitus or high blood pressure.

Hypertension, however, is relatively infrequent in most southwestern Indian tribes except, perhaps, in the Apache (23, 24). Malignant hypertension is a rarity, no cases having been seen in the Phoenix Public Health Service Indian Hospital during an 8-year period.

Skeletal fluorosis. In certain areas, including various regions of the Apache, Papago, Hopi, and Colorado River reservations, the sole water supply has an elevated fluoride content (25). X-ray studies of adults from these regions occasionally show increased density of bones. Skeletal fluorosis is responsible for this development, as chemical analysis has substantiated. X-ray results frequently present diagnostic difficulties to physicians unfamiliar with the specific cause of the bone density. Clinicians have considered and investigated diagnoses varying from osteopetrosis to osteoblastic metastatic carcinoma. Skeletal fluorosis is apparently a benign condition (25) requiring recognition but no further diagnostic or therapeutic measures.

Blood groups and erythroblastosis. About 45 percent of the white population have blood group O, and 40 percent have blood group A (26). Southwestern Indians average 83 percent with group O and 17 percent with group A (1). Only the Apache (1, 27) and Navajo (1) tribes have a larger representation of blood group A. Although the blood of 15 percent of the white population is Rh negative (1), apparently 100 percent of southwestern Indians are Rh positive, the rare Rh negative blood invariably being found in persons of mixed races. Therefore fetal erythroblastosis due to Rh incompatibility is neither expected nor observed among southwestern American Indians.

Miscellaneous threats to health. Trauma is a constant threat to reservation Indians. Subdural hematomas are common in infants, and fractures are frequent at all ages. The underlying causes include automobile accidents, alcoholism, and the occupational riding of horses.

Cannon (28) noted that umbilical hernia was considerably more frequent than inguinal hernia among southwestern Indians, in contrast to the experience of the white population. The explanation for this difference is unknown.

A recent survey of Pima Indians (29) revealed an unexpected prevalence of rheumatoid arthritis. Clinical evidence from many reservation hospitals also suggests a high occurrence rate among most southwestern tribes.

In 1964, Herxheimer (30) discovered only a small number of cases of bronchial asthma among various southwestern Indian tribes. The incidence he found was much less than for the white population. This result substantiates previous opinion.

Congenital lesions occur frequently in many tribes. Albinism, polydactylism, hemorrhagic telangiectasia, congenital heart disease, and dysplasia of the hip are often encountered. One contributing factor may be the tendency for marriages to be confined to the tribe, so that spouses are often closely related. Further study of some of these conditions is proposed or in progress.

Summary

Among southwestern Indians, duodenal ulcer is rare, but cholelithiasis is prevalent, accounting for most laparotomies. Diabetes mellitus occurs frequently, especially in tribes whose members tend to be obese. Gastric and biliary cancer are the leading types of malignancy among southwestern Indians. Breast and lung carcinoma are less frequent than among white people. The infrequency of atherosclerosis may reflect low blood cholesterol levels. Myocardial infarction seldom occurs in these Indians without diabetes, hypertension, or other definite precipitating factors. Hypertension is apparently less frequent than among white persons.

A high rate of tuberculosis persists among southwestern Indians, and this "second great imitator" must always be considered in any obscure illness among them. Coccidioidomycosis occurs only in Indians who reside within, or visit, the area where *Coccidioides immitis* infests the soil. Skeletal fluorosis due to a high fluoride content of drinking water has been noted in Indians in certain southwestern reservation areas and requires recognition but no other diagnostic or therapeutic procedures. For unknown reasons, Indians apparently do not develop primary open-angle glaucoma, but trachoma is a common ocular disease. Since the Rh negative blood type probably does not exist among southwestern Indians, erythroblastosis fetalis due to Rh incompatibility is neither expected nor observed. Alcoholism, dietary deficiency, Laennec's cirrhosis, and bleeding esophageal varices are major health problems of most tribes.

The high rate of traumatic lesions among southwestern Indians may relate to alcoholism, automobile accidents, and the occupational riding of horses. Umbilical hernia has been noted much more often than inguinal hernia. Rheumatoid arthritis is fairly prevalent. Bronchial asthma is infrequent. A significant number of congenital lesions occur, perhaps because of the frequent consanguineous marriages in many southwestern American Indian tribes.

REFERENCES

(1) Sievers, M. L., and Marquis, J. R.: Duodenal ulcer among southwestern American Indians. Gastroenterology 42: 566–569, May 1962.

(2) Sievers, M. L.: A study of achlorhydria among southwestern American Indians. Amer J Gastroent 45: 99–108, February 1966.

(3) Lam, R. C.: Gallbladder disease among American Indians. Lancet 74: 305–309, August 1954.

(4) Gilbert, J.: Absence of coronary thrombosis in Navajo Indians. California Med 82: 114–115, February 1955.

(5) Hesse, F. G.: Incidence of cholecystitis and other diseases among Pima Indians of southern Arizona. JAMA 170: 1789–1790, Aug. 8, 1959.

(6) Sievers, M. L., and Marquis, J. R.: The southwestern American Indian's burden: biliary disease. JAMA 182: 570–572, Nov. 3, 1962.

(7) Moore, R. A.: A textbook of pathology. W. B. Saunders Company, Philadelphia, 1945, pp. 783–793.

(8) Kirshbaum, J. D., and Kozell, D. D.: Carcinoma of the gallbladder and extrahepatic bile ducts. A clinical and pathological study of 117 cases in 13,330 necropsies. Surg Gynec Obstet 73: 740–754, November 1941.

(9) Watson, C. J.: Diseases of the gallbladder and bile ducts. In A textbook of medicine, edited by R. L. Cecil and R. F. Loeb. W. B. Saunders Company, Philadelphia, 1955, pp. 945–961.

(10) Darby, W. J., et al.: Dietary background and nutriture of the Navajo Indian. J Nutr 60: 63–85, Supp. 2, November 1956.

(11) Page, I. H., Lewis, L. A., and Gilbert, J.: Plasma lipids and proteins and their relationship to coronary disease among Navajo Indians. Circulation 13: 675–679, May 1956.

(12) Kraus, B. S.: Indian health in Arizona. Ch. 6. The disease picture. University of Arizona Press, Tucson, 1954.

(13) Miller, M., Burch, T. A., Bennett, P. H., and Steinberg, A. G.: Prevalence of diabetes mellitus in American Indians: results of glucose tolerance tests in the Pima Indians of Arizona. Diabetes 14: 439–440, July 1965.

(14) Sievers, M. L.: The second "great imitator"—tuberculosis. JAMA 176: 809–810, June 3, 1961.

(15) Maddy, K. T., Crecelius, G. H., and Cornell, R. G.: Where can coccidioidomycosis be acquired in Arizona? Arizona Med 18: 184–194, July 1961.

(16) Sievers, M. L.: Coccidioidomycosis among southwestern American Indians. Amer Rev Resp Dis 90: 920–926, December 1964.

(17) Smith, C. E.: Public health significance of coccidioidomycosis. Arizona Public Health News 52: 6–9, March-April 1959.

(18) Sievers, M. L., and Cohen, S. L.: Lung cancer among Indians of the southwestern United States. Ann Intern Med 54: 912–915, May 1961.

(19) Derman, H., et al.: Are gallstones and gallbladder carcinoma related? JAMA 176: 450–451, May 6, 1961.

(20) Smith, R. L., Salsbury, D. G., and Gilliam, A. G.: Recorded and expected mortality among the Navajo with special reference to cancer. J Nat Cancer Inst 17: 77–89, July 1956.

(21) Ackerman, L. V., and del Regato, J. A.: Cancer diagnosis, treatment and prognosis. C. V. Mosby Company, St. Louis, Mo., 1954, pp. 966–1024.

(22) Fulmer, H. S., and Roberts, R. W.: Coronary heart disease among the Navajo Indians. Ann Intern Med 59: 740–764, November 1963.

(23) Clifford, N. J., Kelly, J. J., Jr., Thomas, F. L., and Eder, H. A.: Coronary heart disease and hypertension in the White Mountain Apache tribe. Circulation 28: 926–931, November 1963.

(24) Cohen, B. M.: Arterial hypertension among Indians of the southwestern United States. Amer J Med Sci 225: 505–513, May 1953.

(25) Morris, J. W.: Skeletal fluorosis among Indians of the American Southwest. Amer J Roentgen 94: 608–615, July 1965.

(26) Sievers, M. L., and Calabresi, P.: Gastric pepsin secretion and ABO blood groups in polycythemia vera. Amer J Digest Dis 4: 515–521, July 1959.

(27) Kraus, B. S., and White, C. B.: Micro-evolution in a human population: a study of social endogamy and blood type distributions among the western Apache. Amer Anthrop 58: 1017–1043, December 1956.

(28) Cannon, R.: A study of Indian hernia operations, 1950–1960. Paper presented at the clinical staff meeting of the Phoenix Public Health Service Indian Hospital, May 23, 1961.

(29) Bunim, J. J., Burch, T. A., and O'Brien, W. M.: Influence of genetic and environmental factors on the occurrence of rheumatoid arthritis and rheumatoid factor in American Indians. Bull Rheum Dis 15: 349–350, September 1964.

(30) Herxheimer, H.: Asthma in American Indians. New Eng J Med 270: 1128–1129, May 21, 1964.

Patient acceptance of oral contraceptives

I. The American Indian

EDWARD E. WALLACH, M.D.

ALAN E. BEER, M.D.

CELSO-RAMON GARCIA, M.D.

THE PAST decade has witnessed a surge of interest in the growth of world population and in problems related to unrestricted population increase. Continuing efforts are being directed toward the development of acceptable fertility regulating agents applicable among indigent groups in underdeveloped areas. Oral agents, intrauterine devices, and ovulation timing have received considerable attention toward this end. It has become apparent that in addition to the intrinsic effectiveness of a contraceptive agent, the ultimate success of any family-planning program depends upon patient acceptance of the method and upon the motivation of the individuals involved. The data presented in this study were collected over a 2 year period from experience with oral contraceptives among American Indians. The study involves to a great extent an illiterate, non–English speaking, indigent group of people. Factors relevant to the applicability of oral contraceptives to such a population in an underdeveloped area were investigated.

The health of the American Indian has been the responsibility of The United States Public Health Service, Division of Indian Health, since 1955. The overall health objective has been to provide the Indian beneficiary with comprehensive Medical care. The Navajo Indian Reservation, the largest single reservation in the United States, covers 25,000 square miles of arid land in northern Arizona, northwestern New Mexico, and southeastern Utah. Approximately 100,000 Navajo Indians inhabit this tract of land, many surviving at less than subsistence levels. Health problems of high priority include: (1) reduction in the incidence of tuberculosis, enteric diseases, and upper respiratory infections; (2) reduction of maternal and infant mortality and morbidity; and (3) improvement of environmental sanitation conditions.[1-4]

Over the past 96 years the population of the Navajo Tribe has risen from 7,111 to over 100,000, representing an annual increase of 3 to 4 per cent. Between July 1, 1963, and June 30, 1964, 4,174 Navajo births occurred in Public Health Service, mission, and contract hospitals. An additional 3.0 to 6.8 per cent of Navajo births were thought to occur outside the hospital producing a birth rate of greater than 42/1,000 population.[5]

Materials and methods

The Public Health Service Indian Hospital at Tuba City is situated on the Navajo Indian Reservation in the Northwest portion of Arizona. The hospital services a population of approximately 20,000 Indians mainly Navajos and Hopis, with small numbers of Apaches, Comanches, Paiutes, and representatives of other tribes. The nearest neighboring hospital is 85 miles away. Communications are poor, with few telephones and no form of public transportation. Dwellings are situated to a great extent in remote areas accessible only by primitive dirt roads. United States Public Health Service field clinics, health centers, and mission clinics are situated in the more remote areas. Obstetric and gynecologic problems are frequently referred from these outlying hospitals, clinics, and health centers to Tuba City for care.

No contraceptive methods have been available commercially on the Navajo Reservation. Traditional belief in herbs, ceremonies, and fetishes for the prevention of conception are an inherent part of the Navajo culture. At the inception of this study, the population had been almost totally uninformed concerning reliable methods of contraception.

In July of 1963, the unofficial incorporation of a family planning service within the realm of the gynecologic and postpartum clinics was undertaken. Women interested in contraception were referred to the weekly clinic, and postpartum patients were individually informed of contraceptive methods available prior to referral to postpartum clinics.

At the inception of the program, methods were limited to oral contraception, intravaginal foam, and instruction in the rhythm technique. After the first 12 months, intrauterine contraceptive devices were also obtainable. Available methods of contraception were discussed with the patient by a Navajo-speaking nurse, or by the physician when the patient could speak and understand English. Each patient was then free to choose the method she found preferable. Oral contraceptives were available as Enovid 10 mg.,* 5 mg.,† and 2.5 mg.‡ dispensed in cycle packages consisting of 28 pills: 21 Enovid tablets and 7 saccharin placebos. A postpartum patient seen at the time of the 6 week visit was instructed to take one pink tablet (Enovid) for 21 consecutive days, then one white tablet (saccharin) for 7 consecutive days, and repeat the sequence in each subsequent cycle. This schedule enabled the patient to take one pill daily, and eliminated the necessity for calculating the fifth day of each menstrual cycle. The schedule also insured the patient's return to the clinic for more medication at 28 day intervals (Fig. 1, B).

Prior to institution of oral contraceptives, pelvic examination, Papanicolaou smear, and thorough breast examination were performed, and weight was recorded. At subsequent outpatient visits, the patient was questioned about possible side effects and influence on lactation. A record of the date of onset and duration of menstrual flow was made, and weight was recorded. After two cycles during which the drug was taken correctly without significant side effects, prescriptions were filled for three cycle intervals. Pelvic examinations and Papanicolaou smears were repeated at approximately 6 to 12 month intervals, or more frequently if indicated. Nonpuerperal patients were given the same schedule of administration, but were started on the fifth day of the menstrual cycle. Only several patients received Enovid according to the customary schedule; namely, one tablet daily for 20 days beginning on the fifth day of the menstrual cycle (Fig. 1, A). Prescription pads were prestamped to facilitate dispensing of the medication.

*Norethynodrel 9.85 mg. with 0.15 mg. ethinyl estradiol 3-methyl ether (mestranol), G. D. Searle & Company.

†Norethynodrel 5.0 mg. with 0.075 mg. mestranol, G. D. Searle & Company.

‡Norethynodrel 2.5 mg. with 0.10 mg. mestranol, G. D. Searle & Company.

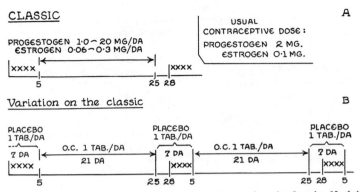

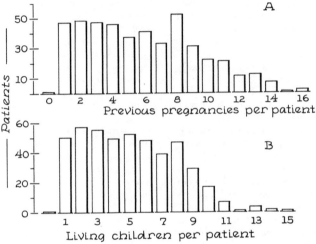

Fig 1. *A*, Classic scheme of administration of oral contraception from day 5 to day 25 of the cycle. *B*, Variation of the classic scheme using 21 days of Enovid and 7 days of placebo.

Fig. 2. *A*, Number of previous pregnancies per patient; *B*, number of living children per patient.

Results

Over the first 20 months of the program, a total of 459 patients were started on Enovid for contraceptive purposes. Patients ranged in age from 17 to 48 years with a mean age of 24.4 and a median of 27 years. Because of frequent transportation difficulties, patients were considered puerperal if medication was initiated within 12 weeks of termination of pregnancy. Of the entire group, 354 women (77 per cent) started Enovid either within the postpartum or postabortal period while Enovid was initiated in 105 (23 per cent) nonpuerperal patients. The number of previous pregnancies per patient ranged from 1 to 16 with a mean of 5.9, and the mean number of living children per patient was 5.1 with a range of 1 to 15 (Fig. 2). The majority of the patients (82 per cent) were Navajo, 16 per cent were

Hopi, and the remaining 10 women represented 7 other Indian tribes.

During the initial 20 months the patients were followed for a total of 2,828 cycles, averaging 6.2 cycles per patient with a range of 1 to 27 cycles (Fig. 3). Dosage breakdown is tabulated in Table I.

A patient was classified as inactive if she failed to return for a scheduled appointment plus an additional 4 week period of grace. Two hundred and sixty-nine patients remained active; 5 women discontinued medication and underwent an operative procedure which resulted in sterilization; 12 patients elected to try a different form of contraception. The remaining 173 patients (38 per cent) became inactive following one to eleven cycles of use (Table II). Ninety-one of these patients were lost to follow-up with only one cycle of use. Eleven patients moved away from the Tuba City area; 9 lacked transportation facilities to return to clinic; 6 were unable to provide a reason for stopping. Four patients discontinued medi-

Table I. Cycles at each dosage level

Dosage (mg.)	No. of cycles
10	207
5	950
2.5	1,671
Total	2,828

Table II. Reasons for discontinuing Enovid in 190 patients

Reason	No.
Lost to follow-up	131
Moved to other area	11
Lack of transportation	9
No reason given	6
Planned pregnancy	4
Nausea	3
Pregnant when started	3
Breakthrough bleeding	1
Physician failure to renew medication	2
Inability to remember to take pills	1
Religious convictions	1
Did not think she would become pregnant	2
Hysterectomy	5
Tubal ligation	2
Preferred to have intrauterine device	7
Preferred intravaginal method	3

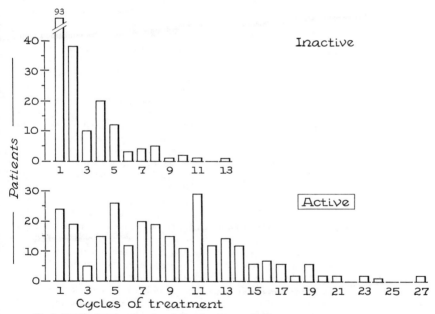

Fig. 3. Distribution of patients by number of cycles completed.

Table III. Correlation of dropout rate with distance traveled

Distance traveled (miles)	Active patients No.	Active patients %	Inactive patients* No.	Inactive patients* %
0-20	103	38.2	54	28.4
21-40	71	26.4	42	22.1
Over 40 (41-120)	95	35.4	106	49.5

*Patients failing to return for a scheduled appointment with an additional 4 week period of grace.

Table IV. Weight change

Weight range (pounds)	No. of patients* Gaining	No. of patients* Losing
> 25	0	0
21-25	0	2
16-20	0	4
11-15	4	12
6-10	17	46
1- 5	82	80
Total	103	144

*No change, 50 patients; insufficient data, 162 patients.

Table V. Side effects while on Enovid in 459 patients

Complaint	Incidence in series No.	Incidence in series %	Reason for dropout No.	Reason for dropout %
Nausea (Total)	20	4.4	3	0.7
First cycle	17	3.7		
Subsequent cycles	3	0.7		
Breakthrough bleeding (Total)	81	17.6	1	0.2
First cycle	28	6.1		
Subsequent cycles	53	11.5		
Hypermenorrhea	3	0.7	0	
Pruritus vulvae	2	0.4	0	
Dysmenorrhea	2	0.4	0	
Hypomenorrhea	1	0.2	0	
Mastalgia	1	0.2	0	

cation in order to establish a planned pregnancy.

Patients in both active and inactive categories were classified into three groups depending upon the approximate distance traveled from home to hospital. Results (Table III) suggest that distance in itself was not the sole factor in the dropout rate. Approximately 35 per cent of the active patients lived in excess of 40 miles from the hospital in comparison with 49.5 per cent of the inactive women.

Weight change was tabulated in 5 pound increments or decrements. Loss or gain of less than one pound was considered as representing no change (Table IV). One hundred and three patients gained weight during treatment while 144 patients experienced weight loss.

A history of nausea was obtained in 20 of the 459 patients followed. In 17 of these women nausea was experienced during the first cycle only. Breakthrough bleeding occurred in 81 patients; however, it is probably significant in this regard that our women were not instructed to double the dosage of medication in the event of breakthrough bleeding.

An episode of superficial thrombophlebitis following trauma to the leg occurred in one patient while on medication. The phlebitis responded favorably to conservative measures within one week; and the patient, who had failed to stop medication as instructed, continued on Enovid for an additional 10 cycles without difficulty. Infectious hepatitis, confirmed histologically by liver biopsy, occurred in one woman who continued Enovid during an uneventful convalescence. Side effects are tabulated in Table V.

Approximately 90 per cent of the postpartum patients nursed their infants. There was no indication of suppression of lactation among patients in this series in which oral contraception was initiated after lactation had been established for at least 6 weeks. Nor was there evidence of gynecomastia or other signs of feminization among the nursing infants, all of whom were seen at 12 week intervals.

A total of 15 pregnancies occurred following discontinuation of Enovid (Table VI). Three patients discontinued medication specifically to establish a pregnancy. Conception had already occurred in 3 patients when medication was initiated. Two pregnancies occurred in women who admittedly took medication sporadically. Pregnancies occurred from 1 to 11 cycles after stopping medication. All infants delivered during the

Table VI. Pregnancies occurring following Enovid administration

Patient	No. cycles completed prior to stopping	Interval between stopping and conception (months)	Pregnancy outcome
M. N.	2	1	Spontaneous abortion
E. B.	10	1	Spontaneous abortion
S. H.	3	Irregular pill taker	Spontaneous abortion
M. S.	5	Irregular pill taker	Normal delivery of normal female
P. H.	8	1	Term delivery of normal male
M. I.	4	2	Term delivery of normal female
M. C.	5	11	Undelivered
L. Y.	2	6	Term delivery of normal male
F. M.	2	2	Term delivery of normal female
B. M.	1	2	Term delivery of normal male
M. N.	2	9	Term delivery of normal female
I. H.	1	2	Term delivery of normal male
M. S.	1	6	Term delivery of normal female
B. W.	3	4	Term delivery of normal female
E. W.	1	2	Term delivery of normal female
N. T.	1	Pregnant when started	Term delivery of normal male
G. C.	1	Pregnant when started	Term delivery of normal male
E. M.	1	Pregnant when started	Undelivered

Table VII. Results of Papanicolaou smears in 459 patients on Enovid, initially and at 6 to 12 month intervals

	Class I	Class II	Class III	Class IV or V	Unsatisfactory	Not reported
Initial smear	443	5	1	0	1	9
Second smear	113	5	0	0	3	4
Third smear	16	0	0	0	0	1

course of the program were carefully examined and found to be normally developed, including 2 female infants whose mothers received one cycle of medication during early pregnancy. No pregnancies occurred during proper adherence to the regimen.

Results of cytologic smears taken from the cervical os and endocervical canal are tabulated in Table VII. None of the follow-up smears performed at 6 to 12 month intervals were abnormal.

Comment

The efficacy of fertility control by oral agents has been well established. The applicability of oral contraception to the developing nations of the world has been questioned. On the one hand, oral agents have been considered to be of special value among the underprivileged and overpopulated areas[6, 7]; while on the other hand, they have been labeled as unsuitable for the great bulk of the world's population because of expense and lack of sustained motivation.[8] Experience with the American Indian suggests that motivation is not uniformly lacking among the underprivileged. Acceptance of the method was apparent in the enthusiastic fidelity of the patients followed during the course of the first 20 months. Of those subjects lost to follow-up, 53 per cent dropped out immediately after the first cycle and 76 per cent by the end of the second cycle. Factors which seemed to influence the outlook for long-term follow-up were: (1) distance traveled and availability of transportation, (2) simplification of method of administration, (3) individualization at the time of clinic visits, and (4) efficiency of a clinic geared toward family planning. Side effects among the respondents did not appear to be a significant cause for discontinuation.

Proximity of the hospital, expressed in terms of mileage, was found to be misleading in that mileage per se had no relationship to the more significant problems of travel such as poor quality of roads and lack of transportation facilities. The presence of a permanent group of physicians and nurse-interpreters created a favorable atmosphere for patient follow-up. Administration of medication by the "21 tablet plus 7 placebo" technique alleviated the necessity for counting days and proved satisfactory from the standpoint of cycle length.

Side effects were of a similar nature to those reported in previous evaluations of oral contraception. The incidence of nausea compared favorably with that of previous studies.[9-14]

The occurrence of breakthrough flow approximated that of recently reported observations,[9, 11-13] in spite of the low dosage used and avoidance of doubled dosage.

Weight gain has frequently been associated with the use of oral contraceptives. Factors which may be responsible for this phenomenon have recently been reviewed.[15] Of interest in the present series was the preponderance of women who failed to experience weight gain. Among those experiencing weight gain, 80 per cent gained only 5 pounds or less.

The absence of inhibition of lactation among the patients studied confirmed the observations of others[16-18] that in the lower dosages oral contraceptives do not significantly affect milk quality or quantity. In reviewing the literature only a single instance of excessive mammary development occurring in a breast-fed infant whose mother had received oral contraception has been reported.[19] No such phenomenon occurred in the present series, and all infants were closely followed by a Board-certified pediatrician. Hormonal content of breast milk with and without the influence of progestins is presently being investigated.[20]

Institution of family planning assistance for the American Indian population has revealed important by-products of such a program. In addition to the intrinsic benefit of an available family planning service, such a program has presented the physician with the opportunity to perform periodic follow-up examinations and to practice fundamentals of preventive medicine. It is significant that oral contraceptives can be accepted and properly employed by the illiterate and the indigent. Motivation studies are required to explore in more detail those factors in any social group which prevent long-term follow-up. These factors are apparently not restricted to proximity or accessibility of the clinic nor to intricacies of the method of administration.

Summary

Oral contraceptives were employed among 459 American Indian women for a total of 2,828 cycles. Medication was dispensed in cycle packages consisting of 28 pills, 21 Enovid tablets followed by 7 placebos, repeated at 28 day intervals. During the initial 20 months, 269 women remained active in spite of frequent hardships endured in traveling to clinic. No inhibition of lactation was noted. Weight gain and nausea during the course of Enovid administration were minimal. Oral contraceptives were considered a satisfactory method of family planning for this indigent and deprived group of American citizens.

We gratefully acknowledge the assistance of Rosemary Goldtooth, Assistant Health Education Aid, Karen Charley, R.N., Cecilia Lopez, L.P.N., and Mrs. Lucille Alfred, without whom this survey could not have been carried out. We are indebted to Dr. Gregory Pincus for his interest and encouragement.

REFERENCES

1. Van Duzen, J. L.: J. Am. M. Women's A. 19: 558, 1964.
2. Adair, J., and Deuschle, K.: Human Organization 16: 19, 1958.
3. McDermott, W., Deuschle, K., Adair, J., Fulmer, H., and Loughlin, B.: Science 131: 197, 280, 1960.
4. United States Department of Health, Educa-

tion and Welfare: Orientation to Health on the Navajo Indian Reservation, Washington, D. C., 1961, United States Government Printing Office.

5. United States Public Health Service Division of Indian Health, Window Rock Field Office Program Plan, July, 1964.

6. Editorial: Obst. & Gynec. Surv. **16:** 411, 1961.

7. Editorial: Obst. & Gynec. Surv. **17:** 164, 1962.

8. Eastman, N. J.: Fertil. & Steril. **15:** 477, 1964.

9. Tyler, E. T., Olson, H. J., Wolf, L., Finkelstein, S., Thayer, J., Kaplan, N., Levin, M. and Weintraub, J.: Obst. & Gynec. **18:** 363, 1961.

10. Rovinsky, J. J.: Obst. & Gynec. **23:** 840, 1964.

11. Goldzieher, J. W.: M. Clin. North America **48:** 529, 1964.

12. Mears, E., and Grant, E. C. G.: Brit. M. J. **2:** 75, 1962.

13. Flowers, C. E., Jr.: J. A. M. A. **188:** 1115, 1964.

14. Garcia, C. R.: Clinical Studies on Human Fertility Control *in* Human Fertility and Population Problems, Cambridge Massachusetts, 1964, Schenkman Publishing Company, Inc., pp. 43-74.

15. Pincus, G.: The Control of Fertility, New York, 1965, Academic Press, Inc., p. 275.

16. Pincus, G.: The Control of Fertility, New York, 1961, Academic Press, Inc., p. 261.

17. Garcia, C. R., and Pincus, G.: Clin. Obst. & Gynec. **7:** 844, 1964.

18. Garcia, C. R., and Pincus, G.: Internat. J. Fertil. **9:** 95, 1964.

19. Curtis, E. M.: Obst. & Gynec. **23:** 295, 1964.

20. Garcia, C. R., Schwarz, R. H., Touchstone, J. C., and Wallach, E. E.: In preparation.

285

INDEX

Neomycin-Resistant Staphylococci, 7
Nephritis, 13
Nitrogen, 172
Norrie's Disease, 39

Oklahoma, 182
Oral Contraceptives, 278
Overfield, Theresa, 67

Paranoid Reactions, 133
Pelner, Louis, 218
Peritonsillar Abscess, 179
Perlman, Lawrence V., 13
Peyote, 218
Phosphorus, 172
Poland, Jack D., 190
Pond, Harry, 149
Prosnitz, Leonard R., 179
Psychosis, 218

Quie, Paul G., 7

Rabin, David L., 224
Respiratory Virus, 190
Rheumatic Diseases, 76
Roentgenographic Evaluation, 122
Roper, Margaret, 149

St. Paul Island, Pribilofs, 62

Scott, Edward M., 212
Seminole Indians, 182
Sievers, Maurice L., 269
Skin Infections, 13
Snow, Clyde, 30
South Dakota Indian, 122
Southwestern Indians, 269
Steele, James P., 122
Sylvatic Helminthiasis, 81

Tarahumara Endurance Runners, 30
Trachoma, 104
Trichinosis, 195
Trisulfapyrimidines, 104

Ungava Indians, 56
Urban Migrants, 158

Vertebral Column, 162

Wallach, Edward E., 278
Wannamaker, Lewis W., 13
Whedon, G. Donald, 172
Wolfe, Dorothy E., 172
Wood, T. Rodman, 104
Woodson, Minnie L., 172
Wulff, Herta, 190

Zrull, Joel P., 133